GLUED IOL

System requirement:
- Operating system—Windows XP or above
- Web browser—Internet Explorer 8 or above, Google Chrome, Mozilla Firefox and Safari
- Essential plugins—Java & Flash player
  - Facing problems in viewing content—it may be your system does not have java enabled.
  - If Videos don't show up—it may be the system requires Flash player or need to manage flash setting
  - You can test java and flash by using the links from the troubleshoot section of the CD/DVD.
- Learn more about flash setting from the link in the troubleshoot section.

Accompanying CD/DVD-ROM is playable only in Computer and not in DVD player.

CD/DVD has Autorun function—it may take few seconds to load on your computer. If it does not works for you then follow the steps below to access the contents manually:
- Click on my computer
- Select the CD/DVD drive and click open/explore—this will show list of files in the CD/DVD
- Find and double click file—"launch.html"

DVD CONTENTS

GLUED IOL

Glued Intrascleral Haptic Fixation of a PC IOL

Editor

Amar Agarwal MS FRCS FRCOphth

Chairman and Managing Director
Dr Agarwal's Group of Eye Hospitals and Eye Research Center
Chennai, Tamil Nadu, India

Foreword

Eric Donnenfeld

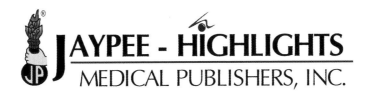

JAYPEE - HIGHLIGHTS
MEDICAL PUBLISHERS, INC.

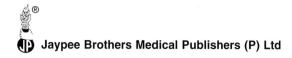

Jaypee Brothers Medical Publishers (P) Ltd

Headquarters

Jaypee Brothers Medical Publishers (P) Ltd
4838/24, Ansari Road, Daryaganj
New Delhi 110 002, India
Phone: +91-11-43574357
Fax: +91-11-43574314
Email: jaypee@jaypeebrothers.com

Overseas Offices

J.P. Medical Ltd.,
83 Victoria Street London
SW1H 0HW (UK)
Phone: +44-2031708910
Fax: +02-03-0086180
Email: info@jpmedpub.com

Jaypee-Highlights Medical Publishers Inc.
City of Knowledge, Bld. 237, Clayton
Panama City, Panama
Phone: +507-301-0496
Fax: +507-301-0499
Email: cservice@jphmedical.com

Jaypee Brothers Medical Publishers (P) Ltd
17/1-B Babar Road, Block-B, Shaymali
Mohammadpur, Dhaka-1207
Bangladesh
Mobile: +08801912003485
Email: jaypeedhaka@gmail.com

Jaypee Brothers Medical Publishers (P) Ltd
Shorakhute, Kathmandu
Nepal
Phone: +00977-9841528578
Email: jaypee.nepal@gmail.com

Website: www.jaypeebrothers.com
Website: www.jaypeedigital.com

Inquiries for bulk sales may be solicited at: jaypee@jaypeebrothers.com

This book has been published in good faith that the contents provided by the contributors contained herein are original, and is intended for educational purposes only. While every effort is made to ensure accuracy of information, the publisher and the editor specifically disclaim any damage, liability, or loss incurred, directly or indirectly, from the use or application of any of the contents of this work. If not specifically stated, all figures and tables are courtesy of the editor. Where appropriate, the readers should consult with a specialist or contact the manufacturer of the drug or device.

Glued IOL

First Edition : **2013**

ISBN: 978-93-5025-996-2

Printed at Ajanta Offset & Packagings Ltd., New Delhi

Dedicated to

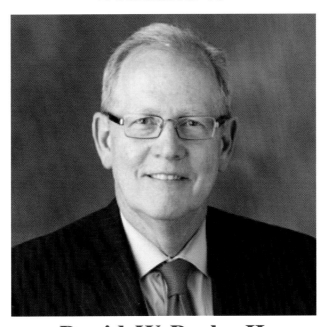

David W Parke II

Executive Vice President and CEO
American Academy of Ophthalmology
USA

Contributors

A SATHIYA PACKIALAKSHMI MSc
Dr Agarwal's Group of Eye Hospitals
and Eye Research Center
Chennai, Tamil Nadu, India

AMAR AGARWAL MS FRCS FRCOPHTH
Chairman and Managing Director
Dr Agarwal's Group of Eye Hospitals and
Eye Research Center
Chennai, Tamil Nadu, India

ANDREW S MCALLISTER MBBS Hons
Princess Alexandra Hospital
Brisbane, Australia

ASHVIN AGARWAL MS
Dr Agarwal's Group of Eye Hospitals
and Eye Research Center
Chennai, Tamil Nadu, India

ATHIYA AGARWAL MD DO
Dr Agarwal's Group of Eye Hospitals
and Eye Research Center
Chennai, Tamil Nadu, India

BALAMURALI AMBATI MD PhD MBA
Moran Eye Center,
University of Utah
Salt Lake City, Utah, USA

BRIAN STAGG MD
Moran Eye Center
University of Utah
Salt Lake City, Utah, USA

BRYCE RADMALL
Moran Eye Center
University of Utah
Salt Lake City, Utah, USA

DHIVYA ASHOK KUMAR MD
Dr Agarwal's Group of Eye Hospitals
and Eye Research Center
Chennai, Tamil Nadu, India

GABOR B SCHARIOTH MD PhD
Aurelios Eye Centers
Recklinghausen, Germany

GAURAV PRAKASH MD
Dr Agarwal's Group of Eye Hospitals
and Eye Research Center
Chennai, Tamil Nadu, India

GEORGE BEIKO BM BCH FRCSC
Assistant Professor
Department of Ophthalmology
McMaster University
Lecturer
University of Toronto
Private Practitioner in St. Catharine's
Ontario, Canada

HIMANSHU SHEKHAR MD
All India Institute of Medical Sciences
RP Center, New Delhi, India

JEEWAN S TITIYAL MD
All India Institute of Medical Sciences
RP Center, New Delhi, India

NAMRATA SHARMA MD
All India Institute of Medical Sciences
RP Center, New Delhi, India

PETER BECKINGSALE FRANZCO
Terrace Eye Center
Princess Alexandra Hospital
Brisbane, Australia

PRIYA NARANG MS
Narang Eye Hospital
Ahmedabad, Gujarat, India

RAJESH SINHA MD FRCS
All India Institute of Medical Sciences
RP Center, New Delhi, India

RASIK B VAJPAYEE MD FRCS
All India Institute of Medical Sciences
RP Center, New Delhi, India

viii

SAMARESH SRIVASTAVA DNB
Iladevi Cataract and IOL Research Center
Raghudeep Eye Clinic
Ahmedabad, Gujarat, India

SMITA NARASIMHAN FERC
Dr Agarwal's Group of Eye Hospitals
and Eye Research Center
Chennai, Tamil Nadu, India

SOM PRASAD MS FRCSED FRCOPHTH FACS
Consultant Ophthalmologist
Eye Department
Arrowe Park Hospital
Wirral, United Kingdom

SOOSAN JACOB MS FRCS Dip NB
Dr Agarwal's Group of Eye Hospitals
and Eye Research Center
Chennai, Tamil Nadu, India

SUNIL GANEKAL FRCS
Nayana Super Speciality Eye Hospital and
Research Center
Davangere, Karnataka, India

SYRIL DORAIRAJ MD
Mayo Clinic
Jacksonville, Florida, USA

TOSHIHIKO OHTA MD PhD
Assistant Professor
Department of Ophthalmology
Juntendo University, Shizuoka Hospital
Shizuoka, Japan

VAISHALI A VASAVADA MS
Iladevi Cataract and IOL Research Center
Raghudeep Eye Clinic
Ahmedabad, Gujarat, India

VIRAJ A VASAVADA MS
Iladevi Cataract and IOL Research Center
Raghudeep Eye Clinic
Ahmedabad, Gujarat, India

VISHAL JHANJI MD
Department of Ophthalmology and Visual Sciences
The Chinese University of Hong Kong
Hong Kong

ZACK OAKEY
Moran Eye Center
University of Utah
Salt Lake City, Utah, USA

Foreword

Dr Amar Agarwal is an international leader in anterior segment surgery who constantly asks and answers the question of how can we improve our surgical techniques to the betterment of our patients. He is one of the most unique thinkers of our time in ophthalmic anterior segment surgery. His videos are masterpieces of innovation that have helped educate an entire generation of ophthalmologists. In addition, he is a prolific writer with over 55 books to his credit. Not only he is a superb surgeon with many innovative instrumentations and surgical techniques to his credit, but most remarkably, he possesses the rarest of all personal attributes. He is an original thinker as well as daring, bold, creative, logical and innovative. His patient care is firmly and well-grounded on the fundamental principle that no matter what we do. 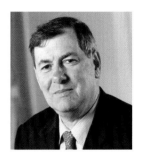 Our patients come first and we should do everything to maximize their visual outcome. No case is too complex for Dr Agarwal. In addition, Dr Agarwal, despite all of his accomplishments, is humble and self-effacing, always giving credit to anyone who has in anyway contributed to his training or surgical idea. If I could send my most demanding surgical cases to only one person or seek consultation from one individual, it would be Dr Amar Agarwal.

One of the most demanding and difficult surgical techniques is to implant an intraocular lens (IOL) in a patient without adequate support for a posterior chamber IOL. An anterior chamber IOL is often a reasonable option but in far too many cases anterior synechiae, glaucoma, or a compromised cornea make this alternative impossible. In addition, anterior chamber IOLs following complex cataract surgery have an increase risk of cystoid macular edema. This left suturing a posterior chamber IOL as the only surgical option prior to Dr Agarwal's glued posterior chamber IOL. Suturing a posterior chamber IOL to the iris or through the pars plana to the sclera are both technically challenging procedures and are associated with late complications. An additional option is quite welcome.

Dr Agarwal's invention of the fibrin glued intrascleral haptic fixation of a posterior chamber IOL is a classic example of the prepared mind investigating a new technology. When Dr Agarwal first learned of the use of fibrin glue in the management of pterygia, he was impressed with the technique like all of us who treat this condition. Most surgeons would have stopped there. However, Dr Agarwal's response was to investigate additional uses for fibrin glue. As a premier anterior segment surgeon, he knew the importance of a new technique for implanting a posterior chamber IOL. However, his additional training in vitreoretinal surgery provided him with the tools for microsurgical implantation through the pars plana under a scleral flap. This approach has been the hallmark of Dr Agarwal's career; never accept the conventional wisdom, employ all of your resources and advance patient care.

Dr Agarwal's new book represents the best of his unique and original approach to anterior segment ocular surgery. The book is a comprehensive analysis of the use of fibrin glue to facilitate intrascleral haptic fixation of a posterior chamber IOL. It summarizes all of the best and most useful and practical pearls that he has developed. Dr Agarwal has brought together an internationally recognized authors and a comprehensive series of videos to demonstrate his signature technique. This book will be widely read by anterior segment surgeons who wish to add to their surgical armamentarium and will be an important contribution to ophthalmology.

Eric Donnenfeld MD
Clinical Professor
Department of Ophthalmology
Trustee Dartmouth Medical School
New York University (NYU)
New York, USA

Preface

The expansion of knowledge in cataract, has been truly remarkable, as evidenced by the advances and new body of literature. With the glued IOL and intrascleral haptic fixation techniques, secondary IOL implantation has gone to another level. The focus of this textbook has been not so much to express one point of view on the science and handling the secondary IOL fixation, but rather to present a balanced view that is pertinent.

The goal was to create a clinically based book and an academic reference that would serve to bring the explosion of new techniques and therapeutic interventions to doctors in trenches who see such patients. This book is non-traditional in several ways. Photos, illustrations and tables are sprinkled liberally throughout the book where appropriate. The book is divided into four sections. An Interactive DVD showcasing surgeries has also been impregnated into this book.

I would like to thank all the authors who contributed to this book and help to make this book a reality. I would also like to thank Shri Jitendar P Vij (Group Chairman), Ms Sunita Katla (Publishing Manager), Ms Chetna Vohra (Senior Manager Business Development) and the entire team of Jaypee-Highlights who have brought out this book. An attempt has been made to create an informative, useful tool for all the surgeons who are interested in this technique. This should ultimately benefit our patients who place their trust in us for proper management.

Editor

Acknowledgments

I wish I could say that I had done extensive research and come out with the concept of a glued IOL. But that would be far from the truth. The actual truth is the idea just came to me from the Lord above and as with all discoveries and inventions, the whole concept of glued IOL are his and his alone.

Nothing in this world moves without him and so also this book was only written by him.

Contents

Section 3: Special Conditions

Section 4: Miscellaneous

1
Section

BASICS

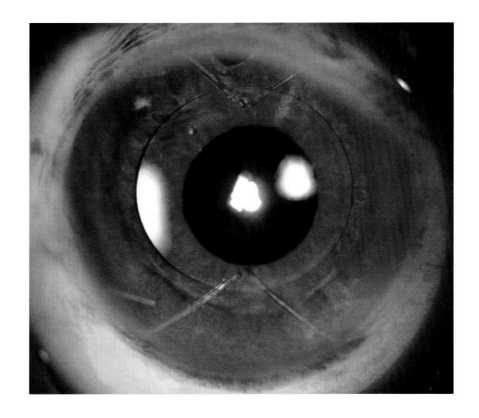

History of Glued IOL: Glued Intrascleral Haptic Fixation of a PC IOL

1

Amar Agarwal

I wish I could say that I had done extensive research and come out with the concept of a Glued IOL. But that would be far from the truth. The actual truth is the idea just came to me from the Lord above and as with all discoveries and inventions the whole concept of Glued IOL are HIS and HIS alone.

If someone had asked me what I would do in aphakic eyes with deficient capsules before 2007, I would have said AC IOL or a sutured IOL. Never in my dreams, I would have thought of the possibility of a Glued IOL or to expand it further a Glued intrascleral haptic fixation of a PC IOL.

Inauguration of a State Conference in India

I was asked to inaugurate the Chattisgarh (a state in India) state ophthalmic conference in India in December 2007. During the conference I heard many lectures and one of the distinguished faculty was talking on pterygium surgery and how it was treated with fibrin glue. To be honest I was not very knowledgable on fibrin glue and whether we were using it in our hospital (Dr Agarwal's Eye Hospital) in Chennai, India. So I called a couple of my doctors while the lecture was going on and asked them why they were not using fibrin glue in pterygium surgery. They informed me they were using it but perhaps not very often. I chided them for not using it enough, disconnected the phone and forgot about fibrin glue. I subsequently inaugurated the conference and the next day took a flight back home.

Message of Glued IOL

I was in the plane and was just thinking of the lovely conference I had just attended. It was at that time a thought struck me. It was as if a message had just entered my head of using fibrin glue to fix a PC IOL in an eye. I had not really done any research on fibrin glue nor worked on a concept. The only knowledge of fibrin glue I had was perhaps even less than what a medical student would have, let alone an ophthalmologist and yet something was telling me to use fibrin glue to fix an IOL in an eye. At that time I knew this message had to be from the Almighty and it shook me. I did not know how to proceed but promised myself to work on it once back in the hospital.

Concept of Using Glue

I started reading up about fibrin glue and understanding its properties, trade names, commercial uses and availability. I realized the only way fibrin glue could be used was if the IOL was fixed onto the sclera and the area kept dry. So obviously the IOL could not be fixed onto the iris or on any other structure.

Subluxated Non-foldable One Piece IOL

By the second week of December, I saw a lady who had been operated elsewhere. She had a one piece non-foldable polymethyl methacrylate (PMMA) IOL implanted in her eye which was lying in the anterior vitreous **(Figures 1A and B)**. I decided to try out the new procedure on her. At that time one of my consultants Dr Chandresh Baid suggested that I create scleral flaps and perform the surgery. It was a very simple but brilliant idea to create scleral flaps.

Plan of Surgery

The basic plan for surgery was to use an infusion cannula in the eye. Being a vitreoretinal surgeon also

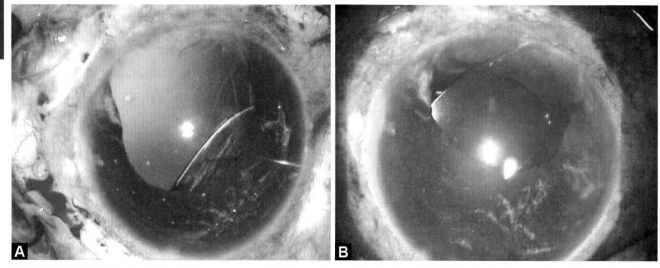

FIGURES 1A AND B: First glued IOL case operated. Case of a subluxated non-foldable single piece polymethyl methacrylate (PMMA) IOL
A. Preoperative
B. Postoperative day one

and quite comfortable in posterior vitrectomy it was not an issue. I decided to create two scleral flaps 180 degrees apart, externalize the haptics, leave them under the scleral flaps and finally glue them down with the fibrin glue. Just before the surgery I emailed a great surgeon, innovator and friend whom I admire a lot- Dr David F Chang from, USA (Discoverer of IFIS- Intraoperative floppy iris syndrome). I informed him that I was going to try out fibrin glue to fix an IOL in an eye, though I was not very sure how the surgery would go.

First Glued IOL Surgery

The surgery was posted on December 14th 2007. I thought the anterior ciliary vessels would trouble me with bleeding so decided to make the two scleral flaps superonasally and inferotemporally. I had to rotate the operating table so that I could work on the flaps with each of my hands. As our operating table is on wheels that was not an issue. I had no space inferotemporally to fix the infusion cannula so I fixed it inferonasally **(Figure 2A)**. I then performed an anterior vitrectomy **(Figure 2B)** as the last thing I wanted was a retinal tear developing due to vitreous traction. I caught the haptic with a microsurgical technology (MST) forceps to prevent it from falling down **(Figure 2C)**. I then made a sclerotomy about 1.5 mm from the limbus using a 22 gauge needle **(Figure 2D)**. I had a microsurgical

technology microrhexis 25 g forceps (designed by Larry Laks). I thought if I had a 22 g opening my 25 g forceps would go through it. Using a forceps in each hand (I had not thought of the handshake technique at that time) I then grasped the haptic and externalized the first haptic **(Figure 2E)**. I subsequently worked on the second haptic **(Figure 2F)**. At that time I did not realize the importance of grasping the extreme tip of the haptic. To externalize a PMMA one piece non-foldable IOL is very tough and doing it through a 22 gauge opening without it breaking that too if you have not caught the extreme tip is even tougher. Fortunately for me the haptics did not break. Once I had externalized the haptics **(Figure 2G)**. I performed some more vitrectomy under the IOL then kept the haptics flush with the sclera. I had made broad scleral flaps at that time so that the haptics would have more surface area to get glued. I kept the area dry, took the fibrin glue which comes with two syringes and a common cannula and applied it under the scleral flaps **(Figure 2H)** and sealed the haptics down. I subsequently used the same glue to seal the conjunctiva.

Subsequent Days

That night I did not sleep too well as I was worried if the IOL would remain stable. The next day I waited to see the patient anxiously **(Figure 1B)**. Postoperatively the patients IOL was very stable. I was delighted to

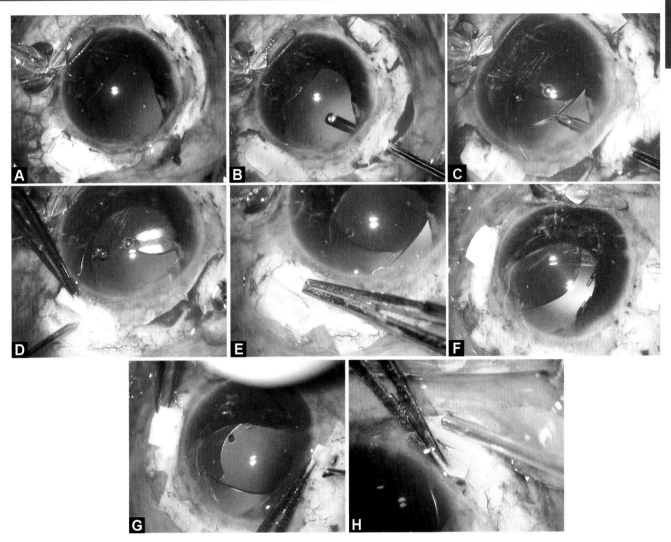

FIGURES 2A TO H: First patient in whom a Glued IOL surgery was performed
A. Scleral flaps made superonasally and inferotemporally. Infusion cannula fixed inferonasally. Surgeon sits temporally
B. Vitrectomy
C. Microsurgical technology (MST) forceps grasping the haptic
D. 22 g sclerotomy under the flap. Notice one hand holding the IOL haptic with the microsurgical technology (MST) forceps
E. Haptic externalized
F. Haptic grasped with a 25 g MST forceps. Note haptic tip not grasped
G. Haptic externalized
H. Haptic flush with the scleral bed and fibrin glue applied

see that there was no great reaction inside the eye though this was a worst case scenario which had been operated. I then did few more cases with the same technique.

Maggi's Pioneering Work

In 1997, Maggi et al published a technique whereby pars plana fixation of a posterior chamber intraocular lens (PCIOL) was achieved by transscleral passage of haptics.[1] They described a special IOL which had three equidistant loops for this procedure.

Gabor Scharioth

Though the IOLs postoperatively were stable, I still was not very convinced. I felt the IOLs though well positioned could be better fixated and made more stable. At that time I thought of the lovely work which my good friend Gabor Scharioth from Germany had done.[2] Gabor is not only a great surgeon but also a great innovator. He had met me once and explained to me his lovely sutureless intrascleral haptic fixation technique which he had started and pioneered in September 2006. He had received a video award for his work and his paper had been accepted in a peer reviewed journal. I thought then of implementing his excellent work in the Glued IOL surgery.

Scharioth Tuck in Glued IOL Surgery

I decided to implement the Scharioth tuck. Once I had externalized the haptics, I created a scleral pocket at the edge of the scleral flap using a 26 gauge needle. This is another area where the scleral flap makes a huge difference. With a scleral flap present it is very easy to create a scleral pocket at the edge of the flap and tuck the haptic inside. Once I had done the Scharioth tuck, I realized the IOL was much more stable.

Live Surgery

The first live surgery of Glued IOL was done in July 2008 at the Indian Intraocular Implant and Refractive Society Conference in Chennai, India. I was only using single piece non-foldable PMMA IOL's and was a bit tense. The problem as one can understand is that if not careful with the PMMA IOL the optic haptic junction can break. The surgery went on very well and a few doctors asked me about the surgery.

Three Piece IOL

It sounds stupid right now but for a year I was using single piece non-foldable PMMA IOLs for glued IOL surgery. A year later one of my doctors Dr Ashvin came to me and asked me why I was not using three piece IOL's. I really had no answer and replied sheepishly that I had not thought of it. Obviously I should have used three piece IOL's (foldable and non-foldable) and subsequently moved into them.

Scleral Markers and AC Maintainer

One of my consultants Dr Smita Narasimhan suggested the use of scleral markers to make sure the scleral flaps were 180 degrees apart. She also suggested the use of an AC maintainer rather than an infusion cannula. Her reasoning was that anterior segment surgeons would not have access to trocar cannulas but would have easy access to AC maintainers. It made sense and so I started using AC maintainers in many of the cases.

White to White

Some cases which had gone smoothly in the surgery, had in the immediate postoperative period a subluxation. I was wondering where the problem was and realized that these cases had a large white to white corneal diameter. Then I analyzed that the normal IOL's are 13 to 13.5 mm. If the white to white is very large lets say 12 mm I would not have enough haptic to tuck and glue. So I started being more careful in such cases by making my sclerotomy 1 mm from the limbus so that I would have more haptic externalized. Dr Jeevan Ladi from India suggested a vertical glued IOL (scleral flaps are at 12 and 6 o'clock) as the vertical cornea would be shorter than the horizontal cornea. This made a lot of sense to me and since then prefer to do vertical glued IOL, especially in eyes with a large white to white diameter.

Terminology

I was wondering what to call this procedure. I knew we had fibrin glue being used with an intrascleral haptic fixation of a PC IOL. So the term was Glued Intrascleral haptic fixation of a PC IOL. Dr Athiya suggested glued IOL as it was a short name taking the first and the last word of the title.

Publication

We published it in the Journal of cataract and refractive surgery under surgical techniques.[3] I entrusted this work to my doctors Dr Dhivya Ashok Kumar, Soosan Jacob and Gaurav Prakash who subsequently published material on glued IOL in other journals.[4-11]

Pediatric Glued IOL

A four-year child from another city had history of injury in her eye while bursting crackers. She underwent emergency surgery for lens removal due to severe injury to the lens and I fixed a sutured IOL in her eye in the last quarter of 2007. At that time the concept of glued IOL had not come through. After a month, when the child came for follow-up, it was found that there was a decenteration of the IOL. The parents noted the child's difficulty in performing activities. Under general anesthesia I then removed the existing sutured IOL and placed a new IOL using the Glued IOL technique. This was the first pediatric Glued IOL done.

Personal: Mother-in-Law

In 2011 Dr Athiya (my wife) and I were invited to Riyadh, Saudi Arabia to give lectures on glued IOL and also to perform some surgeries in Jeddah. At that time I was thinking of my mother-in-law who was 85 years old and had been operated on by Dr (Mrs) T Agarwal (my mother) 30 years back. Intracapsular cataract extraction was done at that time and no IOL was implanted. I suggested to my wife we should do a glued IOL on her. I thought she would divorce me immediately. To my surprise she agreed. When we returned we examined her and noticed she had an endothelial cell count of 1400. Both eyes were aphakic but she was 20/20 with aphakic glasses. I still decided to go ahead with the surgery with my wife watching through the operating microscope side scope and glued in a three piece foldable IOL **(Figures 3A to D)**.

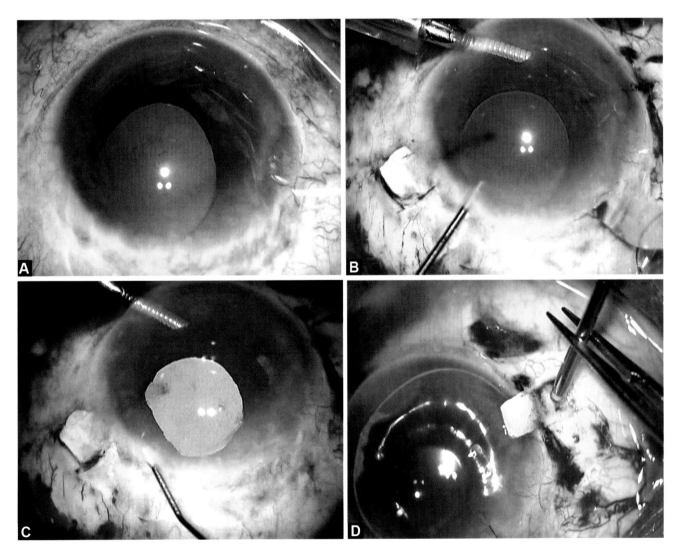

FIGURES 3A TO D: Mother-in-law's glued IOL surgery
A. Intracapsular cataract extraction done. Eye is aphakic. Preoperative 20/20 with aphakic glasses
B. Three piece foldable IOL implantation. Note the AC maintainer and the scleral flaps
C. PC IOL in place and haptics tucked
D. Fibrin glue applied on the scleral bed of the flaps. Note the intrascleral haptic tuck in the Scharioth pocket. Also note the air in the AC which would help the sclerotomy area to be dry and also prevent any hypotony postoperatively. Postoperative vision was 20/20 without aphakic glasses

Luckily the surgery went on very well and she was postoperative 20/20 and was finally rid of those thick aphakic glasses. The reason I mention this case is to explain that if I did not have the confidence in glued IOL I would never have done it on my own mother-in-law. I had never thought of an AC IOL or a sutured IOL in all these years for her.

Conclusion

Science contunues to evolve, so also with the glued IOL technique. From the first case of sutureless scleral fixation done by Maggi in 1997 to the intrascleral haptic fixation done by Gabor Scharioth in 2006 to the glued IOL in 2007 till today so many surgeons have brought in new ideas to refine this procedure started by the Almighty. All we can do is thank HIM for giving us an opportunity to help our patients see better.

References

1. Maggi R, Maggi C. Sutureless scleral fixation of intraocular enses. J Cataract Refract Surg. 1997;23:1289-1294.
2. Gabor SG, Pavilidis MM. Sutureless intrascleral posterior chamber intraocular lens fixation. J Cataract Refract Surg. 2007;33(11):1851-4.
3. Agarwal A, Kumar DA, Jacob S, Baid C, Agarwal A, Srinivasan S. Fibrin glue-assisted sutureless posterior chamber intraocular lens implantation in eyes with deficient posterior capsules. J Cataract Refract Surg. 2008;34(9):1433-8.
4. Kumar DA, Agarwal A, Prakash G, Jacob S, Saravanan Y, Agarwal A. Glued posterior chamber IOL in eyes with deficient capsular support: a retrospective analysis of 1-year postoperative outcomes. Eye (Lond). 2010;24(7):1143-8.
5. Prakash G, Kumar DA, Jacob S, Kumar KS, Agarwal A, Agarwal A. Anterior segment optical coherence tomography-aided diagnosis and primary posterior chamber intraocular lens implantation with fibrin glue in traumatic phacocele with scleral perforation. J Cataract Refract Surg. 2009;35(4):782-4.
6. Prakash G, Jacob S, Kumar DA, Narsimhan S, Agarwal A, Agarwal A. Femtosecond assisted keratoplasty with fibrin glue-assisted sutureless posterior chamber lens implantation: a new triple procedure. J Cataract Refract Surg. J Cataract Refract Surg. 2009;35(6):973-9.
7. Nair V, Kumar DA, Prakash G, Jacob S, Agarwal A, Agarwal A. Bilateral spontaneous in-the-bag anterior subluxation of PC IOL managed with glued IOL technique: A case report. Eye Contact Lens. 2009;35(4):215-7.
8. Agarwal A, Kumar DA, Prakash G, et al. Fibrin glue-assisted sutureless posterior chamber intraocular lens implantation in eyes with deficient posterior capsules [Reply to letter]. J Cataract Refract Surg. 2009;35(5):795-6.
9. Kumar DA, Agarwal A, Jacob S, Prakash G, Agarwal A, Sivagnanam S. Repositioning of the dislocated intraocular lens with sutureless 20-gauge vitrectomy retina. 2010;30(4):682-7.
10. Kumar DA, Agarwal A, Prakash G, Jacob S. Managing total aniridia with aphakia using a glued iris prosthesis. J Cataract Refract Surg. 2010;36(5):864-5.
11. Kumar DA, Agarwal A, Gabor SG, et al. Sutureless sclera fixated posterior chamber intraocular lens. Letter to editor. J Cataract Refract Surg. 2011;37(11):2089-90.

2 | Posterior Capsular Rupture

Dhivya Ashok Kumar, Amar Agarwal

Introduction

Any breach in the continuity of the posterior capsule is defined as a posterior capsule tear. Intrasurgical posterior capsule tears are the most common and can occur during any stage of cataract surgery.[1-3] The incidence of posterior capsule complications is related to the type of cataract and conditions of the eye, increases with the grade of difficulty of the case, and furthermore is influenced by the level of experience of the surgeon. Timely recognition and a planned management, depending upon the stage of surgery during which the posterior capsule tear has occurred, is required to ensure an optimal visual outcome.

Common Risk Factors for Posterior Capsular Rupture (PCR)

1. Intraoperative factors causing variation in anterior chamber depth
2. Type of cataract
3. Extended rhexis

Intraoperative Factors Causing Variation in Anterior Chamber Depth

Intraoperative shallow anterior chamber could be due to various reasons. It may be a tight lid speculum, tight drapes, or pull from the collecting bag. In all the above cases, remove the precipitating factor (Remove the speculum pressure, remove the tight drapes and collecting bags). Variation in the amount of space in the anterior and posterior chambers may result from changes in the intraocular pressure (IOP) due to an alteration in the equilibrium between inflow and outflow of fluid. Diminished inflow may be secondary to insufficient bottle height, tube occlusion or compression, bottle emptying, too tight incisions compressing

the irrigation sleeve, or the surgeon moving the phaco tip out of the incision, making the irrigation holes come out of the incision. Excessive outflow may be caused by too high vacuum/flow parameters, or too large incisions with leakage. Another cause is the post-occlusion surge. Use of air pump or gas forced infusion solves most of these problems of intraoperative shallow anterior chamber.[1]

Type of Cataract

A higher incidence of posterior capsule tear with vitreous loss is associated with cataract with pseudo-exfoliation, diabetes mellitus, and trauma. Missing the diagnosis in a posterior polar cataract **(Figure 1)** can be catastrophic to the surgeon and the patient. It is frequently associated with a weakened or deficient posterior capsule. Posterior lenticonus, cataracts with

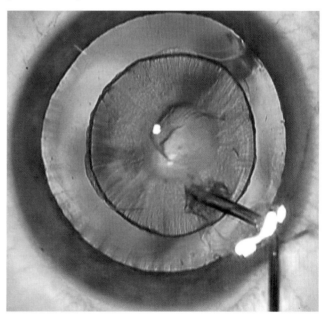

FIGURE 1: Hydrodelineation being performed in a posterior polar cataract

persistent primary hyperplastic vitreous, cataracts following vitreoretinal surgery and morgagnian cataracts are some of the other types. In any intraoperative diagnosis of posterior polar cataract, avoid hydrodissection with balanced salt solution (BSS). Hydrodissection may cause hydraulic perforation at the weakened area of the capsule, hence only a careful controlled hydrodelineation is preferred. One can also make multiple pockets of viscoelastic injection around the nucleus. If a capsular tear does occur, a closed system should be maintained by injecting viscoelastic before withdrawing the phaco tip. This helps to tamponade the vitreous backwards where a capsular dehiscence is present.

Extended Rhexis

Extension of the anterior capsule can occur as a complication in microincision cataract surgery (MICS) also. During capsulorhexis, anterior capsular tears can cause posterior capsule tear by extending to the periphery. In a new method of managing this situation, a nick is made from the opposite side of the rhexis using a cystitome or vannas and the capsulorhexis is completed. The viscoelastic in the anterior chamber (AC) is then expressed out to make the globe hypotonous, following which a gentle hydrodissection is done at 90 degrees from the tear while pressing the posterior lip of the incision to prevent any rise in intraocular pressure (IOP). No attempt is made to press on the center of the nucleus to complete the fluid wave. The fluid is usually sufficient to prolapse one pole of the nucleus out of the capsular bag; else it is removed by embedding the phacoemulsification probe, making sure not to exert any downward pressure and then gently pulling the nucleus anteriorly. The whole nucleus is brought out into the AC and no nuclear division techniques are tried in the bag. The entire nucleus is prolapsed into the anterior chamber and emulsified.

Steps for Management of PCR

The surgeon should be aware of the signs **(Table 1)** of posterior capsular tear. Posterior capsule tears can occur during any stage of phacoemulsification surgery. They occurred most frequently during the stage of nuclear emulsification, as reported by Mulhern et al[4] (49%) and Osher et al,[5] and during irrigation-aspiration, as reported by Gimbel et al.[6]

TABLE 1: SIGNS OF POSTERIOR CAPSULAR RUPTURE

1. Sudden deepening of the chamber, with momentary expansion of the pupil.
2. Sudden, transitory appearance of a clear red reflex peripherally.
3. Apparent inability to rotate a previously mobile nucleus.
4. Excessive lateral mobility or displacement of the nucleus.
5. Excessive tipping of one pole of the nucleus.
6. Partial descent of the nucleus into the anterior vitreous space.
7. 'Pupil snap sign'—sudden marked pupil constriction after hydrodissection

Three possible situations can happen in a posterior capsule rent namely:[7]
1. Posterior capsule tear with hyaloid face intact and nuclear material present.
2. Posterior capsule tear with hyaloid face ruptured without luxation of nuclear material into vitreous.
3. Posterior capsule tear with hyaloid face ruptured and luxation of nuclear material into vitreous.

Immediate precautions are to be taken not to further hydrate the vitreous and not to increase the size of the PCR. The conventional management consists of prevention of mixture of cortical matter with vitreous, dry aspiration, and anterior vitrectomy, if required. In addition, during phacoemulsification low flow rate, high vacuum, and low ultrasound are advocated if a posterior capsule tear occurs.

Reduce the Parameters

Lowering aspiration flow rate and decreasing the vacuum will control surge and will allow the bottle to be lowered, diminishing turbulence inside the eye. If the nucleus is soft, only a small residual amount remains, and there is no vitreous prolapse, the procedure may be continued. If vitreous is already present, special care must be taken for preventing additional vitreous prolapse into the anterior chamber or to the wound. Small residual nucleus or cortex can be emulsified by bringing it out of the capsular bag and can be emulsified in the anterior chamber with viscoelastic underneath the corneal endothelium. In case of a small PCR and minimal residual nucleus **(Figure 2)**, a dispersive viscoelastic is injected to plug the posterior capsule tear. Subsequently the nuclear material is moved into the anterior chamber with a spatula and emulsified. The recommended parameters are low bottle height (20-40 cm above the patient's head), low flow rate

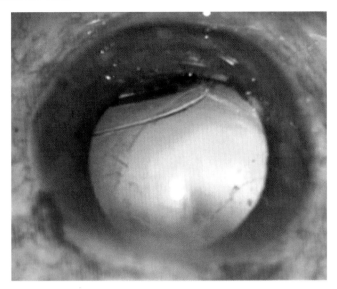

FIGURE 2: Posterior capsular rupture
Note the IOL sinking into the vitreous cavity. The white reflex indicates nuclear fragments also in the vitreous cavity. This patient was managed by vitrectomy, FAVIT (removal of the nuclear fragments) and the IOL repositioned in the sulcus

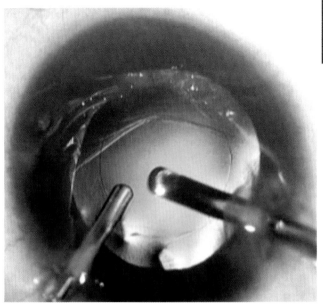

FIGURE 3: Bimanual vitrectomy is being performed in a posterior capsular tear with vitreous prolapse

(10-15 cc/min), high vacuum (120-200 mm Hg) and low ultrasound (20-40%).

Dry Cortical Aspiration

If there is only a small amount or no vitreous prolapse in the presence of a small capsular rent, a dry cortical aspiration with 23 G cannula can be performed.

Viscoexpression

It is a method of removal of the residual nucleus by injecting viscoelastic underneath the nucleus to support it and the nucleus is expressed along with the viscoelastic.

Conversion to ECCE

If there is sizeable amount of residual nucleus, it is advisable to convert to a large incision ECCE to minimize the possibility of a dropped nucleus.

Anterior Bimanual Vitrectomy

Bimanual vitrectomy **(Figure 3)** is done in eyes with vitreous prolapse. Use a 23 G irrigating cannula via side port after extending the side port incision. The irrigation bottle is positioned at the appropriate height to maintain the anterior chamber during vitrectomy. Vitrectomy should be performed with cutting rate (500 to 800 cuts per minute), an aspiration flow rate of 20 cc/min, and a vacuum of 150-200 mm Hg.

Anterior Chamber Cleared of Vitreous

Vitrectomy is continued in the anterior chamber and the pupillary plane. A rod can be introduced into the anterior chamber to check the presence of any vitreous traction and the same should be released. Complete removal of the vitreous from the anterior chamber can be confirmed if you see a circular, mobile pupil **(Figures 4A and B)** and complete air bubble in the anterior chamber. The usage of the fiber of an endoilluminator, dimming the room lights and microscope lights, may be useful in cases of doubt, in order to identify vitreous strands. Another useful measure is the use of purified triamcinolone acetate suspension (Kenalog) to identify the vitreous described by Peyman.[8] Kenalog particles remain trapped on and within the vitreous gel, making it clearly visible.[9]

Suture the Wound

In cases with vitreous loss with PCR, it is recommended to suture the corneal wound as a prophylaxis to prevent infection. Remove any residual vitreous in the incision site in the main and side port with vitrector or manually with vannas scissors. If necessary insert a rod via the side port, and pass it over the surface of the iris, to release them.

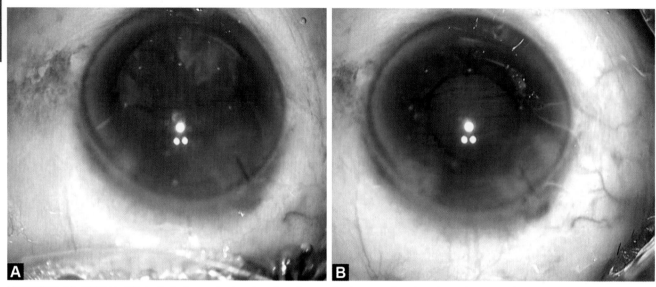

FIGURES 4A AND B: Clinical photograph showing the change in the anterior chamber after complete removal of the vitreous from the anterior chamber
A. Before vitrectomy
B. After vitrectomy

IOL Implantation

Depending upon the state of the capsular bag and rhexis, an IOL is implanted **(Table 2)**.

TABLE 2: IOL IMPLANTATION IN PCR

1. Insertion and rotation of IOL should always be away from the area of capsule tear.
2. The long axis of the IOL should cross the meridian of the posterior capsule tear.
3. Eyes with (< 6 mm) PCR with no vitreous loss, IOL can be placed in the capsular bag.
4. In the presence of a posterior capsule tear (> 6 mm) with adequate anterior capsule rim, an IOL can be placed in the sulcus.
5. In deficient capsules, Glued IOL is a promising technique without complications of sutured scleral fixated or anterior chamber IOL.

In the Bag

In the presence of a posterior capsule tear with good capsular bag, the IOL can be placed in the bag. Small PCR with no vitreous loss and good capsular bag, foldable IOL can be placed.

In the Sulcus

If the rent is large, if the capsular rim is available, then the IOL can be placed in the sulcus. The rigid IOL can be placed in the sulcus in large PCR over the residual anterior capsular rim with Mc Person forceps holding the optic. The "chopstick technique" is another method of placing IOL

in sulcus. In this new chopstick forceps namely, 'Agarwal-Katena forceps' **(Figures 5A and B)** is used for IOL implantation. This chopstick technique refers to the IOL being held between two flangs of the forceps. The advantage is the smooth placement of the IOL in the sulcus without excess manipulation. Moreover the IOL implantation is more controlled **(Figures 6A to D)** with the forceps as compared to other methods. In a small PCR with no vitreous loss and good capsular bag, a foldable IOL can be placed **(Figures 7A and B)**. In eyes with intraoperative miosis with PCR, IOL can be implanted with the pupil expansion with "Agarwal's modified Malyugin ring" method **(Figures 8A and B)**. In this method,[10] a 6-0 polyglactic suture is placed in the leading scroll of the Malyugin ring and injected into the pupillary plane **(Figures 9A and B)**. The end of the suture stays at the main port incision. Once in place, the ring produces a stable mydriasis of about 6.0 mm. Hereby the IOL can be implanted easily in the sulcus with visualization and this prevents the inadvertent dropping of the iris expander into the vitreous during intraoperative manipulation.

Deficient Posterior Capsule

Now recently Glued IOL[11-13] is easily performed in such cases with deficient posterior capsules. Scleral fixated posterior chamber lenses and anterior chamber IOLs[14,15] can also be implanted when the posterior capsule tear is large.

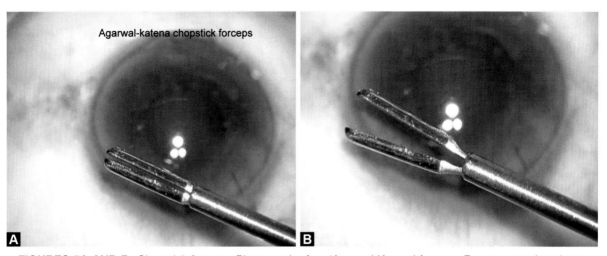

FIGURES 5A AND B: Chopstick forceps. Photograph of an 'Agarwal-Katena' forceps. Reverse opening shown (right) (Katena, USA)

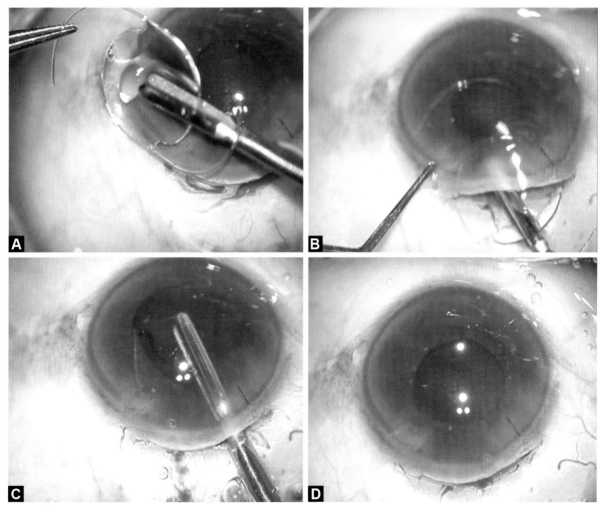

FIGURES 6A TO D: Chopstick technique
A. The 6.5 mm PMMA rigid IOL being held between two flangs of the forceps
B. IOL is being introduced through the limbal incision
C. IOL is positioned in the sulcus
D. IOL is well centered

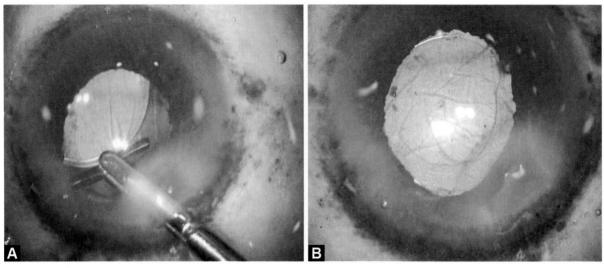

FIGURES 7A AND B: Chopstick technique for a foldable IOL
A. Foldable IOL is placed with 'Agarwal-Katena' forceps into the sulcus
B. IOL well centered on the capsular rim

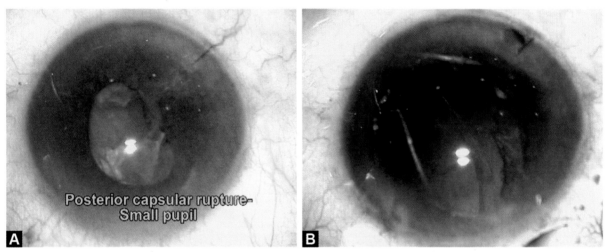

FIGURES 8A AND B: Agarwal modification of the Malyugin ring in cases of PC rupture
A. Intraoperative miosis with posterior capsular tear
B. Agarwal's modification of the Malyugin ring iris expansion
   A 6-0 polyglactic vicryl suture passed in the leading scroll of the ring and injected. The end of the suture stays at the main port incision.

Sequelae after Posterior Capsular Rupture

Vitreous Traction

Incomplete vitrectomy can produce dynamic traction on the retina leading to retinal breaks.

Retinal Detachment

Undetected long-standing vitreous traction progresses to retinal break and detachment.

Macular Edema

Manipulation of vitreous will increase not only the traction transmitted to the retina but also the inflammation in the posterior segment, and the risk of macular edema.

Vitritis

Over enthusiastic use of viscoelastic into the vitreous can lead to sterile inflammation. Dropped minimal residual cortex can also present with postoperative vitritis.

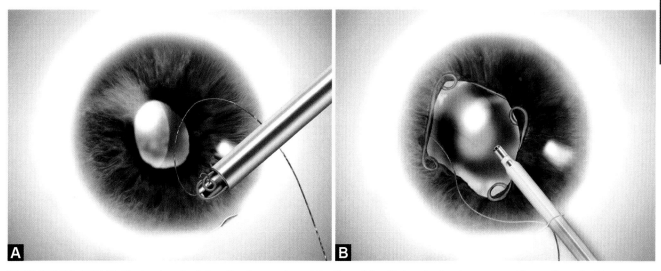

FIGURES 9A AND B: Illustration depicting the Agarwal modification of the Malyugin ring for cases with small pupil with a posterior capsular rupture
A. 6/0 suture tied to the ring
B. Malyugin ring in place in the pupil. The suture can be pulled at if the ring begins to fall into the vitreous

IOL Related Complications

Improperly placed IOL in the sulcus can lead to lens induced astigmatism and tilt.

Conclusion

The occurrence of a posterior capsule tear during cataract surgery is one of the most serious complications. It is important for a surgeon to diagnose the occurrence of a posterior capsule tear at an early stage to avoid further enlargement of the tear and associated vitreous complications. The primary goal of all the maneuvers is to remove the remaining nucleus, epinucleus, and as much cortex as possible without causing vitreoretinal traction.

References

1. Agarwal A. Phaco Nightmares; Conquering cataract catastrophes; Slack Inc, 2006, USA.
2. Agarwal S, Agarwal A, Agarwal A. Phacoemulsification, 2 volumes set, Third edition, Jaypee Brothers Medical Publishers, New Delhi, India, 2004.
3. Fishkind WJ. Facing Down the 5 Most Common Cataract Complications Review of Ophthalmology. October 2001.
4. Mulhern M, Kelly G, Barry P. Effects of posterior capsular disruption on the outcome of phacoemulsification surgery. Br J Ophthalmol 1995;79:1133-7.
5. Osher RH, Cionni RJ. The torn posterior capsule: its intra-operative behaviour, surgical management and long term consequences. J Cataract Refract Surg 1990;16:490-4.
6. Gimbel HV. Posterior capsular tears during phacoemulsification—causes, prevention and management. Eur J Refract Surg. 1990;2:63-9.
7. Vajpayee RB, Sharma N, Dada T, et al. Management of posterior capsule tears. Surv Ophthal 2001;45:473-88.
8. Peyman GA, Cheema R, Conway MD, Fang T. Triamcinolone acetonide as an aid to visualization of the vitreous and the posterior hyaloid during pars plana vitrectomy. Retina 2000; 20:554.
9. Burk SE, Da Mata AP, Snyder ME, Schneider S, Osher RH, Cionni RJ. Visualizing vitreous using Kenalog suspension. J Cataract Refract Surg. 2003;29:645.
10. Agarwal A, Malyugin B, Kumar DA, Jacob S, Agarwal A, Laks L. Modified Malyugin ring iris expansion technique in small-pupil cataract surgery with posterior capsule defect. J Cataract Refract Surg. 2008;34(5):724-6.
11. Agarwal A, Kumar DA, Jacob S, et al. Fibrin glue-assisted sutureless posterior chamber intraocular lens implantation in eyes with deficient posterior capsules. J Cataract Refract Surg. 2008;34:1433-8.
12. Agarwal A, Kumar DA, Prakash G, et al. Fibrin glue-assisted sutureless posterior chamber intraocular lens implantation in eyes with deficient posterior capsules [Reply to letter]. J Cataract Refract Surg. 2009;35:795-6.
13. Prakash G, Kumar DA, Jacob S, et al. Anterior segment optical coherence tomography-aided diagnosis and primary posterior chamber intraocular lens implantation with fibrin glue in traumatic phacocele with scleral perforation. J Cataract Refract Surg. 2009;35:782-4.
14. Bleckmann H, Kaczmarek U. Functional results of posterior chamber lens implantation with scleral fixation. J Cataract Refract Surg. 1994;20:321-6.
15. Numa A, Nakamura J, Takashima M, Kani K. Long-term corneal endothelial changes after intraocular lens implantation. Anterior vs posterior chamber lenses. Jpn J Ophthalmol. 1993; 37:78-87.

3 Tissue Adhesives in Ophthalmology: Current Scenario and Future Prospects

Sunil Ganekal, Syril Dorairaj, Vishal Jhanji

Introduction

Tissue adhesives were initially developed as suture adjuncts and alternatives for sealing wounded tissues. The application of tissue adhesives in ophthalmology started in the early half of the 19th century.[1] The drive towards the development of an adhesive came from the complications associated with suturing, including postoperative discomfort, prolonged healing time, as well as the risk of infection. Tissue adhesives have gained popularity in the recent years due to their ease of use and postoperative comfort. With increasing popularity of sutureless treatment by both clinicians and patients, there is a great need for improved standardization of preparation and application techniques for both existing and emerging adhesives.

Classification

Tissue adhesives can be categorized into two main classes, **Synthetic** (e.g. cyanoacrylate and acrylic-based polymers), and **biological** (e.g. fibrin glue and biodendrimers). Each of these adhesives have their own advantages and disadvantages. An ideal tissue adhesive should be easy to use and have a short setting time, biocompatibility, transparency and high tensile strength.

Synthetic Tissue Adhesives

Cyanoacrylate and Acrylic-based Tissue Adhesives

Characteristics

Cyanoacrylate glue is one of the oldest glues used in ophthalmic surgeries. Cyanoacrylates are esters of cyanoacrylic acid **(Figure 1)**, formed through the condensation of cyanoacetate with formaldehyde in the

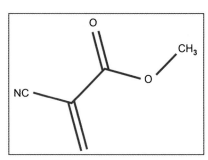

FIGURE 1: Cyanoacrylate

presence of a chemical catalyst.[2] The polymerization of the glue on the surface of any tissue is achieved via a hydroxylation reaction where the cyanoacrylate monomers rapidly polymerize in the presence of water or weak bases.[3,4] The toxicity of the glue depends on the length of alkyl side chains. Shorter side chains have greater toxic effects on the tissue whereas longer side-chain adhesives have a slower degradation rate as well as lower toxicity.[4,5] The bonding strength of various cyanoacrylate derivatives has been found to be higher in dry conditions. It was also found that tensile strength decreased with an increase in alkyl side chains.[6,7] Eiferman et al showed the bacteriostatic effects of butyl-2-cyanoacrylate *in vitro* and *in vivo* against Gram-positive microorganisms.[8] Antibacterial analysis of ethyl-cyanoacrylate also showed bacteriostatic and bactericidal nature against Gram-positive microorganisms and Gram-negative organisms.[9]

Bioadhesives: Fibrin Glue Characteristics

Purified fibrin has been reported to treat parenchymal bleeding since the early 19th century and the combination of fibrin and thrombin has been used for skin graft adhesion.[10] The sealer protein generally has two major components, fibrinogen and thrombin, two coagulating factors, aprotinin (fibrinolysis inhibitor) and calcium chloride. The setting time of the mixture is usually dependent on the thrombin concentration. A fast-setting mixture sets within 30 seconds and a slow-setting mixture sets within 1-2 minutes. Fibrin glue is designed to mimic the last stage of blood coagulation. Factor XIIIa is a transglutaminase that catalyzes the final steps in the formation of a fibrin clot. The enzyme stabilizes the fibrin clot through crosslinking (CXL) of fibrin monomers to each other, as well as CXL of fibronectin and a2-plasmin inhibitor to fibrin.[11-13]

Fibrin glue clot formation starts with the activation of Factor XIII by thrombin. The activated Factor XIII then hydrolyzes prothrombin to thrombin. Thrombin converts fibrinogen into fibrin. Fibrin self-assembles into fibers to form a 3D matrix. Thrombin also activates Factor XIIIa (present in the fibrinogen component of the glue), which stabilizes the clot by crosslinking fibrin fibers as well as by inducing polymerization of the fibers in the presence of calcium ions. The main disadvantages of fibrin glue include long preparation time for thrombin-induced activation of the enzyme, proteolytic degradation, and low adhesion strength. Also, there is a latent risk of viral transmission, although various strategies have been developed to reduce this risk.

Commercially Available Fibrin Glue

Fibrin glue was developed in 1972 by Matras et al. Fibrin sealant has been available in Europe since 1978 and blood bank or laboratory-derived fibrin sealants have been used in the USA since the 1980s. Tisseel® (Baxter Immuno, Vienna, Austria) was the first fibrin sealant approved by the US FDA. Fibrin sealant is now FDA approved for use as a topical hemostat, sealant and adhesive.[14]

All fibrin sealants in use have two major ingredients, purified fibrinogen and purified thrombin derived from human or bovine blood. Many sealants have two additional ingredients, *human blood Factor XIII and aprotinin,* which is derived from cows' lungs.

In India **ReliSeal**® (Fibrin sealant, Relaince life sciences) is commercially available.

There are currently four available FDA-approved commercial fibrin sealants distributed by US companies: **Tisseel and Artiss** (Baxter, CA, USA), **Evicel™** (Johnson & Johnson, NJ, USA), **Cryoseal**® (Thermogenesis, CA, USA) and **Vitagel™** (Orthovita, PA, USA).

- **Tisseel and Evicel** fibrin sealants are prepared from human pooled plasma.
- **Cryoseal** is prepared from individual units of plasma.
- **Vitagel** is prepared from individual units of plasma, bovine collagen, and bovine thrombin.

In Europe, **Tisseel/Tissucol™**, **Beriplast**® (Aventis Behring) and **Quixil** (Johnson & Johnson Wound Management/Omrix Biopharmaceuticals) are approved for use. *Tisseel* and *Beriplast* both utilize aprotinin (fibrinolysis inhibitor) derived from bovine sources. *Quixil* on the other hand uses a synthetic fibrinolysis inhibitor (tranexamic acid) to eliminate the risk of immunological response.

The following are the most commonly used and approved commercially available fibrin glue products.

Tisseel/Tissucol Fibrin Sealant

The commercially available Tisseel is manufactured by Baxter Immuno. It is FDA approved and is utilized in surgical procedures worldwide for hemostasis in general surgery. The kit contains fibrinogen, thrombin, aprotinin and calcium chloride. It can be stored up to 6 months. Viral transmission risk is reduced by a combination of cryoprecipitation, adsorption, vapor heating and freeze-drying.

Evicel (Johnson & Johnson) Fibrin Sealant

Evicel is manufactured by Omrix Biopharmaceuticals (Ramat-Gan, Israel) and marketed by Johnson & Johnson. Evicel has been FDA approved for hemostasis in liver surgery. Viral disease transmission risk is reduced by cryoprecipitation, pasteurization, solvent detergent cleansing and nanofiltration. Unlike Tisseel, Evicel does not require an antifibrinolytic agent.

Vitagel (Orthovita) Surgical Hemostat

The Vitagel kit (Orthovita, Inc., PA, USA) is intended for use with plasma derived from the patient's own blood and has been FDA approved for surgical procedures excluding neurosurgery and eye surgery. The use of autologous derived fibrinogen eliminates risk of viral transmission. Bovine thrombin, however, poses a risk as it elicits elevated production of IgG antibody which interacts with human coagulation protein leading to thromboembolism.[15]

ReliSeal® (Fibrin Sealant)

Biological glue and haemostatic agent ReliSeal is marketed in India by Reliance Life Sciences. It can be used in a variety of surgical procedures to arrest bleeding, seal tissues and as an adjunct to wound healing. The kit is available in 0.5 ml and 1 ml pack sizes. Application involves preparation of fibrinogen and thrombin in separate syringes and mixing both in the applicator system.

Application Techniques

The two components of fibrin glue, fibrinogen and thrombin, can either be applied simultaneously or sequentially, depending on the physician's preference. When simultaneous application is preferred, both the components are loaded into two syringes **(Figure 2)** with tips forming a common port (e.g. Duploject® syringe). When injected, the two components are mixed in equal volumes at the point of delivery. The setting time is dependent on the concentration of the thrombin component.[16] For sequential application, thrombin is first applied on to the area of interest, followed by a thin layer of fibrinogen. When apposition is required between two surfaces, thrombin solution may be applied to one and fibrinogen to the other surface. Spray applicators comprising of gas-pressurized devices (e.g. the Tisseel EasySpray system) have also been developed for fibrin glue application.

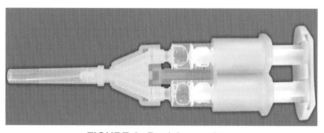

FIGURE 2: Duploject syringe

Safety of Fibrin Glue

The greatest possible hazard of fibrin glue is the risk of viral transmission especially in formulations comprising fibrinogen extracted from multiple donors.[17] Hino et al reported three cases of parvovirus B19 transmission from the use of commercial fibrin sealants.[18] Further methods have been developed to minimize this risk including the use of combination of gamma-radiation, cryoprecipitation, vapor heating, pasteurization and nanofiltration. Although, the safest source would be the patient's own blood, it must be borne in mind that the biological activity of fibrinogen itself also poses a risk.[19] Therefore, reduced amounts of fibrinogen for surgical procedures are recommended to prevent additional inflammatory reactions. Despite the above-mentioned risks, fibrin glue is being extensively used in ophthalmic procedures. It has been shown to cause minimal inflammation in most cases. It causes significantly less postoperative discomfort compared to the use of sutures and cyanoacrylate glue.

Potential Adhesives in Future

Recent years have witnessed the introduction of various adhesives that are being developed for use in surgical fields. The following are some of the novel bioadhesives that have not yet been approved for clinical use but show promise as sutureless alternatives in ophthalmic surgery.

Photo-activated Dendritic Polymers

Carnahan and coworkers have demonstrated the use of the dendritic bioadhesive ([G1]-PGLSA-MA)2-PEG in numerous ocular applications including corneal lacerations, cataract incisions, LASIK flaps and penetrating keratoplasties.[20] Berdahl et al also tested the same polymer adhesive to evaluate clinical and histological healing of corneal lacerations in an *in vivo* chicken model.[21] Crosslinking of this biodendrimer polymer is activated by an argon ion laser. Advantages of photo-activated biodendritic adhesive include faster repair time, transparency, and minimal inflammation. The disadvantages include the added time and equipment that is required for photopolymerization. Another novel chemically derived bioadhesive (CDB), composed of aldehyded dextrans and e-poly (l-lysine) solution was developed by Araki et al[22] Takaoka et al also demonstrated the use of CDB glue in sutureless automated lamellar therapeutic keratoplasty in rabbit eyes.[23] No significant difference was observed in corneal clarity, epithelialization, and inflammatory response between sutureless and suture models.

Gelatin Resorcinol

Gelatin-resorcinol-aldehyde comprises of gelatin and resorcinol and aldehydes. Although studies have demonstrated that its bonding strength to tissues is higher than that of fibrin glue,[24] the major deterrence to using gelatin-resorcinol-formaldehyde in ophthalmic surgery is the high toxicity of formaldehyde.

Albumin-glutaraldehyde Adhesive

The most common formulation of serum albumin and glutaraldehyde is a commercially available product, BioGlue (Cryoline Inc., GA, USA) that was approved by the FDA in 1999 as an adjunct to sutures for aortic dissections. Engel et al reported a case where BioGlue was applied in addition to sutures to a jagged scleral rupture.[25] Use of BioGlue in ophthalmic surgeries has not been popular mainly due to the safety concerns with glutaraldehyde. Also, since serum albumin is derived from bovine products, allergic reaction is also a potential hazard.

Hyaluronic Acid-based Photocatalytic Glue

Miki et al have developed a photocrosslinkable adhesive composed of hyaluronic acid modified with methacrylate groups with ethyl eosin as photo-initiator and triethanolamine as co-catalyst.[26] Upon irradiation with a low-intensity argon laser beam, the viscous polymer solution turns into a flexible transparent hydrophilic hydrogel. The solution has been successfully used on corneal lacerations in an *in vivo* study using rabbits.

Laser Welding and Soldering

Laser welding utilizes photochemical or thermal reactions to induce tissue fusion. The first use of the laser for tissue welding in eye was for the treatment of retinal detachment. Precise control of temperature is the greatest challenge of the laser-induced tissue fusion technique. Matteini and coworkers have reported successful tissue welding at a very low laser power (12-16 W/cm^2).[27] In a retrospective study, Menabuoni et al performed an *in vivo* study on rabbit eyes to evaluate the effect of laser welding on the healing process.[28] In a follow-up study, Menabuoni et al[29] evaluated laser-assisted closure of the corneal wounds by diode laser welding of the stroma in patients undergoing phacoemulsification and extracapsular cataract extraction. Surgeries were followed by laser-assisted closure of the corneal wounds by diode laser welding of the stroma using a technique established in animal models. Seidel test was negative during the follow-up examinations, and endothelial cell loss was similar to that published for standard surgical cataract procedures.

Current Uses of Tissue Adhesives in Ophthalmic Surgery

- Pterygium surgery
- Amniotic membrane transplantation
- Corneal perforations
- Sealing corneal cataract wounds
- Epithelial ingrowth and other laser-assisted *in situ* keratomileusis complications

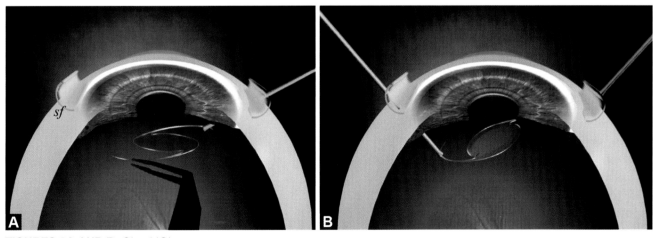

FIGURES 3A AND B: Glued IOL
Image showing sclerotomy made with 20/22G needle beneath the flaps
Haptics exteriorized by 23/25G forceps beneath the scleral flaps (*sf*)

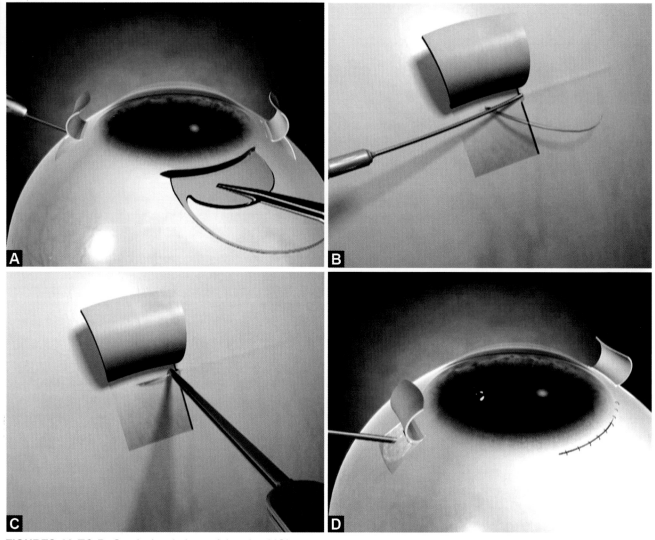

FIGURES 4A TO D: Surgical technique of the glued IOL
A. IOL haptic grasped with a glued IOL forceps (Microsurgical technology, MST, USA)
B. 26 gauge needle creates a Scharioth scleral pocket at the edge of the flap
C. IOL haptic tucked into the scleral pocket
D. Fibrin glue applied under the scleral flaps
.

- Penetrating keratoplasty
- Limbal cell transplantation
- Scleral fixation of intraocular lens **(Figures 3 and 4)**
- Glaucoma surgery and bleb leaks
- Retinal detachment surgery for sealing retinal breaks
- Macular hole surgery
- Attachment of muscles to porous orbital implants
- Total socket reconstruction surgery to stabilize the mucous membrane graft.

References

1. Coover H Jr, Joyner FB, Shearer NH Jr,Wicker TH Jr. Chemistry and performance of cyanoacrylate adhesives 1959; SPE Tech. Papers 5;92.
2. Ellis RA, Levin AM. Experimental sutureless ocular surgery. Am J Ophthalmol. 1963;55:733.
3. Kilpikari J, Lapinsuo M, Tormala P, Patiala H, Rokkanen P. Bonding strength of alkyl-2-cyanoacrylates to bone *in vitro*. J Biomed Mater Res. 1986;20:1095-1102.
4. Vote BJT, Fraco EMJ. Cyanoacrylate glue for corneal perforations: a description of a surgical technique and a review of the literature. Clin Exp Ophthal. 2000;28:437-42.

5. Leggat PA, Smith DR, Kedjarune U. Surgical applications of cyanoacrylate adhesives: a review of toxicity. ANZ J Surg. 2007;77:209-13.

6. Refojo MF, Dohlman CH, Ahmad B, Caroll JM, Allen JC. Evaluation of adhesives for corneal surgery. Arch Ophthalmol. 1968;80:645-56.

7. Refojo MF, Dohlman CH. The tensile strength of adhesive joints between eye tissues and alloplastic materials. Am J Ophthalmol. 1960;68:248-55.

8. Eiferman RA, Snyder JW. Antibacterial effect of cyanoacrylate glue. Arch Ophthalmol 1983;101:958-60.

9. de Almeida Manzano RP, Naufal FC, Hida RY, et al. Antibacterial analysis *in vitro* of ethyl-cyanoacrylate against ocular pathogens. Cornea. 2006;25:350-1.

10. Jackson MR, MacPhee MJ, Drohan WN, Alving BM. Fibrin sealant: current and potential clinical applications. Blood Coagul. Fibrinolysis. 1996;7:737-46.

11. Chung SI. Comparative studies on tissue transglutaminase and Factor XIII. Ann NY Acad Sci. 1972;202:240-55.

12. Iwanaga S, Suzuki K, Hashimoto S. Bovine plasma cold-insoluble globulin: gross structure and function. Ann NY Acad Sci. 1978;31256-73.

13. Sakata Y, Aoki N. Significance of crosslinking of a2-plasmin inhibitor to fibrin in inhibition of fibrinolysis and in hemostasis. J Clin Invest. 1982;69:536-42.

14. Spotnitz WD. Fibrin sealant: past, present, and future: a brief review. World J Surg. 2010;34:632-4.

15. Ortel TL, Mercer MC, Thames EH, Moore KD, Lawson JH. Immunologic impact and clinical outcomes after surgical exposure to bovine thrombin. Ann Surg. 2001;233:88-96.

16. Goessl A, Redl H. Optimized thrombin dilution protocol for a slowly setting fibrin sealant in surgery. Acta Chirurgica Austriaca. 2005;37:43-51.

17. Wilson SM, Pell P, Donegan EA. HIV-1 transmission following the use of cryoprecipitate fibrinogen as gel/adhesive. Transfusion. 1991;31:51.

18. Hino M, Ishiko O, Honda KI, et al. Transmission of symptomatic parvovirus B19 infection by fibrin sealant used during surgery. Br J Haematol 2000;108:194-5.

19. Rubel C, Fernandez GC, Dran G, Bompadre MB, Isturiz MA, Palermo MS. Fibrinogen promotes neutrophil activation and delays apoptosis. J Immunol 2001;166:2002-10.

20. Carnahan MA, Grinstaff MW. Synthesis and characterization of poly(glycerolsuccinic acid) dendrimers. Macromolecules. 2001; 34:7648-55.

21. Berdahl JP, Johnson CS, Proia AD, Grinstaff MW, Kim T. Comparison of sutures and dendritic polymer adhesives for corneal laceration repair in an *in vivo* chicken model. Arch Ophthalmol. 2009;127:442-7.

22. Araki M, Tao H, Nakajima N, et al. Development of new biodegradable hydrogel glue for preventing alveolar air leakage. J Thorac Cardiovasc Surg. 2007;134:1241-8.

23. Takaoka M, Nakamura T, Sugai H. Novel sutureless keratoplasty with a chemically defined bioadhesive. Inv Ophthalmol Visual Sci. 2009;50(6):2679-85.

24. Braunwald NS, Gay W, Tatooles CJ. Evaluation of crosslinked gelatin as a tissue adhesive and hemostatic agent:an experimental study. Surgery. 1966;59:1024-30.

25. Engel HM, Chechik D, Burde RM. Repair of a traumatic scleral rupture with sclera imbrication and BioGlue. Retina 2007;27: 505-8.

26. Miki D, Dastgheib K, Kim T, et al. A photopolymerized sealant for corneal lacerations. Cornea. 2002;21:393-9.

27. Matteini, P, Rossi F, Menabouni L, Pini R. Microscopic analysis of structural changes in diode-laser-welded corneal stroma. Proc SPIE Int Soc Optical Eng. 2007;6426:14.

28. Menabuoni L, Minicione F, Minicione GP, Pini R. Laser welding to assist penetrating keratoplasty: *in vivo* studies. Proc SPIE Int Soc Optical Eng. 1998;3195:25.

29. Menabuoni L, Pini R, Rossi F, Lenzetti I, Yoo SH, Parel JM. Laser-assisted corneal welding in cataract surgery: retrospective study. J Cataract Refract Surg. 2007;33:1608-12.

4 Preoperative Evaluation of a Patient for Glued IOL

Priya Narang, Amar Agarwal

Introduction

Glued IOL is a technique which is aimed at ensuring pseudophakia in eyes with posterior capsular dehiscence. Preoperative evaluation of any patient undergoing this surgery is a must; as all these eyes have had their episode of surgical insult. The postoperative outcome of this surgery depends a lot on the proper preoperative evaluation of the case. Many times these eyes are associated with an element of vitritis and cystoid macular edema; or are at times associated with corneal decompensation following an eventful phacoemulsification surgery. The role of preoperative evaluation cannot be underestimated or over-ruled as it helps to explain the visual prognosis to the patient.

Vision

The uncorrected visual acuity (UCVA) and the best corrected visual acuity (BCVA) of the patient should be recorded diligently on Snellen's chart. The pinhole vision should also be assessed so that the macular function is also scrutinised. The pin hole vision gives an idea as to the level of acuity that can be achieved postoperatively and also the current status of the eye.

Intraocular Pressure

It should always be recorded with an applanation tonometer. Pre-existing secondary glaucoma should always be ruled out as it often leads to altered surgical outcome. Raised IOP should be well controlled before the surgery with the use of oral and topical drugs. At times the IOP refuses to go down due to presence of vitreous in the anterior chamber or due to traumatic disruption of the anterior chamber angle structures. One should be careful of an angle recession glaucoma **(Figure 1)**.

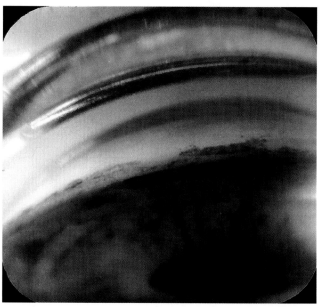

FIGURE 1: Gonioscopy of a patient with angle recession glaucoma

Slit Lamp Examination (SLE)

All the ocular structures should be examined properly as a careful SLE reveals the saga that the eye has undergone intraoperatively. The following things should be especially looked for during slit lamp examination.

Status of Cornea

While assessing cornea **(Figure 2)**, look for striaes and bullaes. Decompensated corneas at times need Glued IOL surgery to be clubbed with any of the corneal procedures like DSEK, DMEK or Boston K Pro **(Figure 3)**; depending on the etiology and the severity of the corneal involvement.

Anterior Chamber

Look out for vitreous strands, anterior chamber depth,

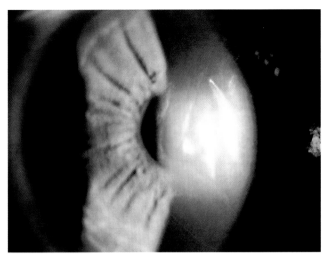

FIGURE 2: Corneal damage after phacoemulsification. Visualization in such a case for glued IOL surgery will be difficult

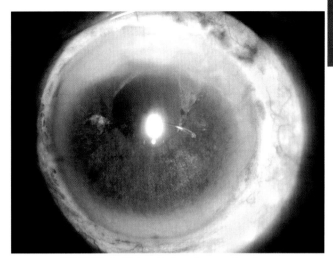

FIGURE 4: Dislocated endocapsular ring. Note the corneal damage superiorly

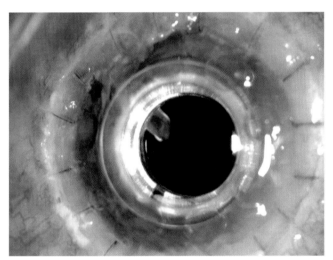

FIGURE 3: Boston keratoprosthesis with Ahmed valve and a glued IOL

element of inflammatory cells, etc. while assessing the anterior chamber. Anterior chamber can be screened with an optical section slit lamp beam at an angle of 60 degrees directed onto the peripheral cornea just inside the limbus. The chamber is considered to be shallow if the distance between the corneal endothelium and the surface of the iris is less than one fourth the thickness of the cornea **(Figure 4)**. Flare refers to the visibility of the slit lamp light beam as it passes through the aqueous humor in the anterior chamber. This occurs when the protein content increases due to intraocular inflammation.

Inflammatory cells when present can be seen as "white dots", rising and falling in the convection currents of the anterior chamber. Blood in the anterior chamber layering inferiorly is usually from trauma.

Assess the Iris Structure

Iris details like its shape, architecture, chaffing, dehiscence, iridodialysis, etc. should also be evaluated in detail. Mild to moderate amount of iridodialysis can be corrected with iris suturing whereas massive iridodialysis or virtually absent iris tissue can be treated with Aniridia Glued IOL procedure which requires the use of special aniridia IOL's.

Assess the Degree of Posterior Capsular Rupture

The extent of rupture, the amount of posterior capsule present, margins of rhexis (if intact) should also be assessed thoroughly. If good amount of anterior capsule is present one can implant the three piece IOL anterior to the rhexis.

Lens

The lenticular assessment is extremely important in cases of traumatic subluxation or dislocation. In subluxation the edge of the lens might be visible in the pupil. In complete dislocation (luxation), the lens displaces into the vitreous or rarely, into the anterior chamber.

White to White (WTW)

One should always measure the white to white corneal diameter as one will have to decide to perform a vertical or horizontal glued IOL. In eyes with horizontal WTW more than 11 mm it is advisable to do a vertical glued IOL and make the flaps at 12 and 6 o'clock.

Specular Microscopy

Endotheliopathy can occur secondary to ocular inflammation following an eventful previous surgery. Specular microscopy is a noninvasive photographic technique that allows you to visualize and analyze the corneal endothelium. Using computer-assisted morphometry, modern specular microscopes analyze the size, shape and population of the endothelial cells. Iridocyclitis can result in endothelial cell loss and reduced endothelial cell function.[1] Specifically, iridocyclitis causes a release of immune response proteins into the anterior chamber that leads to endothelial cell death.[2]

Glaucoma-induced endotheliopathy is also a well-known term. Long-term exposure to elevated intraocular pressure can produce an abnormal reduction in endothelial cell density. One study suggested that the mechanism of cell loss is not the result of increased intraocular pressure, but rather some other physiological alteration in the glaucomatous eye, such as abnormal aqueous outflow or decreased oxygen concentration in the aqueous.[3]

Gonioscopy

There are six ocular structures normally available for observation. The appearance of the anterior chamber angle varies according to congenital individual differences and with acquired changes due to age, injury or disease. Always look out for traumatic angle recession in cases of trauma with raised intraocular pressure **(Figure 1)**.

Other indications for gonioscopy include:
- Narrowness or closure of the anterior chamber angle as observed with Van Herick's technique
- Historical evidence of angle closure
- History of previous attack of angle closure
- Evidence suggesting possible anterior chamber neovascularization
- Recent or previous central or branch vein occlusion
- Active or past inflammation in the chamber
- History or evidence of trauma
- History or signs of penetrating ocular foreign body
- Degenerative conditions affecting the anterior segment.

Ophthalmoscopy

Fundus examination is an integral part of the routine ophthalmic examination and should always be done.

Indirect ophthalmoscopy is a useful technique to allow a wide angle view of the fundus, to screen for retinal disease, and to examine the peripheral retina **(Figures 5 and 6)**. It provides a better view of the fundus in patients with lens opacities than is allowed by direct ophthalmoscopy. The patient may have a retinal detachment which might be missed. Retinal new vessels can be checked better with fluorescein angiography **(Figures 7 to 9)**. Retinal examinations may reveal the presence of vitreous and retinal diseases and even contribute to the detection of nonocular diseases.

Ultrascan

B-scan ultrasonography is an important adjuvant for the clinical assessment of various ocular diseases. With understanding of the indications for ultrasonography and proper examination technique, one can gather a vast amount of information not possible with clinical examination alone. B-scan ultrasound of the eye is a vital part of an ophthalmologist's diagnostic armamentarium.

B-scan ultrasound is most useful when direct visualization of intraocular structures is difficult or impossible. Situations that prevent normal examination include corneal opacities (e.g. scars, severe edema), hyphema, hypopyon, miosis, pupillary membranes, dense papillary membrane or vitreous opacities (e.g. hemorrhage, inflammatory debris). In such cases, diagnostic B-scan ultrasound can accurately image intraocular structures and give valuable information on the status of the retained lenticular fragments following a posterior capsular rupture, vitreous, retina, choroid, and sclera.

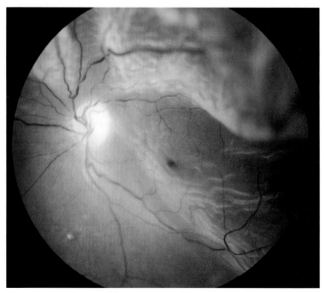

FIGURE 5: Retinal detachment

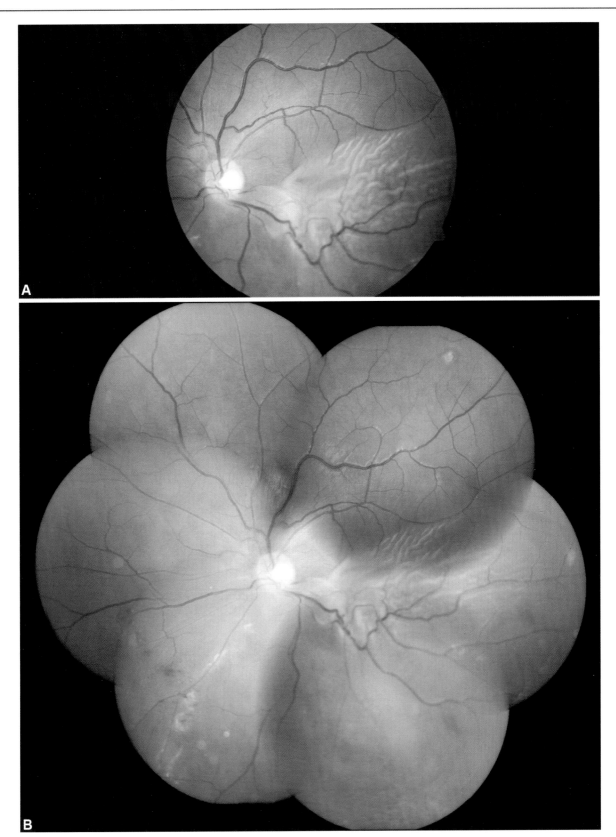

FIGURES 6A AND B: Retinal detachment
A. Close fundus view showing the retinal detachment
B. Montage showing the extent of the retinal detachment

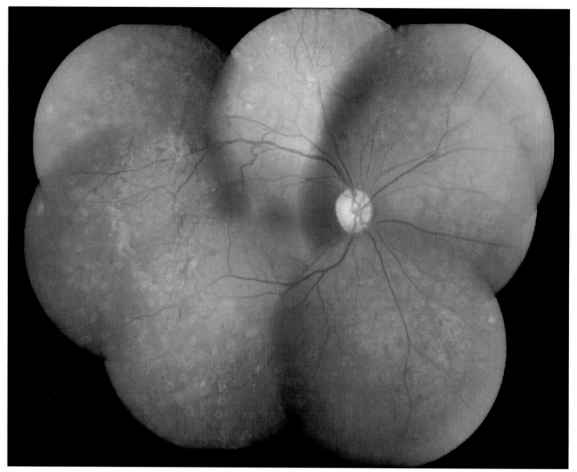

FIGURE 7: Proliferative diabetic retinopathy

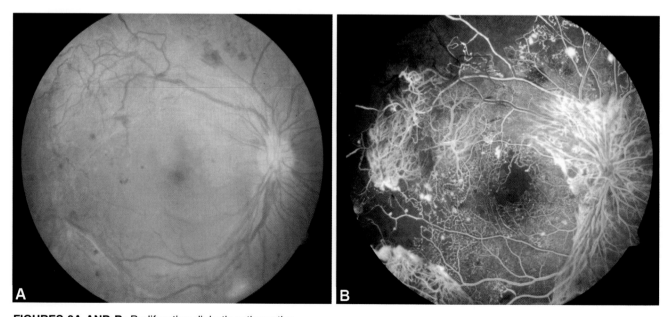

FIGURES 8A AND B: Proliferative diabetic retinopathy
A. Fundus picture. Note the new vessels
B. Fundus fluorescein angiography

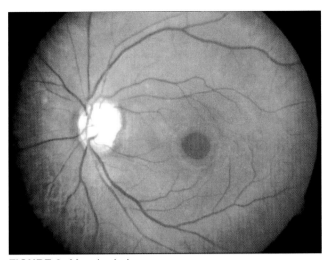

FIGURE 9: Macular hole

Trauma can give a varied picture depending on the severity. The ciliary body is visualized best with high-resolution scanning. A ciliary body detachment can extend into the peripheral choroid and can be seen on contact B-scan, although it is displayed best on high-resolution scanning. A low-to-medium reflective cleft is seen in the subciliary space.

However, in many instances, ultrasound is used for diagnostic purposes even though pathology is clinically visible. Such instances include differentiating iris or ciliary body lesions; ruling out ciliary body detachments; serous versus hemorrhagic choroidal detachments, rhegmatogenous versus exudative retinal detachments.

Optical Coherence Tomography (OCT)

For patients undergoing glued IOL surgery adequate assessment of the macula and its function is very important. Preoperatively existing cystoid macular edema (CME) should be ruled out **(Figures 10A and B)**. Clinical cystoid macular edema (CCME) produces a variable degree of eyesight deterioration, in a percentage between 0.2 and 13% of patients operated for cataract[4-7] with or without complications.

Quantitative measurement of retinal thickness is possible because of the well-defined boundaries in optical reflectivity at the inner and outer margins of the neurosensory retina. Optical coherence tomography appears useful for objectively monitoring retinal thickness with high resolution in patients with macular edema. It may eventually prove to be a sensitive diagnostic test for the early detection of macular thickening in patients with diabetic retinopathy. Aphakic cystoid macular edema (CME) is a relatively frequent complication of cataract surgery. It has been described with greater frequency after complicated surgery or in patients with eye diseases, but also in normal eyes after uncomplicated surgery.

Systemic Illness

A detailed patient history of systemic illness should also be evaluated. According to some studies, patients with

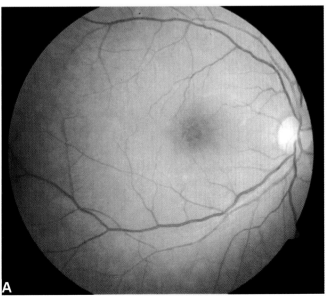

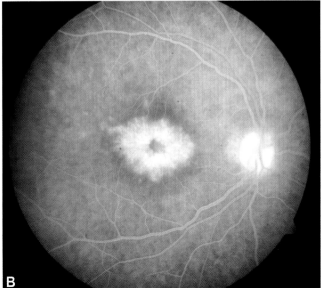

FIGURES 10A AND B: Cystoid macular edema
A. Fundus picture
B. Fundus fluorescein angiography

diabetes mellitus are at greater risk of developing aphakic CME.[8,9] Eyes with certain autoimmune disorders and infections are prone to anterior uveitis. A history of autoimmune disorders like juvenile rheumatoid arthritis, ankylosing spondylosis, Reiter's syndrome, inflammatory bowel disease, psoriasis and a history of infections like syphilis, TB, herpes zoster, herpes simplex, adenovirus should be evaluated.

References

1. Taravella M, Walker M. Emedicine: Postoperative corneal edema. Available at: www.emedicine.com/oph/topic64.htm (Accessed May 6, 2009).
2. Samudre SS, Lattanzio FA, Willimas PB, Sheppard JD. Comparison of topical steroids for acute anterior uveitis. J Ocul Pharmacol Ther. 2004;20(6):533-47.
3. Phillips C, Laing R, Yee R. Specular Microscopy. In: Krachmer JH, Mannis MJ, Holland EJ (Eds). Cornea, 2nd edition. Philadelphia: Elsevier Mosby. 2005;261-77.
4. Taylor DM, Sachs SW, Stern AL. Aphakic cystoid macular edema. Longterm clinical observations. Surv Ophthalmol. 1984; 28:437-41.
5. Norregard JC, Bernth-Petersen P, Bellan L, Alonso J, Black C, Dunn E, et al. Intraoperative clinical practice and risk of early complications after cataract extraction in the United States, Canada, Denmark and Spain. Ophthalmology. 1999;106:42-8.
6. Collins JF, Gaster RN, Krol WF, Colling CL, Kirk GF, Smith TJ, et al. A comparison of anterior chamber and posterior chamber intraocular lenses after vitreous presentation during cataract surgery: the Department of Veterans Affairs Cooperative Cataract Study. Am J Ophthalmol. 2003;136:1-9.
7. Collins JF, Krol WF, Kirk GF, Gaster RN. VA Cooperative Cataract Study Group. The effect of vitreous presentation during extracapsular cataract surgery on the postoperative visual acuity at one year. Am J Ophthalmol. 2004;138:536-42.
8. Pollack A, Leiba H, Bukelman A, Oliver M. Cystoid macular oedema following cataract extraction in patients with diabetes. Br J Ophthalmol. 1992;76:221-4.
9. Dowler JG, Sehmi KS, Hykin PG, Hamilton AM. The natural history of macular edema after cataract surgery in diabetes. Ophthalmology. 1999;106:663-8.

SURGICAL TECHNIQUE

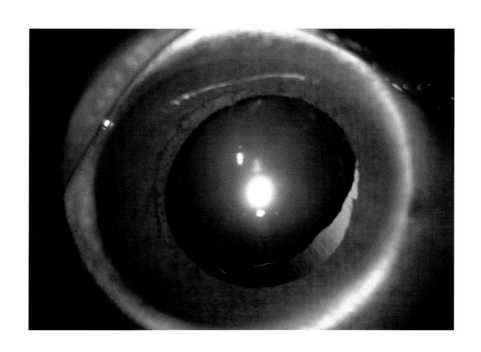

Som Prasad

Introduction

Intrascleral haptic fixation techniques have gained increasing popularity in recent years. The idea was first introduced by Maggi,[1] but later refined and popularized by Scharioth[2] as 'intrascleral haptic fixation' and by Agarwal and colleagues as the 'Glued IOL'.[3] Further modifications have been suggested by Prenner[4] from a posterior segment approach and Yotan and Karadag from an anterior approach.[5] All these techniques represent variations on the theme of fixating haptics into the sclera to allow for long-term stability with good centration and no tilt. They are equally suitable for the management of aphakia by implantation of posterior chamber three-piece IOLs or refixation of a subluxed or dislocated three-piece IOL in an 'IOL rescue' scenario. They offer potentially early rehabilitation with good visual outcomes. The presentation of these cases can be very varied, ranging from aphakia with contact lens intolerance, traumatic cataracts with zonular loss, subluxated lenses in syndromes like Marfan's, or iatrogeneic damage from complicated cataract surgery amongst others.[6] The surgical approach has to be varied to meet the very variable pathology the surgeon is faced with.

Indications

In essence, there are three settings in which this technique can be deployed effectively as part of the surgical armamentarium. Firstly, if a three piece intraocular lens is already in the eye but subluxated or dislocated it can be secured in the sclera using this method, if necessary by lifting it out of the posterior segment by a standard 3 port pars plana vitrectomy as a first step. Second, for subluxed lenses either from trauma or congenital conditions such as Marfan's syndrome, a pars plana vitrectomy and lensectomy can

be followed by scleral fixation of IOL using this technique. Finally, in eyes where cataract surgery is complicated with loss of the capsular bag or massive zonular loss, this is a good method of securing an IOL in the posterior chamber. This may be done at the primary operation or as a secondary procedure, making it equally applicable to eyes which have been left aphakic in the past.

Vitrectomy

Irrespective of the presentation, one of the essential prerequisites is that all surgical maneuvers involving the IOL and associated surgery such as iris repair, etc. must be carried out in a vitreous free environment. Remember that even in an eye with a complete PVD (Posterior vitreous detachment), the vitreous is still attached to the vitreous base **(Figure 1)**, which is the region in which most retinal tears occur in pseudophakic eyes and as many of the surgical maneuvers required to manipulate scleral fixated IOLs have to be done in the ciliary sulcus in close proximity to the vitreous base, there exists a potential for causing retinal traction and possibly tears leading to further complications. The force required to cause a tear in the retina is quite small, of the order of 200 dynes/cm^2, which is only about three times the surface tension of water (72 dynes/cm^2).[7] It is thus essential to reduce the risk of retinal traction and tears while performing vitrectomy and it is also important to remove as much vitreous as safely possible as the first step in this kind of surgery. As a general principle, procedures, like making scleral flaps or tunnels, are best done before doing the vitrectomy, or if the eyes open already then a continuous infusion either through an anterior chamber maintainer or a pars plana infusion should be running as a firm eye facilitates scleral dissection.

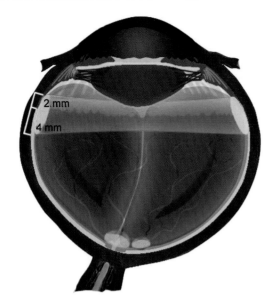

FIGURE 1: Diagrammatic representation of vitreous still attached to the area of the vitreous base straddling the ora serrata, in a eye with complete vitreous detachment

Cut Rate in Vitrectomy

One should use the highest cut rate that your machine is capable of, as it is well-known that high cut rate reduces retinal traction and thus the risk of retinal tears. Therefore, although it may be counterintuitive to put 'foot to metal' that is what needs to be done. Vacuum (100-150 mm Hg) and flow levels should only be moderate if a conventional 20 G cutter is being used. With smaller gauge systems, higher vacuum levels (400-600 mm Hg) are required to ensure efficient removal of vitreous.

Anterior Vitrectomy through a Limbal or Clear Corneal Approach

Anterior vitrectomy is an essential skill for any cataract surgeon as posterior capsule (PC) rupture occurs in approximately 2% of cases in large series.[8] However, when this is done as an initial step, prior to fixating a glued IOL, or any scleral fixated lens there are some important points to keep in mind. "Full function" anterior vitrectomy probes with an irrigating sleeve over the cutter should be avoided. Older phacoemulsification machines often come with this for anterior vitrectomy, however, it is easy to remove the irrigating sleeve and attach the irrigating line to a separate cannula. More modern machines, already come with packs which have infusion cannulas and vitreous cutter's. It is useful to

use the separate irrigation line which is placed through a sideport incision (or an anterior chamber maintainer) and the vitreous cutter used to remove the vitreous placed through a separate incision. Bimanual anterior vitrectomy offers very good surgical control and avoids softening of the eye during vitrectomy. It is useful to inject a small amount of triamcinolone into the anterior chamber at this stage. The triamcinolone (Kenalog) crystals adhere to any vitreous that has presented, thus greatly facilitating visualization **(Figure 2)**.[9] The use of the bimanual approach also allows the two instruments to be swapped from one port to the other, which facilitates access to all parts of the anterior chamber helping complete vitreous removal **(Figure 3)**. If the eye is already open, for example, if a corneal scleral incision has been made for phacoemulsification and it is felt that this incision is unstable, it should be secured with a suture to avoid hypotony and iris prolapse during vitrectomy. The infusion line is placed through a sideport with a low bottle height, with the fluid flow directed toward the anterior chamber angle. The cutter goes through the second sideport, establishing a stable closed system. A high cut rate and low flow are advisable; the cutting rate should be set at the highest rate allowable on that machine, which ranges from 600 to 5000 cuts/min on various models and vacuum of 150 to 200 mm Hg. This minimizes the risk of retinal traction while the vitreous is cut and removed. The cutter is placed fairly deep, going behind an IOL when the IOL is already *in situ* with the cutting port

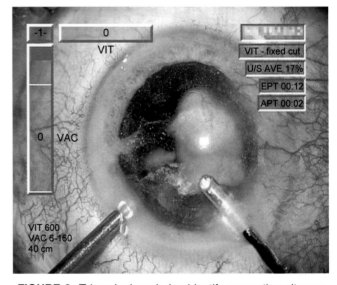

FIGURE 2: Triamcinolone helps identify presenting vitreous and any vitreous strands to guide anterior vitrectomy

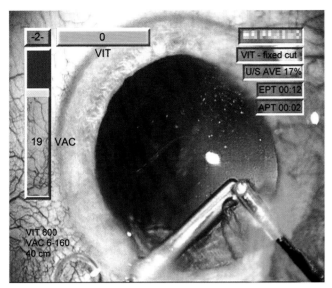

FIGURE 3: The instruments can be swapped during anterior vitrectomy to facilitate access to all parts of the anterior chamber

orientated anteriorly so that it is always visible. Most of the anterior vitreous is drawn backward and efficiently removed. The cutter is then moved forward to deal with any remaining vitreous strands which may be extending forward to previous corneal incisions; any peaking of the pupil indicates that there are vitreous strands extending anteriorly still present. Triamcinolone will obviously highlight these as well. It is important to perform very deep and generous anterior vitrectomy in this setting as further maneuvers to place the IOL and secure it to the sclera can disturb any vitreous which remains close behind the iris. Because of this, techniques such as dry anterior vitrectomy, which are designed to shave away the minimum amount of vitreous required to clear the anterior chamber are not recommended when planning to put in a scleral fixated lens.

Pars Plana Approach to Anterior Vitrectomy

Whilst bimanual anterior vitrectomy is usually the standard approach to remove vitreous in complex anterior segment surgery, a conceptually more attractive approach is to use a single pars plana incision for the vitrectomy part of the procedure. The attraction of the pars plana approach, is that vitreous moves in an anterior to posterior direction (as opposed to an anterior approach which is used in bimanual anterior vitrectomy whether vitreous may be drawn forwards)

to be removed. One also achieves enhanced and much more controlled access to the anterior part of the posterior segment, and can also separate iris adhesions and synechiae in a controlled manner. There are also certain situations where a pars plana incision offers unique advantages such as a very crowded eye with a very shallow anterior chamber. Removal of some vitreous allows reformation of the anterior chamber. Access through the pars plana incision can also facilitate manipulation of the haptics should that be required at a later part of the procedure when the IOL is being secured. Briefly, the technique is to use an infusion through the sideport and make a single pars plana incision 3.5 mm behind the limbus. This is done after reflecting the conjunctiva with a MVR blade for a 20-gauge cutter or transconjunctivally using a 23 or 25-gauge trocar cannula system for a high-speed 23 or 25-gauge cutter. This allows the flow to move in one direction—from anterior to posterior—making removal of vitreous more efficient. Many anterior segment surgeons may not be familiar or comfortable with pars plana incisions, and therefore, I highlight some of the nuances and surgical pearls which will allow the deployment of this technique in a safe and predictable manner.

Steps of Surgery

As with any surgical technique, it is essential to learn the steps of the procedure. The first principle is to maintain a 'closed chamber' at all times. Hypotony must be avoided throughout. If there is any doubt about the competency of any other incisions, such as corneal scleral incisions which have already been made it should be closed with temporary suture prior to pars plana incision being made. This avoids hypotony, and also facilitates the pars plana incision which requires a firm eye. If performing surgery under topical anesthesia, remember that the pars plana incision will be uncomfortable and it is, therefore, advisable to administer a small amount of subconjunctival anesthetic in the area of the planned incision. The importance of constantly explaining the situation to the patient, sometimes termed 'vocal anesthesia' cannot be over emphasised. With a firm eye and adequate anesthesia, one can either use an MVR blade after taking the conjunctiva down (try to minimize use of diathermy as this permanently weakens the sclera[10]) or a transconjunctival approach. Incisions should always be bevelled, to allow better

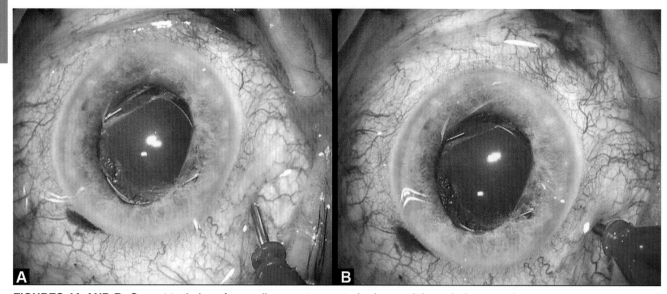

FIGURES 4A AND B: Correct technique for small gauge trocars to be inserted through the pars plana
A. The conjunctiva is displaced and the trocar enters the pars plana, 3.5 mm behind the limbus, initially at an acute angle
B. Once the cannula has engaged sclera, the direction of approach is changed to a perpendicular direction. This results in a two plane bevelled incision in the sclera which self-seals nicely when the cannula is removed at the end of the procedure

sealing at the end of the procedure **(Figures 4A and B)**. The highest cut rate possible should be used. Small gauge transconjunctival incisions self-seal when the port is removed, but it is necessary to suture a 20 G scleral incision and also closed the conjunctiva over it.

Because small gauge cannula systems are designed to self seal, wound construction is critically important to achieve this. The conjunctiva is displaced using a cotton applicator or forceps. Trocar-guided cannulas are passed through conjunctiva and sclera into the vitreous cavity. The angle of entry into the sclera influences the sealing of the sclerotomy after removal of cannulas. More oblique the path through the sclera, the better the re-apposition of the edges after the removal of cannulas, and lesser the leakage from sclerotomies.[11] Some favor a biplanar scleral incision, with a more oblique initial and a more perpendicular final entry into the vitreous to create a two-step incision in cross-section **(Figures 4A and B)**. Newer entry systems have a blade like configuration, rather than the older needle like design, which allows improved wound configuration.

Again vitrectomy is to be generous, and as much vitreous is can be removed safely under direct visualization should be removed to avoid problems with vitreous strands emerging later during the procedure when the IOL is being secured.

Three Port Posterior Vitrectomy for Dislocated IOL

If the IOL is dislocated into the posterior segment **(Figure 5)**, it is necessary to perform a formal three port pars plana vitrectomy to remove vitreous completely and then rescue the IOL from the posterior segment into the anterior chamber following which it can be fixated to the sclera. Traditionally, 20 gauge vitrectomy systems have been used for this as they offer relatively more rigid instruments (forceps, et cetera) and the conjunctiva has to be opened for scleral fixation anyway. However, more recently small gauge systems are being increasingly used for this. This allows the area of conjunctival peritotomy to be limited to the areas needed for scleral fixation of haptics. Also, the use of cannulas through which pars plana instruments pass potentially reduces the risk of entry site tears to the retina in the area of the sclerostomy.[12] There is decreased pain and inflammation postoperatively as scleral sutures are not required and the need for conjunctival suturing is reduced.

Wide angle illumination systems which remains fixed to the cannula without the need for suture placement (a chandelier type illumination) has enabled the execution of bimanual surgery and provides wide illumination of the vitreous cavity greatly facilitating the removal of

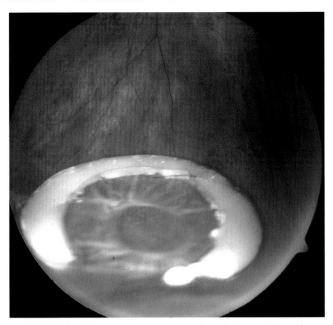

FIGURE 5: IOL capsular bag complex dislocated into the inferior vitreous cavity

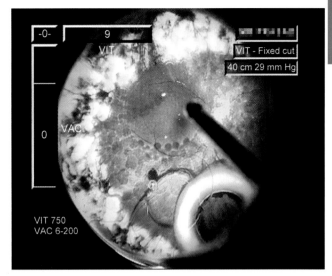

FIGURE 7: A small amount of perfluorocarbon liquid is covering the macular area and displacing the intraocular lens and lens material onto the mid-peripheral retina from where it can be safely grasped

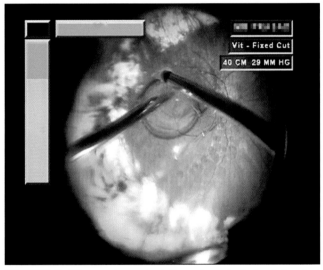

FIGURE 6: Bimanual manipulation of posteriorly dislocated IOL and lens tissue using chandelier illumination in an eye with a previously treated retinal detachment

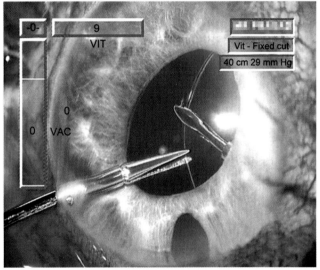

FIGURE 8: The haptic of the intraocular lens is lifted to the area behind the pupil and handed over to another pair of forceps passed through a paracentesis using the 'hand-shake' technique

intraocular lenses **(Figure 6)**. It is important to do a complete vitrectomy including induction of a PVD (Posterior vitreous detachment), and shaving of the vitreous base, as this will avoid the risk of retinal traction if parts of the IOL or haptics engage any bits of remaining vitreous and pull on it while the IOL is being lifted. A small amount of perfluorocarbon liquid may be used to cover the macular area before manipulating the intraocular lens as this acts as a cushion and reduces the risk of instruments or parts of the IOL

damaging the macular area **(Figure 7)**. The IOL can then be grasped with forceps and lifted into the anterior chamber **(Figure 8)**. Once IOL fixation has been achieved, the posterior segment is accessed again to remove any perfluorocarbon liquid that may have been used and also to ensure that there are no fragments of lens matter remaining **(Figure 9)**. It is also important to do a full peripheral indentation and search at the end of the procedure so that no retinal tears or suspicious areas are left untreated with retinopexy **(Figure 10)**.

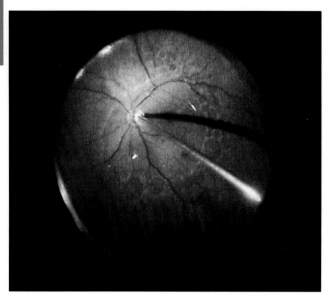

FIGURE 9: Once IOL fixation has been done, the posterior segment is revisited to remove any perfluorocarbon liquid, which may have been used or any lens fragments which may remain

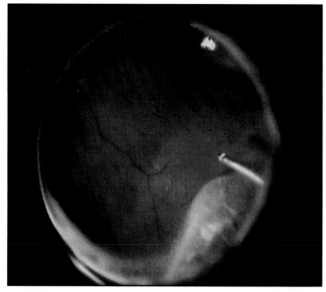

FIGURE 10: A full peripheral retinal search is done at the end of the procedure to ensure that there are no retinal tears or areas needing retinopexy left untreated

Endophthalmitis

Initial concerns of an increased risk of postoperative endophthalmitis after transconjunctival sutureless vitrectomy and discourage surgeons using this approach. Earlier retrospective series reported rates ranging from 0.04 to 0.84%, more recently published large retrospective studies do not indicate that sutureless small gauge vitrectomy is associated with higher rates of endophthalmitis than in 20 G vitrectomy.[13,14]

Finishing Steps and Postoperative Care

Once the intraocular lens has been securely placed using the glued IOL or a similar technique, it is useful to then constrict the pupil with an agent such as Miochol (Novartis Pharmaceutical, Basel, Switzerland). It is often useful to place a small amount of triamcinolone in at this point again to identify any errant strands of vitreous, which may have come forward during the manipulations required to secure the lens. The triamcinolone is flushed out with irrigation and aspiration. If wound integrity is in any doubt, one can put a suture in. It is important to manage post-operative inflammation and intraocular pressure adequately. Finally, a detailed fundus and full peripheral examinations must be obtained before the patient is discharged. This may be done a few days or even weeks after the surgery to allow time for any postoperative inflammation to settle and the wound to be secure.

References

1. Maggi R, Maggi C. Sutureless scleral fixation of intraocular lenses. Journal of cataract and refractive surgery. 1997;23(9): 1289-94. Epub 1998/01/10.
2. Gabor SG, Pavlidis MM. Sutureless intrascleral posterior chamber intraocular lens fixation. Journal of cataract and refractive surgery. 2007;33(11):1851-4. Epub 2007/10/30.
3. Agarwal A, Kumar DA, Jacob S, Baid C, Agarwal A, Srinivasan S. Fibrin glue-assisted sutureless posterior chamber intraocular lens implantation in eyes with deficient posterior capsules. Journal of Cataract & Refractive Surgery. 2008;34(9):1433-8.
4. Prenner JL, Feiner L, Wheatley HM, Connors D. A novel approach for posterior chamber intraocular lens placement or rescue via a sutureless scleral fixation technique. Retina. 2012; 32(4):853-5. Epub 2012/02/09.
5. Yotan Y, Karadag R. Trocar-assisted sutureless intrascleral posterior chamber foldable intraocular lens fixation. Eye. 2012; 26:788-91. doi:10.1038/eye.2012.19; published online 2 March 2012.
6. Bastawrous A, Parkes C, Prasad S. Choices in correction of aphakia during vitrectomy. Ophthalmologica Journal international d'ophtalmologie International journal of ophthalmology Zeitschrift fur Augenheilkunde. 2011; 226Suppl 1:46-52. Epub 2011/08/04.
7. Teixeira A, Chang LP, Matsuoka N, et al. Vitreoretinal Traction Created by Conventional Cutters during Vitrectomy. Ophthalmology. 2010;117(7):1387-92.
8. Lundström M, Behndig A, Kugelberg M, Montan P, et al. Capsule complication during cataract surgery: Background, study

design, and required additional care: Swedish Capsule Rupture Study Group report 1. J Cataract Refract Surg. 2009;35(10): 1679-87.

9. Burk E, Da Mata AP, Snyder ME, Schneider S, et al. Visualizing vitreous using kenalog suspension 1. J Cataract Refract Surg. 2003; 29(4):645-51.

10. Schwartz A, Rathbun E. Scleral strength impairment and recovery after diathermy. Arch Ophthalmol. 1975;93(11):1173-7.

11. Hsu J, Chen E, Gupta O, et al. Hypotony after 25-gauge vitrectomy using oblique versus direct cannula insertions in fluid-filled eyes. Retina. 2008;28:937-40.

12. Scartozzi R, Bessa AS, Gupta OP, Regillo CD. Intraoperative sclerotomy-related retinal breaks for macular surgery. 20- vs. 25-gauge vitrectomy systems. Am J Ophthalmol 2007;143: 155-6.

13. Hu Ay, Bourges JL, Shah SP, et al. Endophthalmitis after pars plana vitrectomy: a 20- and 25-gauge comparison. Ophthalmology. 2009;116:1360-5.

14. Chen JK, Khurana RN, Nguyen QD, Do DV. The incidence of endophthalmitis following transconjunctival sutureless 25- vs 20-gauge vitrectomy. Eye (Lond). 2009;23:780-4.

6

Sutureless Intrascleral PC IOL Fixation

Gabor B Scharioth

Introduction

A surgeon could be faced with three main scenarios. The patient could be aphakic after complicated phacoemulsification, trauma, vitreoretinal surgery or years after intracapsular cataract extraction. Second, the patient could be pseudophakic with a dislocated intraocular lens or even dislocated capsular bag-intraocular lens-complex, sometimes with a capsular tension ring in place. Even more complicated would be if a previous secondary implantation with an intraocular (transiridal or transscleral) suturing was performed. Finally, the surgeon could recognize the dislocation during surgery (preexisting or caused by the surgeon himself) complicating the surgery and may require an intraoperative repair. Fixation of intraocular lenses in such cases of insufficient or no capsular support is challenging and requires a large armamentarium of techniques to solve different situations.[1-22]

Scleral Location

I am convinced that the best place for fixation of intraocular lens in the absence of sufficient zonular/capsular support is the sclera. It is the strongest intraocular tissue, mainly avascular and does not tend to inflammation. Vitreoretinal surgeons know for decades that implants and explants for retinal procedures are well tolerated over a long period.

Alternate Techniques

In moderately damaged zonular apparatus we are using for many years capsular bag refixation techniques with modified capsular tension rings (Cionni rings) or Ahmed segments (both Morcher, Germany). These implants are positioned in the capsular bag and have an extra eyelet which is positioned on the anterior surface of the anterior capsule and fixed with a 10 × 0 or 9 × 0 Prolene suture transsclerally into the ciliary sulcus. This technique is difficult and needs an intact capsulorrhexis. For more severe luxated capsular bags or for fixation of intraocular lenses in the absence of sufficient support the haptic of the intraocular lens could be knotted to a 10 × 0 or 9 × 0 Prolene suture and fixed to the scleral wall. Many variations of transscleral suture fixation are reported and these techniques are used worldwide because small incision techniques can be used, the intraocular lens is positioned more physiologically in the posterior chamber and standard lenses could be used. In cases of dislocated intraocular lens this could be refixated by intraoperative haptic externalization for knot fixation to the haptic and transsclerally suture fixation without the need for intraocular lens explantation. A fibrosed capsular bag especially with a capsular tension ring in place can easily be refixated with a double armed 10 × 0 or 9 × 0 Prolene suture to the ciliary sulcus. The first needle is passed through the capsule catching the haptic and/or capsular tension ring and passed through the sclera while the second needle is just placed above the bag through the sclera. The created suture loop will hold the bag after knotting to the sclera. Usually more than one scleral fixation is necessary to stabilize the whole bag.

Hoffmann's Scleral Pocket Technique

Recently Richard Hoffmann reported a technique for transscleral suture fixation without the opening of the conjunctiva.[22] Here the pockets for suture knots are prepared from the limbus intrasclerally. A double armed suture is used and stitched 1.5 mm postlimbal through the scleral pockets and conjunctiva. The needles are cut off and the sutures are caught with a hook from the limbus. Then the suture is knotted and the ends buried into the scleral pocket.

Problems with Alternate Techniques

However centration of suturefixated intraocular lenses is difficult and lens tilt are a common problem. This will result in internal astigmatism and inconvenient refractive outcome. Fixation into the ciliary sulcus without capsular and zonular support is difficult and malpositioning may result in chronic irritation to ciliary body and/or iris with secondary complications. Good long term stability is reported but late dislocations due to suture biodegradation may occur and require reinterventions.[23-27] There is a long learning curve for suture fixation techniques and the outcome depends on the surgeons experience. Furthermore there could be a need for a special intraocular lens, which may not be available everywhere.

Sutureless Intrascleral Posterior Chamber IOL Fixation

For these reasons we were searching for a technique for intraocular lens fixation in the absence of sufficient capsular support which used a standard foldable intraocular lens. The scleral fixation should be independent from iris changes and the amount of zonular/capsular damage. It should be sutureless and reduce the contact to uveal tissue and be standardized. In 2006 I performed the first intrascleral haptic fixation of a standard three piece intraocular lens and reported the surgical technique in 2007.[28] This sutureless technique for fixation of a posterior chamber intraocular lens uses permanent incarceration of the haptics in a scleral tunnel parallel to the limbus.

Surgical Technique

After peritomy the eye is stabilized either by a pars plana infusion (i.e. 25G) or by an anterior chamber maintainer (**Figure 1**). We try to prevent any diathermy of episcleral vessels to reduce the risk of scleral atrophy. Two straight sclerotomies *ab externo* are prepared with a sharp 23G cannula or 23G MVR blade about 1.5 mm postlimbal exactly 180° from each other and directed towards the center of the globe (**Figures 2 and 3**). Then new cannulas are used to create a limbus-parallel tunnel at about 50% of scleral thickness, starting from inside the ciliary sulcus sclerotomies and ending with externalization of the cannula after 2.0 to 3.0 mm (**Figures 4 to 6**). A standard 3-piece IOL with a haptic design fitting to the diameter of the ciliary sulcus is implanted with an injector, and the trailing haptic is kept out of the corneal incision (**Figures 7 and 8**). The leading haptic is then grasped at its tip (**Figure 9**) with a special straight 25G forceps (Scharioth IOL fixation forceps 1286.SFD, DORC Int., The Netherlands), pulled through the sclerotomy and left externalized (**Figures 10 and 11**). With the curved Scharioth forceps then the haptic is grasped at its tip, introduced into the intrascleral tunnel and pushed through (**Figure 12**). Then the haptic is released, forceps is turned, closed and pulled back (**Figure 13**) leaving the haptic (**Figure 14**) in the sclera (pushing technique). Alternatively one can introduce the Scharioth forceps from the distal end of the intrascleral tunnel until it becomes visible in the sclerotomy, then the haptic tip is grasped and pulled in the scleral tunnel (pulling technique). The same maneuvers are performed with the trailing haptic (**Figures 15 and 16**). The ends of the haptic are left in the tunnel to prevent foreign body sensation, erosion of the conjunctiva and to reduce the risk for inflammation. The sclerotomies are checked for leakage and if necessary sutured (**Figure 17**).

Results

I have used this technique in more than 200 eyes over the past six years (**Figures 18 and 19**). Our standard IOL were Sensar AR40e (AMO, USA) and Acrysof (Alcon, USA) but any three piece IOL sufficient for sulcus fixation should work. I have also used multifocal IOL (ReZoom and Tecnis, AMO, USA) in young patients.[29] In 2010 we reported our interim results of a European multicenter study. We had four haptic dislocations which could be reimplanted and one transient vitreous hemorrhage. These complications occurred in the first ten cases and in the first four postoperative weeks.[30] Some young patients with floppy iris showed postoperative recurrent iris capture which disappeared after NdYAG laser iridotomy. If this condition is anticipated I suggest intraoperative iridectomy with the vitreous cutter. For PCIOL calculation I use the SRK-T formula and the same A-constant as for in-the-bag implantation. Meanwhile a variation of our technique under scleral flap intrascleral haptic fixation and use of fibrin glue was published by Agarwal et al.[31]

Discussion

Management of secondary implantation or refixation of dislocated intraocular lenses with the use of scleral

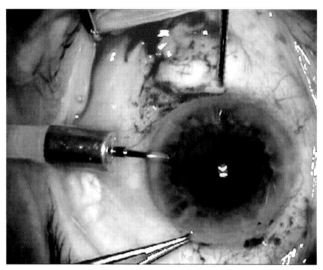

FIGURE 1: 25G infusion cannula as AC maintainer, conjunctiva opened, ciliary sulcus sclerotomy at 6 o´clock with a sharp 23G or 24G cannula

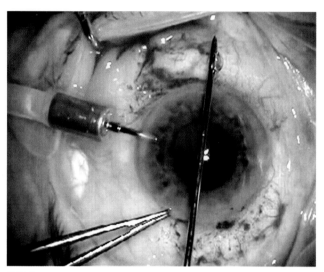

FIGURE 2: Second sclerotomy should be made exactly 180°. This could be estimated like shown or marked with special marker

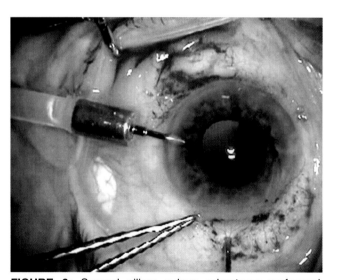

FIGURE 3: Second ciliary sulcus sclerotomy performed exactly on the opposite side 1.5 to 2.0 mm postlimbal, cannula is directed towards the center of eye to prevent iridodialysis

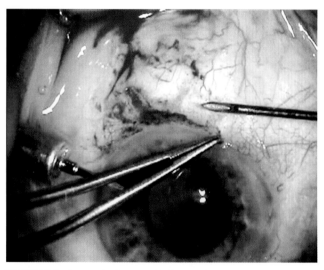

FIGURE 4: A new 23G cannula is used to create a 2-3 mm a long intrascleral limbus parallel tunnel staring from inside the sclerotomy, the direction is counterclockwise, colibri forceps is used for counter pressure

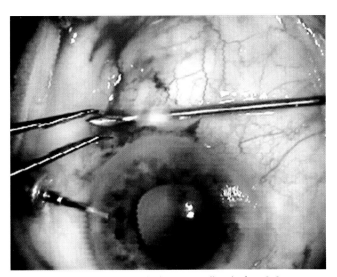

FIGURE 5: The cannula is externalized after 2-3 mm

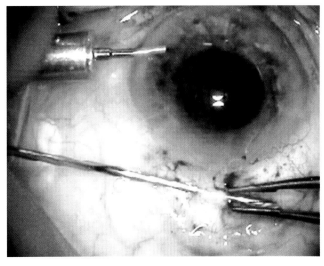

FIGURE 6: Same tunnel is created on the opposite side for the second haptic incarceration. The direction is counter-clockwise

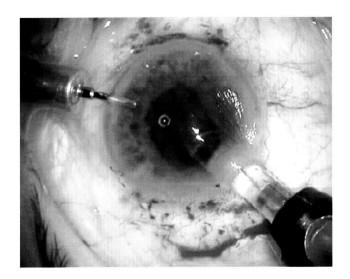

FIGURE 7: Implantation of a foldable three piece IOL with the injector through 2.6 mm incision. No additional OVD is placed into the eye. Continuous infusion is mandatory

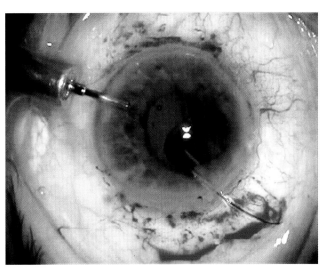

FIGURE 8: After implantation the trailing haptic is left in the corneal incision to prevent dislocation into the vitreous cavity

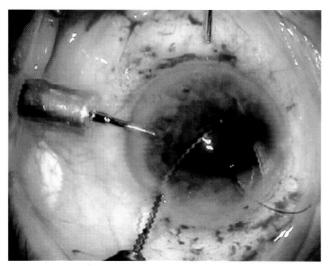

FIGURE 9: With the handshake technique the leading haptic is grasped near its tip and presented towards 6 o´clock, special Scharioth forceps (DORC, The Netherlands) is used. A curved Scharioth forceps (DORC, The Netherlands) holds the haptic through paracentesis, straight Scharioth forceps is introduced through the ciliary sulcus sclerotomy and grasps the leading haptic at its very tip

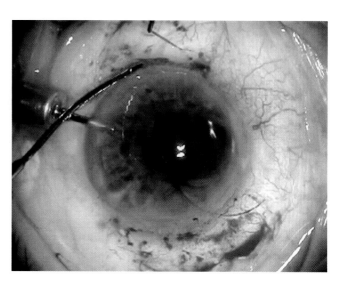

FIGURE 10: Leading haptic is externalized with the straight Scharioth forceps while the trailing haptic is still in the corneal incision

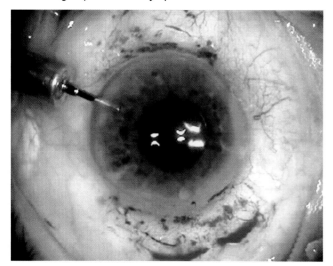

FIGURE 11: Same handshake technique is used to introduce the trailing haptic, then it is grasped and externalized. Both IOL haptics are externalized and the IOL is already well centered. Infusion is on to prevent collapse of the eye

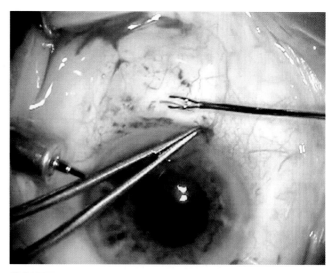

FIGURE 12: With the curved Scharioth forceps (DORC, The Netherlands) the very tip of the haptic is grasped, now the haptic is pushed backward through the sclerotomy and then the forcpes with the haptic is introduced into the intrascleral tunnel until it externalizes

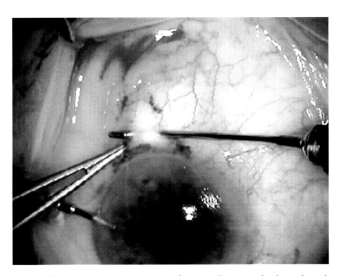

FIGURE 13: Haptic is released, forceps is turned, closed and pulled back. If needed the tip of the haptic could be held with a forceps to prevent retraction

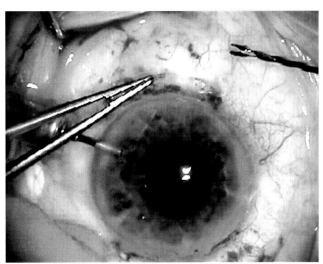

FIGURE 14: To prevent late erosion it is important to ensure that the haptic end is intrascleral. It could be pushed from outside into the tunnel or pulled from inside (e.g. with a Sinskey hook)

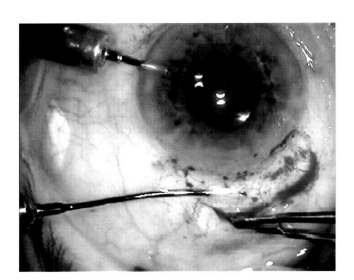

FIGURE 15: Same maneuver is performed on the opposite side

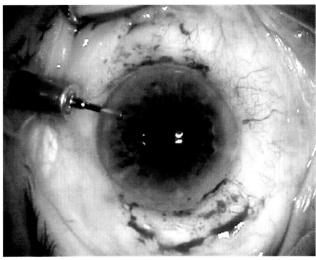

FIGURE 16: PCIOL is well centered with both haptics fixed intrasclerally. Infusion is reduced and incisons are checked for leakage before closing the conjunctiva. In case of leakage sclerotomies are sutured with Vicryl 8/0

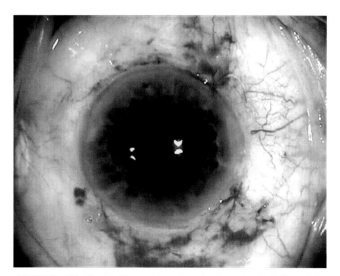

FIGURE 17: Finally the conjunctiva is closed with 8/0 or 9/0 Vicryl sutures and the paracentesis is hydrated

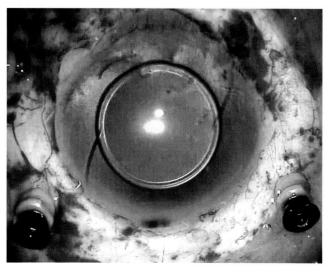

FIGURE 18: Intraoperative view in an aniridic eye with sutureless intrascleral haptic fixation. Note 25G pars plana sclerotomies

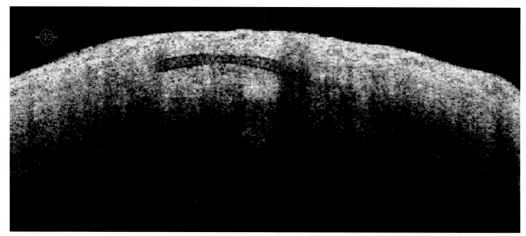

FIGURE 19: Postoperative OCT image of the intrascleral position of the incarcerated IOL haptic

tunnel fixation of the haptic is less technically demanding because it stabilizes the intraocular lens in the posterior chamber without difficult suturing procedures and uses a real microsurgical approach if injector assisted IOL implantation is used in combination with 25G or even a 27G vitrectomy system. Incarcerating a longer part of the haptic stabilizes the axial position of the PC IOL, which should decrease the incidence of IOL tilt. Up to six years follow up with only minimal complication after the early postoperative period seems to indicate the excellent long term stability of the intraocular lenses fixated with this technique. In our opinion the only possible contraindications are chronic, scleritis or scleromalacia, but these are very rare conditions.

Conclusion

Surgeons should be familiar with this new technique for fixation of intraocular lenses because we will be faced with a situation where an intraocular lens is already implanted and requires secondary intervention. In future urgent phacoemulsification problems like dropped nucleus will need revision and we will also see eyes with late dislocation of the entire capsular bag after primary uneventful cataract surgery because of a chronic ongoing disease like a pseudoexfoliation syndrome. We should be then able to select a less demanding and traumatizing technique which gives a great chance so that no further intervention is necessary.

References

1. Anand R, Bowman RW. Simplified technique for suturing dislocated posterior chamber intraocular lens to the ciliary sulcus [letter]. Arch Ophthalmol. 1990;108:1205-6.
2. Azar DT, Wiley WF. Double-knot transscleral suture fixation technique for displaced intraocular lenses. Am J Ophthalmol. 1999;128:644-6.
3. Bloom SM, Wyszynski RE, Brucker AJ. Scleral fixation suture for dislocated posterior chamber intraocular lens. Ophthalmic Surg. 1990;21:851-4.
4. Chan CK. An improved technique for management of dislocated posterior chamber implants. Ophthalmology. 1992;99:51-7.
5. Chang S. Perfluorocarbon liquids in vitreoretinal surgery. Int Ophthalmol Clin. 1992;32(2):153-63.
6. Chang S, Coll GE. Surgical techniques for repositioning a dislocated intraocular lens, repair of iridodialysis, and secondary intraocular lens implantation using innovative 25-gauge forceps. Am J Ophthalmol. 1995;119:165-74.
7. Fanous MM, Friedman SM. Ciliary sulcus fixation of a dislocated posterior chamber intraocular lens using liquid perfluorophenanthrene. Ophthalmic Surg. 1992;23:551-2.
8. Friedberg MA, Pilkerton AR. A new technique for repositioning and fixating a dislocated intraocular lens. Arch Ophthalmol. 1992;110:413-5.
9. Kokame GT, Yamamoto I, Mandel H. Scleral fixation of dislocated posterior chamber intraocular lenses;temporary haptic externalization through a clear corneal incision. J Cataract Refract Surg 2004;30:1049-56.
10. Little BC, Rosen PH, Orr G, Aylward GW. Trans-scleral fixation of dislocated posterior chamber intraocular lenses using a 9/0 microsurgical polypropylene snare. Eye. 1993;7:740-3.
11. Maguire AM, Blumenkranz MS, Ward TG, Winkelman JZ. Scleral loop fixation for posteriorly dislocated intraocular lenses; operative technique and long-term results. Arch Ophthalmol. 1991;109:1754-8.
12. Nabors G, Varley MP, Charles S. Ciliary sulcus suturing of a posterior chamber intraocular lens. Ophthalmic Surg. 1990;21:263-5.
13. Schneiderman TE, Johnson MW, Smiddy WE, et al. Surgical management of posteriorly dislocated silicone plate haptic intraocular lenses. Am J Ophthalmol. 1997;123:629-35.
14. Shin DH, Hu BV, Hong YJ, Gibbs KA. Posterior chamber lens implantation in the absence of posterior capsular support [letter and reply by WJ Stark, GL Goodman, JD Gottsch]. Ophthalmic Surg. 1988;19:606-7.
15. Smiddy WE. Dislocated posterior chamber intraocular lens;a new technique of management. Arch Ophthalmol. 1989;107:1678-80.
16. Smiddy WE, Flynn HW Jr. Needle-assisted scleral fixation suture technique for relocating posteriorly dislocated IOLs [letter]. Arch Ophthalmol. 1993;111:161-2.
17. Smiddy WE, Ibanez GV, Alfonso E, Flynn HW Jr. Surgical management of dislocated intraocular lenses. J Cataract Refract Surg. 1995;21:64-9.
18. Thach AB, Dugel PU, Sipperley JO, et al. Outcome of sulcus fixation of dislocated posterior chamber intraocular lenses using temporary externalization of the haptics. Ophthalmology. 2000;107:480-4;discussion by WF Mieler, 485.
19. Koh HJ, Kim CY, Lim SJ, Kwon OW. Scleral fixation technique using 2 corneal tunnels for a dislocated intraocular lens. J Cataract Refract Surg. 2000;26:1439-41.
20. Lewis JS. Ab externo sulcus fixation. Ophthalmic Surg. 1991;22:692-5.
21. Mohr A, Hengerer F, Eckardt C. Retropupillare Fixation der Irisklauenlinse bei Aphakie;Einjahresergebnisse einer neuen Implantationstechnik. [Retropupillary fixation of the iris claw lens in aphakia; 1 year outcome of a new implantation technique.] Ophthalmologe. 2002;99:580-3.
22. Hoffman RS, Fine I, Packar M. Scleral fixation without conjunctival dissection. J Cataract Refract Surg. 2006;32:1907-12.
23. Teichmann KD, Teichmann IAM. The torque and tilt gamble. J Cataract Refract Surg. 1997;23:413-8.
24. Por YM, Lavin MJ. Techniques of intraocular lens suspension in the absence of capsular/zonular support. Surv Ophthalmol. 2005;50:429-62.

25. Wagoner MD, Cox TA, Ariyasu RG, et al. Intraocular lens implantation in the absence of capsular support;a report by the American Academy of Ophthalmology. (Ophthalmic Technology Assessment) Ophthalmology. 2003;110:840-59.

26. Gross JG, Kokame GT, Weinberg DV. In-the-bag intraocular lens dislocation;the Dislocated In-the-Bag Intraocular Lens Study. Am J Ophthalmol. 2004;137:630-5.

27. Jehan FS, Mamalis N, Crandall AS. Spontaneous late dislocation of intraocular lens within the capsular bag in pseudoexfoliation patients. Ophthalmology. 2001;108:1727-31.

28. Gabor SG, Pavlidis MM. Sutureless intrascleral posterior chamber intraocular lens fixation. J Cataract Refract Surg. 2007; 33:1851-4.

29. Pavlidis M, de Ortueta D, Scharioth GB Bioptics in sutureless intrascleral multifocal posterior chamber intraocular lens fixation J Cataract Refract Surg. 2011;27:386-8.

30. Scharioth GB, Prasad S, Georgalas I, Tatru C, Pavlidis M. Intermediate results of sutureless intrascleral posterior chamber intraocular lens fixation. J Cataract Refract Surg. 2010; 36:254-9.

31. Agarwal A, Kumar DA, Jacob S, Baid C, Agarwal A, Srinivasan S. Fibrin glue-assisted sutureless posterior chamber intraocular lens implantation in eyes with deficient posterior capsules. J Cataract Refract Surgery. 2008;34(9):1433-8.

7

Surgical Technique of Glued IOL

Ashvin Agarwal, Amar Agarwal

Introduction

Posterior capsular rent (PCR)[1,2] can occur in the early learning curve in Phacoemulsification.[1-15] Intraoperative dialysis or a large PCR will prevent IOL implantation in the capsular bag. Implantation of an IOL in the sulcus will be possible in cases of adequate anterior capsular support. The first glued PC IOL implantation in an eye with a deficient capsule was done on 14th December 2007. In eyes with inadequate anterior capsular rim and deficient posterior capsule, the new technique of IOL implantation is the fibrin glue-assisted **(Figures 1A to C)** sutureless IOL implantation with scleral tuck.[3-7] Since 2007, a large number of cases have been done with this technique. The technique has also evolved since then and extended its application to many different scenarios and as part of combined surgeries. The scleral tuck and intrascleral haptic fixation of a PC IOL was first started by Gabor Scharioth from Germany.[8] Maggi had done previously a sutureless scleral fixation of a special IOL.[9]

White to White Measurement

One should always measure the corneal white to white (WTW) diameter. If the horizontal WTW is about 11 mm then one can do a horizontal glued IOL. This means the flaps can be made at 3 and 9 o'clock positions. If the WTW is more then it would be better to do a vertical glued IOL which means the scleral flaps are made at 12 and 6 o'clock positions. The reason this is performed is that the vertical cornea will always be shorter than the horizontal so one will have more haptic to tuck and glue **(Figures 2A and B)**. This idea was suggested by Jeevan Ladi from India.

Conjunctival Peritomy

If one is performing a manual non-phaco technique or a non-foldable glued IOL implantation, then it is better to have the superior rectus secured as exposure is better. In such cases one should prepare the conjunctival peritomy in the areas where the scleral flaps are to be made. Adequate but not over

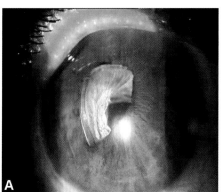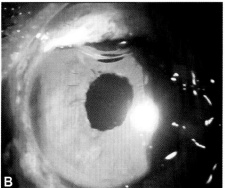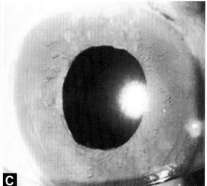

FIGURES 1A TO C: Subluxated IOL explanted and glued IOL implanted
A. Preoperative slit lamp image showing anterior subluxated IOL
B. Day one postoperative period
C. Three months after surgery

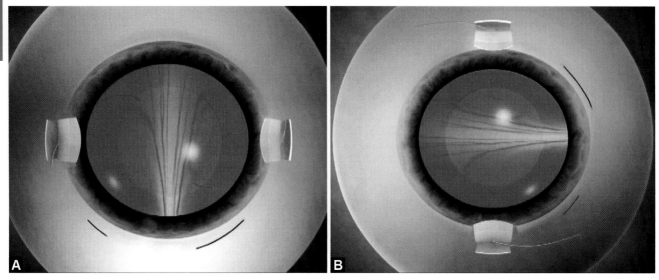

FIGURES 2A AND B
A. Horizontal glued IOL. Note the amount of haptic available to tuck and glue is less
B. Vertical glued IOL. Note the amount of haptic available to tuck and glue is more

excessive cautery should be done to stop any bleeding vessels.

Scleral Marking

It is imperative that the scleral flaps are 180 degrees apart. If not, the IOL will be decentered. For this reason it is better to use a scleral marker which creates marks on the cornea to see that the scleral flaps created are diagonally opposite **(Figures 3A to D)**. One of the scleral markers is designed by one of the authors **(Figure 4)**.

Scleral Flap Preparation

The size of the flaps should be 2.5 mm × 2.5 mm with the base at the limbus. Too large a flap is not ideal as the haptic has to traverse a longer distance to get tucked. There are many ways by which the scleral flap can be prepared just like one prepares a trabeculectomy flap. Sometimes it is cumbersome to create these flaps as one might have to use the non-dominant hand. A simple way by which we perform the scleral flaps **(Figures 5A to E)** is to first use a knife to create a mark on the sclera to up to half thickness **(Figure 5A)**. One should be careful not to make it too deep or too shallow. Once the marks are made, then one should take the hockey flap dissector (same one which one uses to make a scleral tunnel) and pass it from one end

of the flap **(Figure 5B)** till it comes out from the other end **(Figure 5C)**. Then move the dissector outwards so that the flap is created **(Figure 5D)**. The flap is then lifted **(Figure 5E)** and any bleeding vessels can be cauterized.

Infusion with a Trocar Cannula

One should get infusion of fluid into the eye. This can be done using a sutureless 23G/25G trocar cannula **(Figures 6A to D)**. The advantage is that there is no disruption of conjunctival integrity, no need for suturing the sclerotomy, and a reduction in surgical time. Insertion and removal of the cannula is faster than with a conventional 20-gauge infusion cannula. The trocar infusion kit is available separately and can be used by anterior segment surgeons in special situations. It contains a scleral guide, an inserter, and an infusion cannula. The scleral guide is inserted into the pars plana about 3.0 mm from the limbus with the help of the inserter **(Figures 6A and B)**, the inserter is removed, and the infusion cannula connected to the infusion bottle is then inserted **(Figures 6C and D)**. During removal of the cannula, the infusion is switched off and the scleral guide removed. No suture is applied in the sclerotomy site. We noted that the surgical time needed to fixate the infusion cannula was reduced when 23-gauge infusion was used. It was also safe and easy in the hands of the anterior segment surgeons as one had

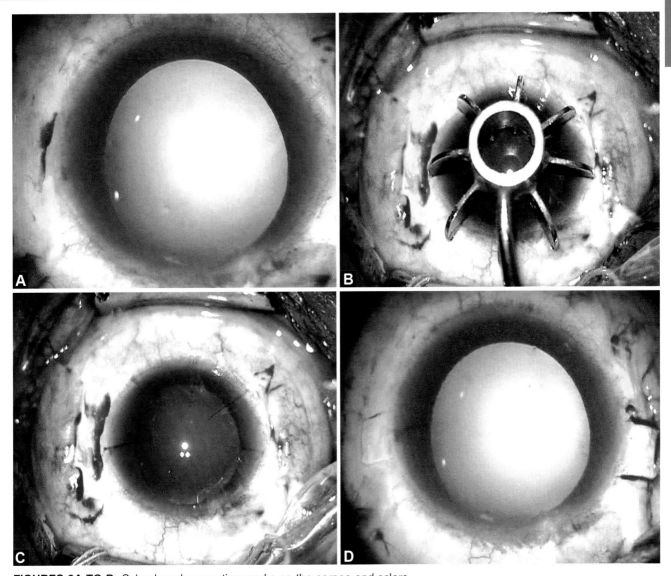

FIGURES 3A TO D: Scleral marker creating marks on the cornea and sclera

A. Aphakic eye
B. Scleral marker
C. Scleral and corneal marks made
D. Scleral flaps made

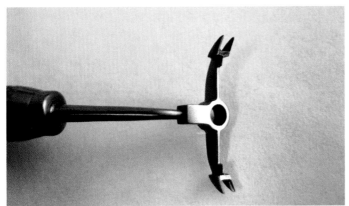

FIGURE 4: Ashvin Agarwal's scleral marker (Epsilon, India). The special feature of this is that it makes marks for the scleral flaps. It also measures 11 mm so one can know immediately if the WTW is too large

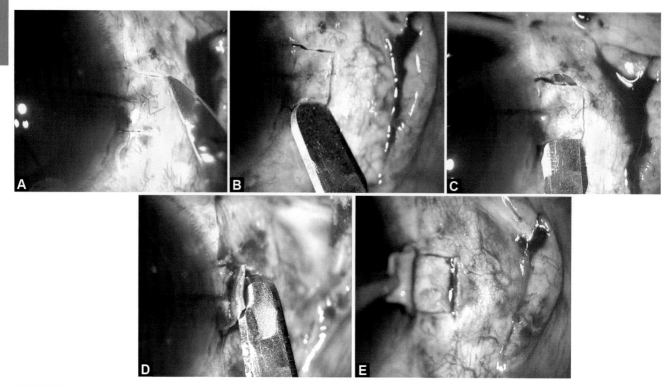

FIGURES 5A TO E: Scleral flap creation
A. Knife first makes half thickness marks
B. The dissector passes from one end of the flap
C. Dissector comes out from the other end
D. The dissector is moved outward to complete the flap
E. Flap is lifted and checked

to insert only the trocar and fixate the infusion cannula. One should always ensure the tip of the infusion cannula is in the vitreous cavity before the infusion is started. If the pupil is miotic, an iris retractor can be used to retract the iris and check that the infusion cannula is in the vitreous cavity. Direct visualization of the cannula during entrance and exit decreases the risk of complications.

Fixating a normal 20-gauge infusion cannula requires time to cut the conjunctiva, perform cautery, and then suture the infusion cannula to the sclera. Compared with the 20-gauge infusion cannula, the 23-gauge cannula causes significantly less postoperative pain and discomfort. In summary, if a 23-gauge trocar cannula kit is readily available in the operating room, it would be easy to use in glued IOL implantation by the anterior segment surgeon.

Infusion with an AC Maintainer

Another alternative is to fix an AC maintainer in the eye. For this one has to make a clear corneal incision with a side port knife and then pass the AC maintainer in the eye. It should be parallel to the iris and in an area which does not affect the surgical view **(Figure 7)**.

Trocar Cannula vs AC Maintainer

Infusion of fluid can be done with either a trocar cannula or an AC maintainer. The advantage of a trocar cannula is that it is in the vitreous cavity so does not hamper the surgical view. It also does not push back the iris or touch the iris. The disadvantage is that an anterior segment surgeon might not have easy access to a trocar cannula compared to a posterior segment surgeon. Another problem is that one should check that the trocar cannula is in the vitreous cavity before turning on the infusion so that the fluid does not go into the subretinal space. Sometimes this may be difficult to visualize in small pupils, etc.

The advantage of an AC maintainer is that it is easily available for an anterior segment surgeon, can be reautoclavable and also there is no issue of one having

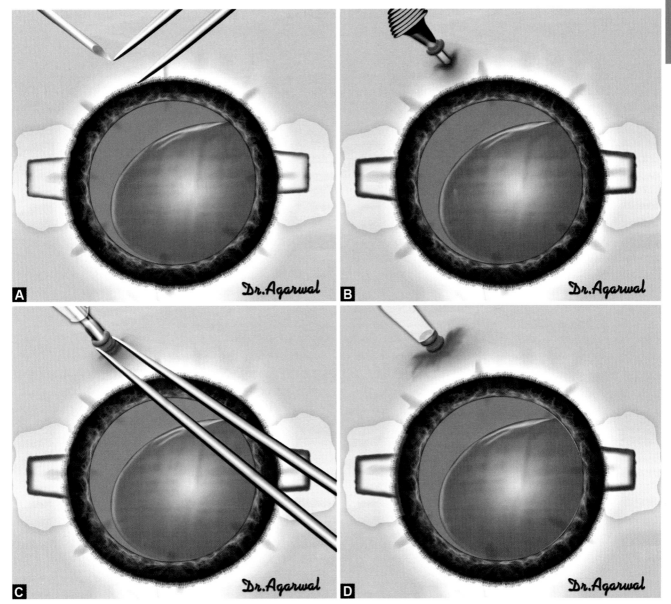

FIGURES 6A TO D: Insertion of 23-gauge trocar and cannula for glued IOL surgery
A. A 23-gauge trocar is placed 3.0 mm from the limbus. The distance is measured using a caliper.
B. The trocar is inserted into the pars plana
C and D. The inserter is removed and an infusion cannula connected to the infusion bottle is inserted

to be careful that the tip is in the subretinal space. The disadvantage of the AC maintainer is that the clear corneal incision does not always match the size of the AC maintainer accurately. This can lead to the AC maintainer coming out in the middle of the surgery and would then have to be refixed. Another issue with the AC maintainer is that when the AC maintainer fluid is turned on it pushes the iris back creating a deep anterior chamber (AC). When one has to make the 20G needle sclerotomy under the scleral flaps one can

hit the iris root as the iris is pushed back by the fluid. A solution to this is to fix the AC maintainer, create the 20G sclerotomies and then turn on the infusion.

Scleral Flaps or Infusion— Which Comes First?

One has to decide whether to create the scleral flaps first or fix the infusion for fluid. If one is operating a fresh case, for example, a patient posted for

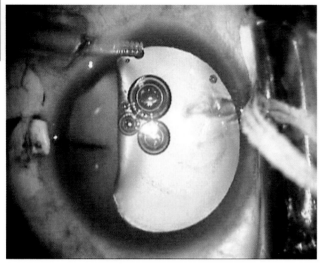

FIGURE 7: AC maintainer

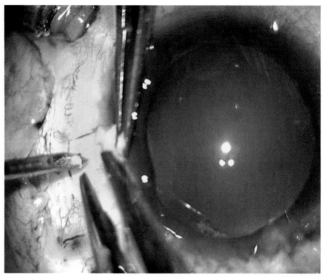

FIGURE 8: Sclerotomy made 1 mm from the limbus under the scleral flap using a 20G needle

secondary IOL in aphakia or a fresh ectopia lentis, it is better to create the scleral flaps first. The reason is that the globe is firm and it is easy to create the scleral flaps. In a case of a posterior capsular rupture where the corneal or scleral tunnel is open and one is preparing for a glued IOL surgery, it is better to first fix the infusion. This way fluid is flowing inside the eye. One can suture the open wound (either clear corneal or scleral tunnel) then fix the infusion for fluid. This way the globe becomes firm. Then it is easy to create the scleral flaps. Creating the scleral flaps in eyes which are open is tricky as the eyeball is soft.

Sclerotomies Under the Flap

Two straight sclerotomies with a 20G needle are made about 1.0 mm from the limbus under the existing scleral flaps **(Figure 8)**. The sclerotomies are to be directed obliquely into the mid-vitreous cavity so that one does not hit the iris which can happen if the sclerotomies are made in a horizontal direction. If one is using a 23G glued IOL forceps one can make a 20G sclerotomy. If one is using a 22G needle for the sclerotomy then one has to use a 25G glued IOL forceps for externalizing the haptics.

Vitrectomy

Vitrectomy is performed using a 20/23/25G vitrectomy probe. A good vitrectomy is crucial so that there is no vitreous traction and chances of retinal breaks and retinal detachments. If one is using a 23/25G vitrectomy probe which are available with posterior

vitrectomy machines one can pass the probe through the sclerotomy under the scleral flap **(Figure 9)**. If one is using the vitrectomy set up of a phaco machine one should remember that those vitrectomy probes are 20G and will not pass through the 20G needle sclerotomies made. In such a case one should make a clear corneal incision **(Figure 10)** and do the vitrectomy through the clear corneal incision.

IOL Types

Glued IOL can be performed well with rigid poly-methylmethacrylate (PMMA) IOL, 3-piece PC IOL, or

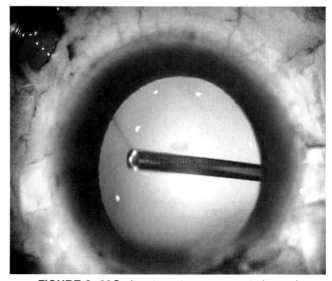

FIGURE 9: 23G vitrectomy to remove anterior and mid-vitreous

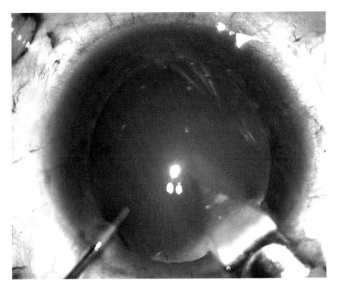

FIGURE 10: Clear corneal incision

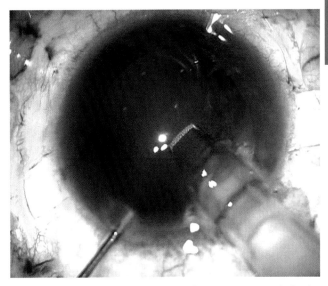

FIGURE 11: Foldable three piece IOL being injected slowly. Note the cartridge is inside the eye. One should not do wound assisted as the injection might happen too fast. This can either break the IOL or push it so fast it might go into the vitreous cavity

IOLs with modified PMMA haptics. One, therefore, does not need to have an entire inventory of special sutured scleral fixated SFIOLs with eyelets. In dislocated PC PMMA IOL or three piece IOLs, the same IOL can be repositioned thereby reducing the need for further manipulation. The one IOL that cannot be glued is the single piece foldable IOL as one needs a firm haptic to tuck and glue.

The best IOL to use is a three piece IOL as the haptics don't break compared to a single piece non-foldable IOL. A foldable three piece IOL **(Figure 11)** is even better for the simple reason the incision does not have to be enlarged. The length of a normal foldable three piece IOL is 13 mm. The Staar surgical lens is 13.5 mm which makes it better for glued IOL surgery as one will have more haptic externalized. The three piece non-foldable IOLs are also 13.5 mm.

Foldable IOL Injectors

It is preferable to have a plunger-type injector for better coordination although a screwing mechanism type injector may also be used. In the latter case, the assistant gently maneuvers the IOL forward as the surgeon holds the injector with one hand and the glued IOL forceps with the other hand. While introducing the injector, it is advisable to have the injector tip within the mouth of the incision and not use wound-assisted injection of the IOL that can lead to a sudden, uncontrolled entry of the IOL into the eye and a consequent IOL drop into the vitreous.

Leading Haptic Externalization

When we are using a foldable IOL one has to take a three piece foldable IOL. Once the lens is loaded see that the haptic is slightly out of the cartridge **(Figures 12A to E)**. The cartridge is passed into the AC **(Figures 13A to D)**. The glued IOL forceps is passed through the sclerotomy and grasps the tip of the haptic. The IOL is then gradually injected into the eye. If the injector is a screwing mechanism one then the assistant screws the injector. One should not externalize the haptic till the optic totally unfolds inside the eye, otherwise the optic can break. Once the optic is unfolded the glued IOL forceps pulls the haptic out and externalizes it. The haptic can then be caught by an assistant.

At this stage George Beiko from Canada has suggested to put the silicone plugs of an iris hook onto the haptic which has been externalized to prevent the haptic from slipping back. Priya Narang from India has suggested a no assistant technique where the trailing haptic is passed into the eye near the inferior portion so that due to physics principles the leading haptic cannot slip back.

When one is injecting the IOL one hand is holding the tip of the haptic. Fear of the IOL falling into the vitreous cavity is not there as:

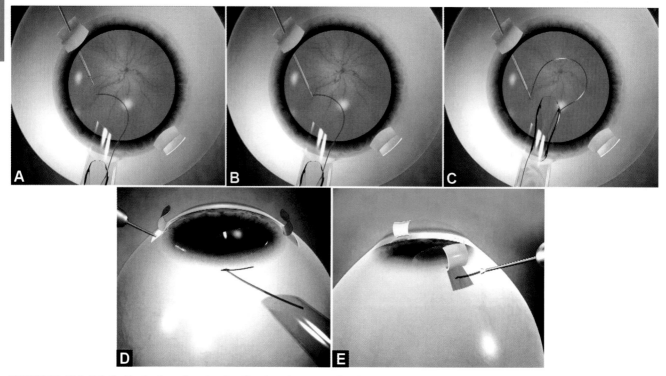

FIGURES 12A TO E: Illustration showing leading haptic externalization
A. Haptic ouside the cartridge. Glued IOL forceps ready to grasp the haptic tip
B. Haptic tip caught with the forceps
C. Injection of the IOL is continued till the optic unfolds inside the AC. One should not externalize the haptic till entire optic has unfolded otherwise the optic can break
D. Haptic externalization started
E. Haptic externalized

1. The tip of the haptic is caught with the forceps so the IOL cannot go down, and
2. The trailing haptic is still outside the eye. If the forceps slips and the haptic is missed the trailing haptic can still be caught and the IOL would not fall into the vitreous cavity.

Trailing Haptic Externalization

The trailing haptic is caught with the first glued IOL forceps and flexed into the AC **(Figures 14A to G)**. The haptic is transferred from the first forceps to the second using the handshake technique. The second forceps is passed through the side port. The first forceps is then passed through the sclerotomy under the scleral flap. The haptic is transferred from the second forceps back to the first using the handshake technique once again. The haptic tip is grasped with the first forceps and pulled towards the sclerotomy and externalized **(Figures 15A and B)**.

Vitrectomy Around the Sclerotomy

While all these maneuvers are being done some vitreous might be in the sclerotomy site. Vitrectomy should be done around the sclerotomy **(Figure 16A)**. Then one should assess the IOL position **(Figure 16B)**. Without anyone holding the IOL the lens must be stable. If the haptic is slipping back then it is possible:
1. The eye is large and has a large WTW in which case a vertical glued IOL would have to be done.
2. The sclerotomy made is too far back so very little haptic has been externalized.

If the haptics are slipping back then a fresh sclerotomy should be made more anterior to the previous one, the haptic pushed back into the vitreous cavity and using the handshake technique again grasped and re-externalized through the fresh anterior sclerotomy. Once again assessment should be made if the IOL is stable without tucking and gluing.

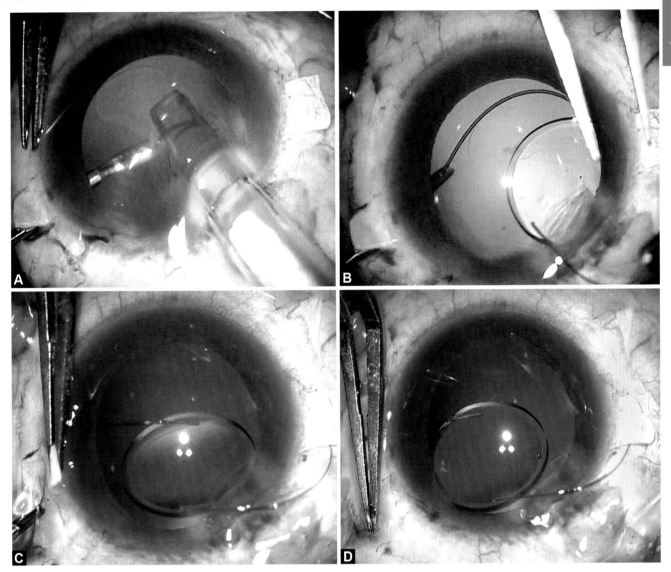

FIGURES 13A TO D: Leading haptic externalization
A. Cartridge inside the AC with the haptic slightly outside. The glued IOL forceps is passed through the sclerotomy and is ready to grasp the haptic tip
B. Haptic tip grasped with the glued IOL forceps. Foldable IOL injection continued with one hand. This injector has a pushing mechanism so one hand can be used. If the injector has a screwing mechanism the assistant continues the injection
C. Forceps pulls the haptic while injection of the foldable IOL is continued
D. Haptic externalized. Assistant then holds the haptic which is externalized

Scharioth Scleral Pocket and Intrascleral Haptic Tuck

Gabor Scharioth from Germany started the first intrascleral haptic fixation in 2006. It is the intrascleral haptic fixation which gives stability to the IOL. A 26G needle is taken and bent so that it is like a keratome **(Figure 17)**. The 26G needle then creates a scleral tunnel at the edge of the flap where the haptic is externalized. The haptic is then flexed and tucked into the scleral pocket. One can also mark the Scharioth scleral pocket and create it even before the eye is opened. The 26G needle is marked with the marker pen to leave a mark in the sclera where the scleral pocket is created **(Figures 18 and 19)**. This can be done adjacent to the area where the sclerotomy will be made. It is now easy to know where the scleral pocket is located. Another way is to pass a rod in the area of the sclera pocket to check its location.

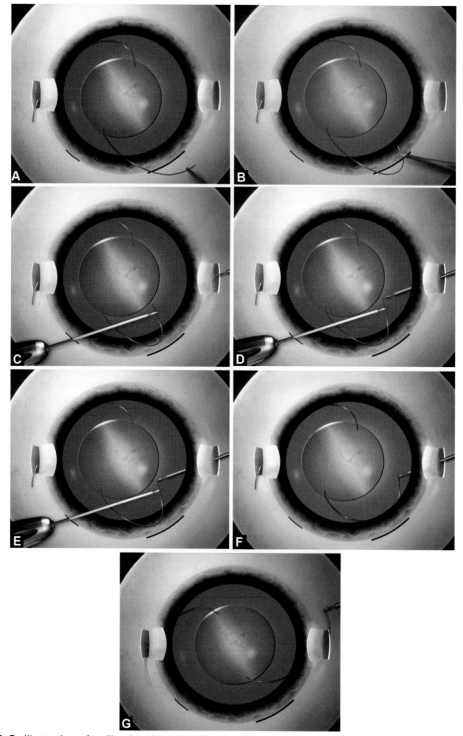

FIGURES 14A TO G: Illustration of trailing haptic externalization

A. The trailing haptic is caught with the first glued IOL forceps
B. Haptic flexed into the AC
C. Haptic is transferred from first forceps to the second using the handshake technique. The second forceps is passed through the side port
D. First forceps is passed through the sclerotomy under the scleral flap
E. Haptic is transferred from second forceps back to the first using the handshake technique
F. Haptic tip grasped with the first forceps
G. Haptic is pulled towards the sclerotomy and the haptic externalized

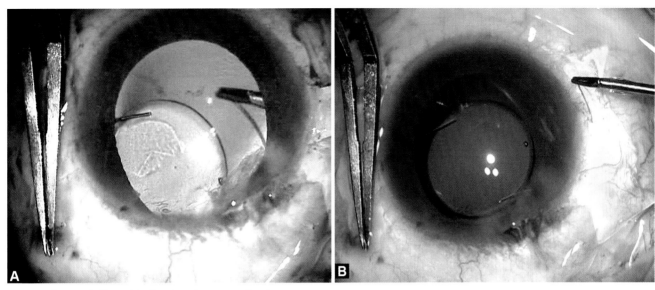

FIGURES 15A AND B: Trailing haptic externalization
A. Trailing haptic caught with the glued IOL forceps
B. Haptic externalized

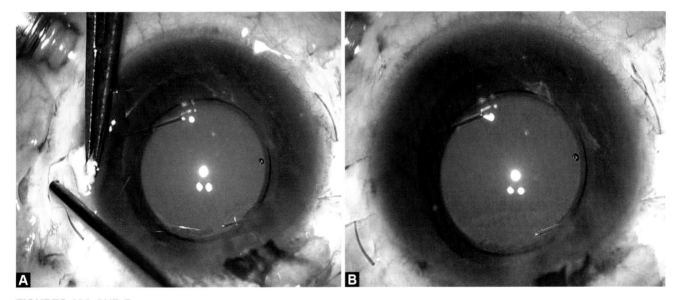

FIGURES 16A AND B
A. Vitrectomy around the sclerotomy site
B. IOL stable without the tuck

Air in the AC

Air is now injected into the AC once the fluid from the infusion cannula is turned off **(Figure 20).** The fibrin glue has to work in a dry area so the fluid has to be turned off. Otherwise fluid might keep on coming from the sclerotomy site. Once fluid is turned off there could be intraoperative and postoperative hypotony. To prevent this we inject air in the AC to have a firm globe intra- and postoperatively.

Fibrin Glue

The fibrin kit we use is Reliseal (Reliance Life Sciences, India) or Tisseel (Baxter, USA). The fibrinogen and thrombin are first reconstituted according to the manufacturer's instructions. The commercially available FG is virus inactivated and is checked for viral antigen and antibodies with polymerase chain reaction; hence, the chances of transmission of infection are very low. The glue is applied over the flaps and after sealing

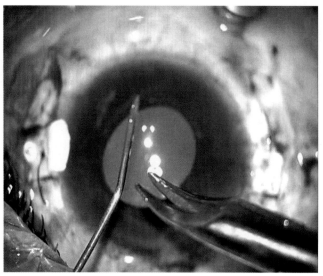

FIGURE 17: 26G needle bent like a keratome

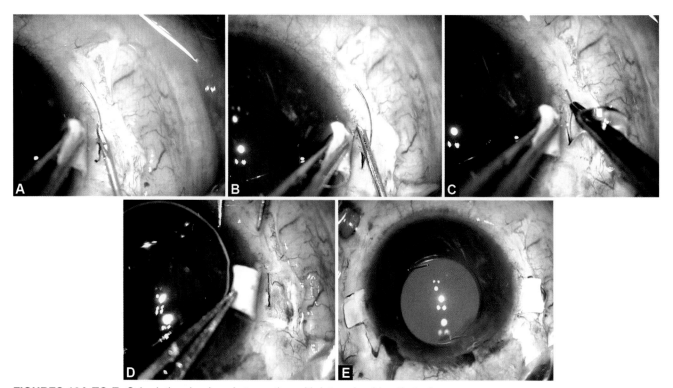

FIGURES 18A TO E: Scharioth scleral pocket creation with intrascleral haptic tuck
A. 26G needle creating a scleral tunnel at the edge of the flap where the haptic is externalized
B. Scharioth scleral pocket
C. Haptic flexed to be tucked into the scleral pocket
D. Haptic tucked in the scleral pocket
E. IOL centered and stable with haptics tucked

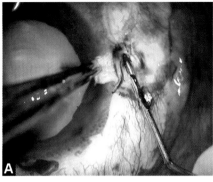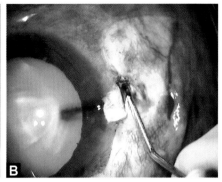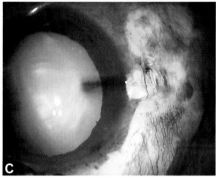

FIGURES 19A TO C: Marked Scharioth scleral pocket creation before IOL implantation
A. 26G needle is marked with the marker pen to leave a mark in the sclera where the scleral pocket is created. This can be done before opening the eye as it will have to be done adjacent to the area where the sclerotomy will be made
B. Marked scleral pocket created by 26G needle
C. Marked scleral pocket created. It is now easy to know where the scleral pocket is located. Another way is to pass a rod in the area of the sclera pocket to check its location

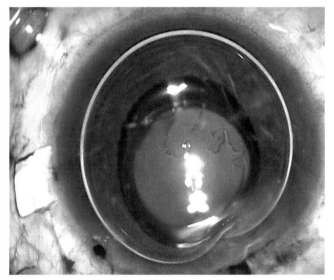

FIGURE 20: Air in the AC

them it can be used over the conjunctiva and clear corneal incisions to seal them too **(Figures 21A to D)**.

Role of Fibrin Glue

The fibrin glue plays a multifactorial role in Glued IOL surgery.
1. The glue helps seal the haptic to the sclera which gives extra support to the intrascleral haptic tuck.
2. The glue seals the flaps so that there is no opening from inside the eye to the outside. This prevents any chances of endophthalmitis even some years later where one could get conjunctivitis leading to endophthalmitis as there is an opening from inside to the outside of the eye.

3. The glue prevents any trabeculectomy opening as the flaps are now firmly stuck.
4. The glue helps seal the cut conjunctiva.
5. The glue helps seal the clear corneal incisions.

Postoperative Regimen

One should keep a watch on the patients postoperatively as these are worst case scenarios being operated upon **(Figures 22A and B)**. They need postoperative antibiotic steroids for 6 weeks. If there is temporary elevation of IOP antiglaucoma medications can be given. If there is a reaction, if necessary, subconjunctival antibiotic-steroids can also be given.

Stability of the IOL Haptic

As the flaps are manually created, the rough apposing surfaces of the flap and bed heal rapidly and firmly around the haptic, being helped by the fibrin glue early on. The major uncertainty here is the stability of the fibrin matrix *in vivo*. Numerous animal studies have shown that the fibrin glue is still present at 4-6 weeks. Because postoperative fibrosis starts early, the flaps become stuck secondary to fibrosis even prior to full degradation of the glue. The ensuing fibrosis acts to form a firm scaffold around the haptic which prevents movement along the long axis **(Figure 23A)**. To further make the IOL rock stable, we tuck the haptic tip into the scleral wall through a tunnel. This prevents all movements of the haptic along the transverse axis as well **(Figure 23B)**. The stability of the lens first comes through the tucking of the haptics in the scleral

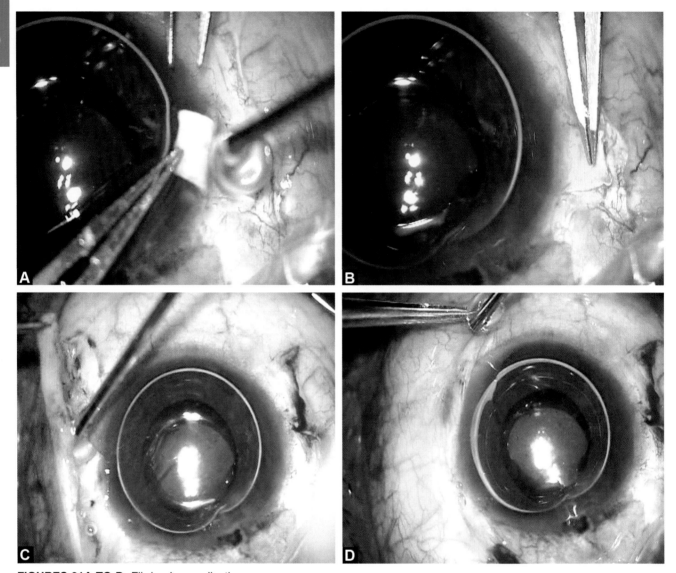

FIGURES 21A TO D: Fibrin glue application
A. Fibrin glue applied under the flaps
B. Scleral flaps stuck
C. Fibrin glue applied to seal the conjunctiva
D. Conjunctiva sealed with the glue

pocket created. The tissue glue then gives it extra stability and also seals the flap down. Externalization of the greater part of the haptics along its curvature stabilizes the axial positioning of the IOL and thereby prevents any IOL tilt.

Advantages

This fibrin glue assisted sutureless PCI OL implantation technique would be useful in a myriad of clinical situations where scleral fixated IOLs are indicated, such

as, luxated IOL, dislocated IOL, zonulopathy or secondary IOL implantation.

No Special IOLs

It can be performed well with rigid PMMA IOL, three piece PC IOL or IOLs with modified PMMA haptics. One therefore, does not need to have an entire inventory of special SFIOLs with eyelets, unlike in sutured SFIOLs. In dislocated posterior chamber PMMA IOL, the same IOL can be repositioned thereby reducing the need for further manipulation.

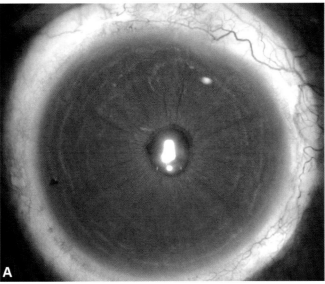

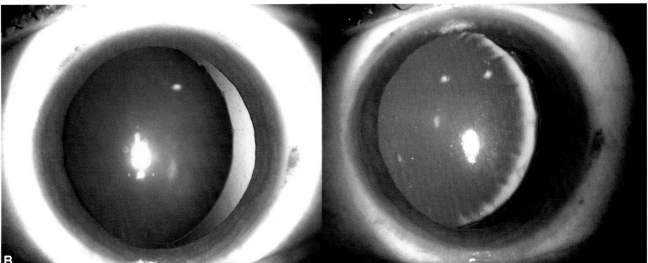

FIGURES 22A AND B: Glued IOL
A. Glued IOL done in right eye one and half year postoperative
B. Subluxated cataract in left eye

No Tilt

Since the overall diameter of the routine IOL is about 12 to 13 mm, with the haptic being placed in its normal curved configuration and without any traction, there is no distortion or change in shape of the IOL optic **(Figure 24)**. Externalization of the greater part of the haptics along its curvature stabilizes the axial positioning of the IOL and thereby prevents any IOL tilt.

Less Pseudophacodonesis

When the eye moves, it acquires kinetic energy from its muscles and attachments and the energy is dissipated to the internal fluids as it stops. Thus, pseudopha-codonesis is the result of oscillations of the fluids in the anterior and posterior segment of the eye. These oscillations, initiated by movement of the eye, result in shearing forces on the corneal endothelium as well as the vitreous motion leads to permanent damage. Since the IOL haptic is stuck beneath the flap, it would prevent the further movement of the haptic and thereby reduce pseudophacodonesis.

Less UGH Syndrome

We expect less incidence of UGH syndrome in fibrin glue assisted IOL implantation as compared to sutured scleral fixated IOL. This is because, in the former the

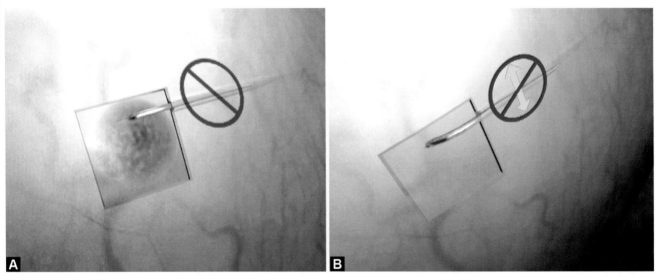

FIGURES 23A AND B: Stability of the IOL
A. Long axis movement is prevented by the tissue glue
B. Transverse axis movement is prevented by the scleral tuck

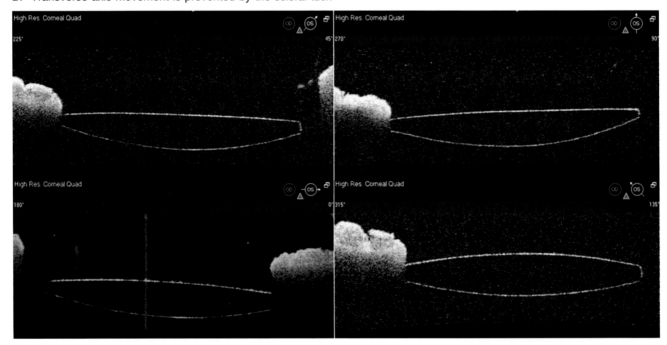

FIGURE 24: Anterior segment OCT showing 360 degrees good centration of the IOL

IOL is well stabilized and stuck onto the scleral bed and thereby, has decreased intraocular mobility whereas in the latter, there is increased possibility of the IOL movement or persistent rub over the ciliary body.

No Suture Related Complications

Visually significant complications due to late subluxation which has been known to occur in sutured scleral fixated IOL may also be prevented as sutures are totally avoided in this technique. Another important advantage of this technique is the prevention of suture related complications like suture erosion, suture knot exposure or dislocation of the IOL after suture disintegration or broken suture.

Rapidity and Ease of Surgery

The time taken in SFIOL for passing sutures into the IOL haptic eyelets, and tying down the knots as well

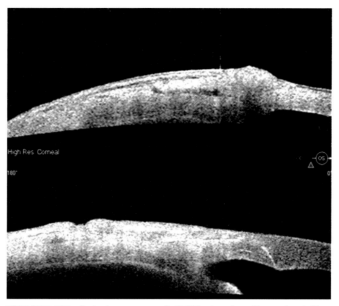

FIGURE 25: Anterior segment OCT showing the scleral flap placement on day 1 (above) and adhesion well maintained till 6 weeks (below)

as time for suturing scleral flaps and closing the conjunctiva are all significantly reduced in glued IOL surgery. The risk of retinal photic injury which is known to occur in SFIOL would also be reduced in our technique due to the short surgical time. Fibrin glue takes less time [Reliseal (20 seconds)/Tisseel (3 seconds)] to act in the scleral bed and it helps in adhesion as well as hemostasis. The preparation time can also be reduced in elective procedures by preparing it prior to surgery as it remains stable up to 4 hours from the time of reconstitution. Fibrin glue has been shown to provide airtight closure and by the time the fibrin starts degrading, surgical adhesions would have already occurred in the scleral bed. This is well shown in the follow up anterior segment OCT **(Figure 25)** where postoperative perfect scleral flap adhesion is observed.

References

1. Vajpayee RB, Sharma N, Dada T, et al. Management of posterior capsule tears. Surv Ophthal. 2001;45:473-88.
2. Wu MC, Bhandari A. Managing the broken capsule. Curr Opin Ophthalmol. 2008;19:36-40.
3. Agarwal A, Kumar DA, Jacob S, et al. Fibrin glue-assisted sutureless posterior chamber intraocular lens implantation in eyes with deficient posterior capsules. J Cataract Refract Surg. 2008;34:1433-8.
4. Prakash G, Kumar DA, Jacob S, et al. Anterior segment optical coherence tomography-aided diagnosis and primary posterior chamber intraocular lens implantation with fibrin glue in traumatic phacocele with scleral perforation. J Cataract Refract Surg. 2009;35:782-4.
5. Prakash G, Jacob S, Kumar DA, et al. Femtosecond assisted keratoplasty with fibrin glue-assisted sutureless posterior chamber lens implantation: a new triple procedure. J Cataract Refract Surg. In press (manuscript no 08-919).
6. Agarwal A, Kumar DA, Prakash G, et al. Fibrin glue-assisted sutureless posterior chamber intraocular lens implantation in eyes with deficient posterior capsules [Reply to letter]. J Cataract Refract Surg. 2009;35:795-6.
7. Nair V, Kumar DA, Prakash G, et al. Bilateral spontaneous in-the-bag anterior subluxation of PC IOL managed with glued IOL technique: A case report, Eye Contact Lens 2009. In Press (manuscript no ECL-07-281).
8. Gabor SGB, Pavilidis MM. Sutureless intrascleral posterior chamber intraocular lens fixation. J Cataract Refract Surg. 2007; 33:1851-4.
9. Maggi R, Maggi C. Sutureless scleral fixation of intraocular lenses. J Cataract Refract Surg. 1997;23:1289-94.
10. Teichmann KD, Teichmann IAM. The torque and tilt gamble. J Cataract Refract Surg. 1997;23:413-8.
11. Jacobi KW, Jagger WS. Physical forces involved in pseudo-phacodonesis and iridodonesis. Albrecht Von Graefes Arch Klin Exp Ophthalmol. 1981;216:49-53.
12. Price MO, Price FW Jr, Werner L, et al. Late dislocation of scleral-sutured posterior chamber intraocular lenses. J Cataract Refract Surg. 2005;31(7):1320-6.
13. Solomon K, Gussler JR, Gussler C, Van Meter WS. Incidence and management of complications of transsclerally sutured posterior chamber lenses. J Cataract Refract Surg. 1993;19: 488-93.
14. Asadi R, Kheirkhah A. Long-term results of scleral fixation of posterior chamber intraocular lenses in children Ophthalmology. 2008;115(1):67-72. Epub 2007 May 3.
15. Lanzetta P, Menchini U, Virgili G, et al. Scleral fixated intraocular lenses: an angiographic study. Retina. 1998;18:515-20.

Athiya Agarwal

Introduction

Glued IOL as a technique for PC IOL fixation in eyes with absent or insufficient capsular support was first described by us in 2007.[1-9] Since then a large number of cases have been done with this technique. The technique has also evolved since then and extended its application to many different scenarios and as part of combined surgeries.[4,7,8] "Handshake" technique is a modification in the glued IOL procedure in which the IOL haptic is bimanually transferred from one end opening forceps to another under direct visualization in the pupillary plane.

Leading Haptic Externalization

One of the greatest changes was the use of foldable IOLs for performing this surgery thus extending all the advantages that a small incision offers. Any three piece foldable IOL can be used for this technique. Depending on surgeon preference, an infusion cannula or AC maintainer is fixed and the flaps and sclerotomies made. A 2.8 mm keratome is used to make a corneal incision. This may be enlarged very slightly so as to allow easy insertion. A side port may also be made to allow the surgeon easier maneuverability and as a future access point if required. The three piece foldable IOL is loaded into the injector. The extreme tip of the haptic is left protruding out to allow the MST forceps to grab it easily. The injector tip is then introduced into the AC (Figures 1A to E). At the same time, a 23G Glued IOL (Microsurgical technology, MST, USA) forceps is then introduced through the sclerotomy under the scleral flap. As the IOL is being injected into the AC, the tip of the haptic is caught with the MST forceps and exteriorized while injection is continued very gently. The injector is then slowly withdrawn so that the second haptic is left trailing outside the wound. The first haptic is then held by an assistant.

Trailing Haptic Externalization

The surgeon now flexes the second haptic into the AC into the jaws of an MST forceps introduced through the second sclerotomy. This haptic is also thus externalized out (Figures 2A to F). In a routine foldable glued IOL, the MST forceps can also be introduced through the side port to grasp the trailing forceps and feed it into the jaws of the second MST forceps. Depending on ease of access, the other MST forceps is introduced through the opposite sclerotomy or through the side-port.

Scharioth Tuck and Glue

A bent 26 gauge needle is then used to create a tunnel in the direction of the exteriorized haptics at the edge of the scleral flap. Vitrectomy is then used to clear up the scleral bed in case any vitreous has prolapsed out. Both haptics are then tucked intrasclerally. Centration of the IOL is checked for and if not well centered, the degree of tuck of the individual haptics is adjusted till the lens becomes well centered. The scleral bed is then dried, fibrin glue applied and the scleral flaps are glued down. Fibrin glue is also used to seal the mainport and the sideport by applying over the incisions. The conjunctiva is also closed with fibrin glue.

Injector

It is preferable to have a plunger type injector for better coordination though a screw mechanism type injector may also be used. In the latter case, the assistant gently maneuvers the IOL forwards as the surgeon holds the injector with one hand and the MST

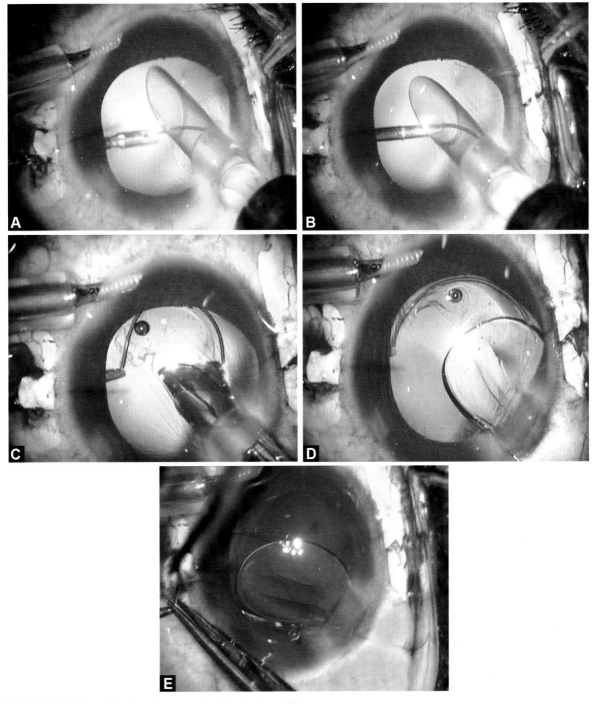

FIGURES 1A TO E: Leading haptic externalization in glued IOL surgery

A. IOL in injector. Note the haptic tip is slightly out of the cartridge. Note also that the cartridge is in the AC. There is no wound assisted injection. Glued IOL forceps (Epsilon, India) is passed through the sclerotomy with the other hand ready to grasp the tip of the haptic. One should not do wound assisted as the injection might happen too fast. This can either break the IOL or push it so fast it might go into the vitreous cavity

B. Tip of the haptic grasped with the glued IOL forceps

C. Injection of the IOL continued. If it is a plunger type injector surgeon can do it, but if it is a screwing mechanism injector, assistant can screw the injector for release of the IOL as both hands of the surgeon are occupied

D. IOL has unfolded inside the eye, then only the cartridge is removed. Note one hand still holding the haptic tip but the tip has not been externalized as yet. If one externalizes the haptic before the IOL has unfolded from the cartridge the IOL can break.

E. Haptic externalized and assistant tries to grasp the haptic so that the haptic does not fall back inside the eye

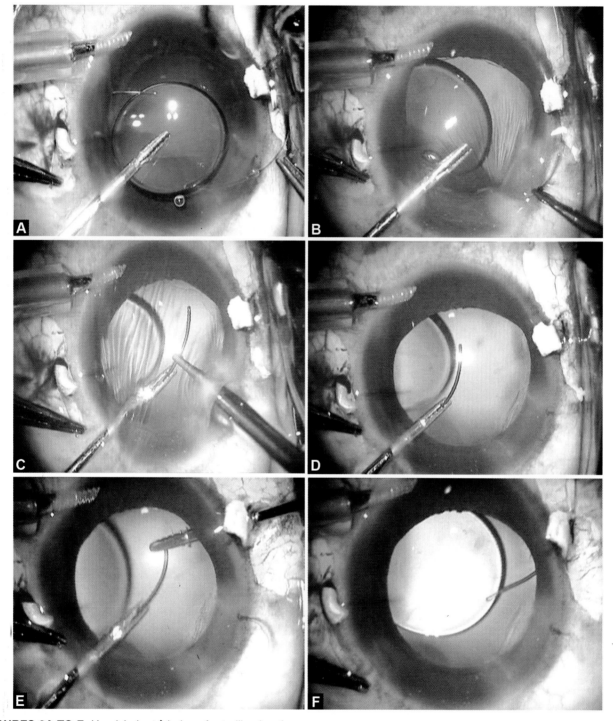

FIGURES 2A TO F: Handshake technique for trailing haptic

A. Glued IOL forceps (Epsilon, India) passed through the side port

B. The trailing haptic grasped with a forceps and flexed to make it enter the AC

C. Trailing haptic passed into the AC and with handshake technique, haptic grasp shifted from one forceps to the other. Note the dimpling on the cornea as the main incision is open due to the forceps passage

D. Trailing haptic caught with forceps passed through the side port. Note no dimpling on the cornea as main port incision is closed. It is now easy to see the tip of the haptic

E. Glued IOL forceps passed through the sclerotomy and tip of the haptic grasped. Once again handshake technique helps pass the haptic from one forceps to the other

F. Trailing haptic externalized

forceps with the other hand. While introducing the injector, it is advisable to have the injector tip within the mouth of the incision and not use wound assisted injection of the IOL which can lead to a sudden, uncontrolled entry of the IOL into the eye and a consequent IOL drop into the vitreous.

Handshake Technique for Foldable Glued IOL

We have seen that exteriorization of the haptics is a key step in performing glued IOL. Since the surgeon is maneuvering with both hands simultaneously, one hand injecting the IOL while the other grasps and exteriorizes the haptics, he/she needs to be familiar with the handshake technique as a means of transferring the haptic from one hand to the other. The handshake technique can be utilized in a variety of situations. For example, it is essential to hold the haptic at its tip before exteriorizing it so that it does not snag on the sclerotomy while being brought out. The handshake transfer of the haptic between the two MST forceps is continued till the tip of the haptic is caught by the forceps on the side to which the haptic is to be exteriorized. Another situation is if one of the haptics is not caught or if it gets released accidentally after grasping it. In this case too, the handshake technique can be used to regrasp the haptic. The MST forceps is introduced through the side port which becomes invaluable in this situation. The handshake technique utilizes two MST forceps, one of which holds one haptic **(Figures 3A to F)**. The other MST forceps is then introduced into the eye and the first hand then transfers the haptic into the second MST forceps such that the first hand now becomes free. This technique is especially useful in subluxated three piece IOLs as it allows easy intraocular maneuverability of the entire haptic or IOL within a closed globe system. The MST forceps is introduced through the sclerotomy to grasp the IOL while a vitrectomy is done all around the IOL to free vitreous traction. Once the IOL is free, an MST forceps **(Figure 4)** is introduced through the other sclerotomy and the IOL is exchanged between hands till

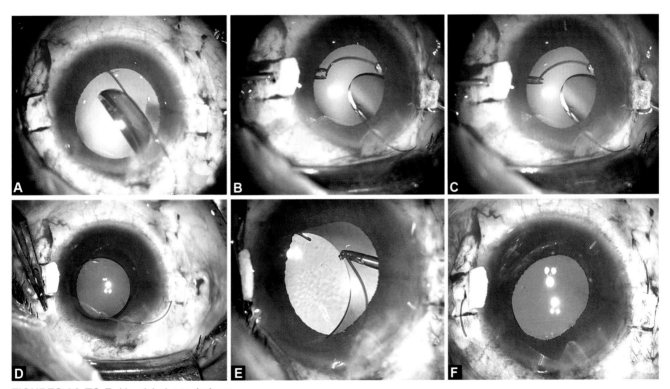

FIGURES 3A TO F: Handshake technique
A. Foldable IOL haptic is below the iris
B. One end opening forceps is passed through the opposite sclerotomy site while other forceps is ready to receive the haptic
C. The leading haptic is grasped with forceps and the haptic tip is fed into another forceps
D. One haptic externalized and assistant holds the haptic
E. Trailing haptic caught with the end opening forceps
F. Both the haptics externalized under the scleral flaps

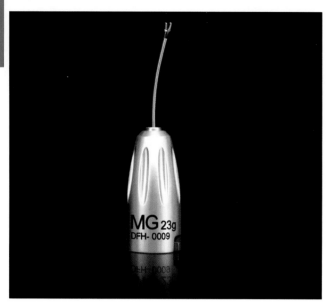

FIGURE 4: Ahmed micrograsper: End opening forceps for glued IOL surgery (Microsurgical technology, MST, USA) (*Courtesy:* Larry Laks, MST, USA)

the tip of the haptic is grasped. This haptic is then exteriorized and held by the assistant while the handshake maneuver is next used for the second haptic in a similar manner. This allows refixation of the same IOL with a closed chamber approach with minimal intervention.

Conclusion

The foldable glued IOL technique and the handshake technique further refine this procedure by the use of smaller incisions and better intraocular maneuverability, making it possible to perform the entire procedure through small self-sealing incisions. This has the intraoperative advantages of having a well-formed globe throughout all the steps of surgery. It eliminates iris prolapse during IOL insertion, wound suturing and also significantly decreases time of surgery as there is no need to suture the corneoscleral section. The risk of

having a large section such as expulsive hemorrhage, etc. are also reduced. This foldable glued IOL also has postoperative advantages of doing away with all complications associated with larger wounds such as postoperative wound leak, shallow AC, etc. as well as decreases the astigmatism associated with a large wound. To be able to perform this technique with ease, it is imperative that the surgeon becomes familiar with the handshake technique.

References

1. Agarwal A, Kumar DA, Jacob S, Baid C, Agarwal A, Srinivasan S. Fibrin glue-assisted sutureless posterior chamber intraocular lens implantation in eyes with deficient posterior capsules. J Cataract Refract Surg. 2008;34(9):1433-8.
2. Kumar DA, Agarwal A, Prakash G, Jacob S, Saravanan Y, Agarwal A.Glued posterior chamber IOL in eyes with deficient capsular support: a retrospective analysis of 1-year post-operative outcomes. Eye (Lond). 2010;24(7):1143-8.
3. Prakash G, Kumar DA, Jacob S, Kumar KS, Agarwal A, Agarwal A. Anterior segment optical coherence tomography-aided diagnosis and primary posterior chamber intraocular lens implantation with fibrin glue in traumatic phacocele with scleral perforation. J Cataract Refract Surg. 2009;35(4):782-4.
4. Prakash G, Jacob S, Kumar DA, Narsimhan S, Agarwal A, Agarwal A. Femtosecond assisted keratoplasty with fibrin glue-assisted sutureless posterior chamber lens implantation: a new triple procedure. J Cataract Refract Surg. 2009;35(6):973-9.
5. Nair V, Kumar DA, Prakash G, Jacob S, Agarwal A, Agarwal A. Bilateral spontaneous in-the-bag anterior subluxation of PC IOL managed with glued IOL technique: A case report. Eye Contact Lens. 2009;35(4):215-7.
6. Agarwal A, Kumar DA, Prakash G, et al. Fibrin glue-assisted sutureless posterior chamber intraocular lens implantation in eyes with deficient posterior capsules [Reply to letter]. J Cataract Refract Surg 2009;35(5):795-6.
7. Kumar DA, Agarwal A, Jacob S, Prakash G, Agarwal A, Sivagnanam S. Repositioning of the dislocated intraocular lens with sutureless 20-gauge vitrectomy Retina. 2010;30(4):682-7.
8. Kumar DA, Agarwal A, Prakash G, Jacob S. Managing total aniridia with aphakia using a glued iris prosthesis. J Cataract Refract Surg. 2010;36(5):864-5.
9. Kumar DA, Agarwal A, Gabor SG, et al. Sutureless sclera fixated posterior chamber intraocular lens. Letter to editor. J Cataract Refract Surg. 2011;37(11):2089-90.

9 IOL Scaffold Technique

Smita Narasimhan, Amar Agarwal

IOL Scaffold

A foldable intraocular lens (IOL) is used as a scaffold for preventing the nucleus fragment from descending into the vitreous in cases of posterior capsular ruptures. After removing the vitreous in the anterior chamber by anterior vitrectomy, a three piece foldable IOL is injected via the existing corneal incision with one haptic above the iris and the other haptic extending outside the incision. The nucleus is emulsified with the phacoprobe above the IOL optic. Cortical cleaning is done and the IOL is then placed over the remnants of the capsule in the ciliary sulcus. This can be performed in eyes with moderate to soft cataracts. It avoids corneal incision extension and there by limits induced astigmatism.

Introduction

Posterior capsular rupture (PCR) is one of the common complications during phacoemulsification.[1-3] PCR with vitreous prolapse and the nucleus still in the capsular bag is an impending situation for a nucleus drop. As a preventive step it is usual for the cataract surgeon to extend the corneal incision and deliver the nucleus.[4-6] Lens glide or Viscoat assisted levitation have also been used to remove the nuclear fragments.[8] Another method is to emulsify the nucleus in the anterior chamber with low flow rate and vacuum.

Scaffold

The word scaffold comes from Medieval Latin scaffaldus. The word means a temporary platform. In the IOL scaffold technique the three piece IOL acts as a temporary platform and prevents the nuclear fragments from falling into the vitreous cavity.

Surgical Technique

When there is a posterior capsule rupture **(Figure 1A)**, an anterior chamber (AC) maintainer is introduced through a 1.2 mm stab microvitreoretinal (MVR) blade incision **(Figure 1B)**. The position of the AC maintainer should be away from the PCR and flow should be kept low. Anterior vitrectomy is done with the vitrectomy cutter to remove the vitreous prolapsed in the anterior chamber. An Agarwal globe stabilization rod (Katena, USA) passed through the side port helps to push the fragment away from the PCR. The fragments are brought into the anterior chamber. A foldable IOL is then injected via the existing corneal wound and is maneuvered below the nucleus **(Figure 1B)**. The leading haptic of the IOL is positioned above the iris and the trailing haptic is placed just outside the incision site **(Figure 1C)**. Using a dialer in the nondominant hand, the junction of the optic haptic junction on the trailing side is maneuvered so that the IOL blocks the pupil. Thus the IOL acts now as a scaffold and prevents the fragments from falling into the vitreous cavity **(Figure 1D)**. The nucleus fragment is then removed with the phacoprobe (low flow and vacuum) **(Figure 1D)**. Cortex is removed with suction and low aspiration using a vitrectomy probe. The non-dominant hand adjusts the trailing optic haptic junction so that the IOL is well centered over the pupil acting as a scaffold while emulsifying the nucleus **(Figures 2 and 3)**. Once cortical cleaning is done, the IOL is placed over the capsular remnants in the ciliary sulcus. The AC maintainer is then removed and wound hydration done. Postoperatively, topical ofloxacin and corticosteroid eye drops are used 4 times daily for 2 weeks. A short acting mydriatic drop twice a day is used for initial 3 days. Postoperative anterior chamber flare is graded by slit lamp examination.

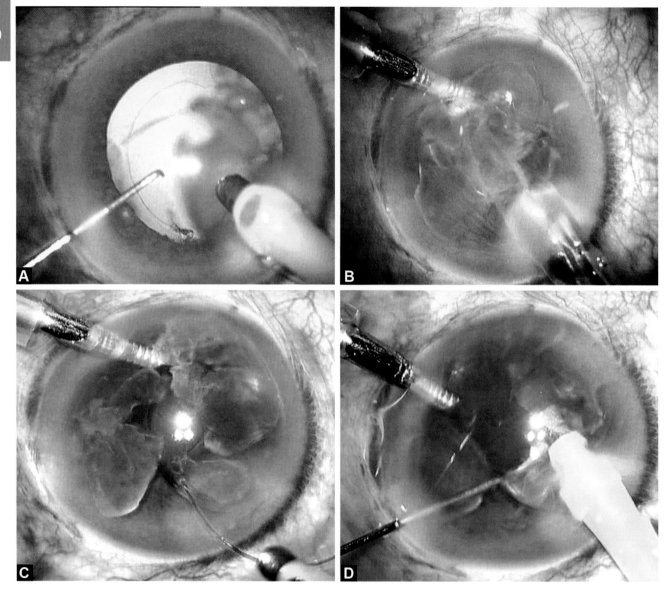

FIGURES 1A TO D: Intraocular lens (IOL) scaffold technique
A. Posterior capsular rupture during epinucleus removal
B. Anterior chamber maintainer placed. Foldable IOL is injected through the clear corneal wound
C. One haptic is placed over the iris and the other outside the incision
D. Epinucleus removed with phaco probe

Instead of an AC maintainer one can use a sutureless trocar cannula also. This technique can be easily done in moderately soft nuclei **(Figures 4A to F)**. In very hard cataracts it might be better to extend the incision and remove the nucleus to avoid corneal damage.

Posterior Capsular Rupture

Posterior capsular rupture (PCR) is known to occur at any stage of phacoemulsification **(Figures 5 and 6)**.[3]

When it happens with the nucleus still left to emulsify, excess manipulation can cause extension of the PCR. The aim of any method at this stage is to prevent the nucleus fragment from dropping into the vitreous. The chances of nucleus drop increases with increasing size of the PCR and vitreous loss. Though a small fragment which descends into the vitreous may be left for observation; larger nucleus fragments always require surgical removal.[9,10] Nucleus drop can induce vitritis and macular edema thereby affecting the best corrected

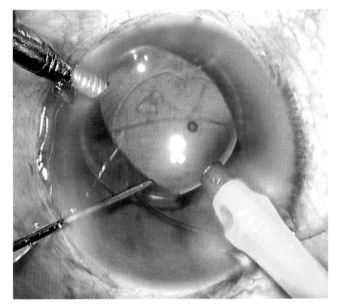

FIGURE 2: Nondominant hand adjusts the optic haptic junction so that the IOL is well centered while emulsifying the epinucleus

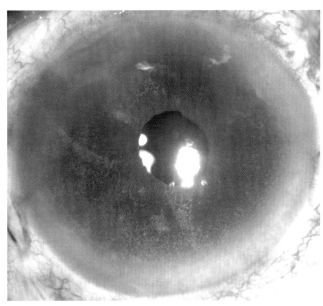

FIGURE 3: One month postoperative clinical photograph of the patient after IOL scaffold procedure

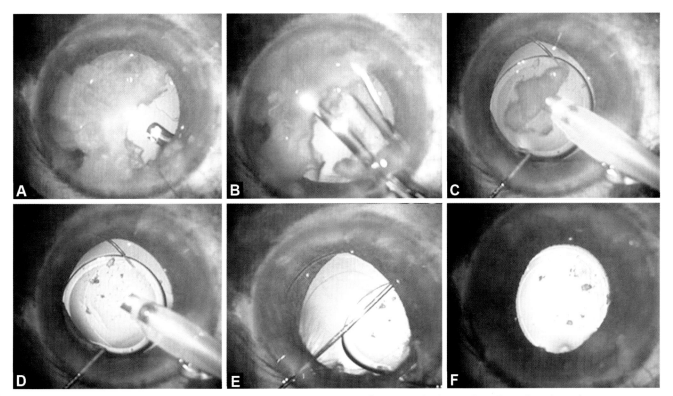

FIGURES 4A TO F: Intraocular lens (IOL) scaffold technique with 23G trocar infusion and moderately soft nucleus

A. Posterior capsular rupture during nucleus removal
B. Foldable IOL is injected through the clear corneal wound
C. Nucleus removed with phacoprobe above the IOL optic
D. Cortical aspiration done
E. IOL pushed into the ciliary sulcus
F. IOL well centered at the end of surgery

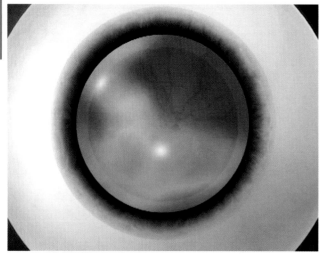

FIGURE 5: Posterior capsular rupture

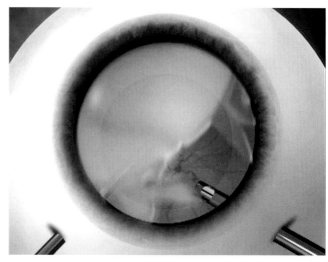

FIGURE 7: Vitrectomy

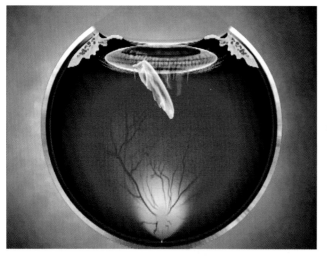

FIGURE 6: Posterior capsular rupture with nucleus sinking

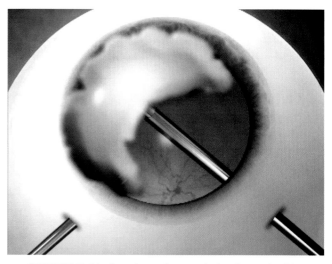

FIGURE 8: Nucleus brought anteriorly above the iris

vision.[10] Moreover, a second surgery for retrieving the dropped nucleus again can cause additional trauma to the eye. Hence, it is always better to prevent the complication from happening by proper management of the PCR.

IOL Scaffold Technique

Though there have been techniques performed to prevent nucleus fragment from descending into the vitreous after intraoperative PCR, this method of using the IOL as a scaffold has not been reported earlier.[11] The IOL scaffold technique comes into play once the nucleus pieces have been brought anteriorly into the anterior chamber **(Figures 7 and 8)**. Conversion of phacoemulsification to extracapsular cataract extraction

(ECCE)[4,5] is done when a large nucleus is still left. Some surgeons prefer to use the Sheet's lens glide to deliver the nucleus. In both methods, corneal wound extension is required and this can increase the risk of postoperative suture induced astigmatism. Another technique used is nucleus removal by phacosandwich method,[6] where a vectis and a spatula are used. However, the incision in a phacosandwich is sclerocorneal and requires extension. In eyes with nucleus displaced in the anterior vitreous, Viscoat posterior assisted levitation[7] is done followed by nucleus emulsification with a phacoprobe above a trimmed sheet's glide[8] after wound extension. With the sheet glide the problem is one has to increase the incision. Then after the nucleus is removed one obviously has to still do vitrectomy and cortical removal for which

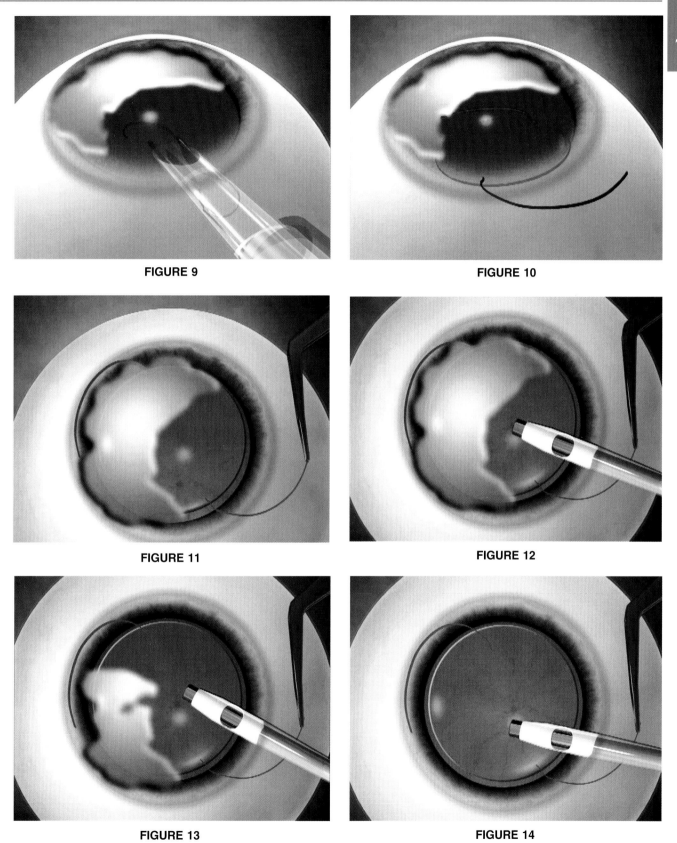

FIGURE 9

FIGURE 10

FIGURE 11

FIGURE 12

FIGURE 13

FIGURE 14

FIGURES 9 to 14: Illustrations depicting the IOL scaffold technique

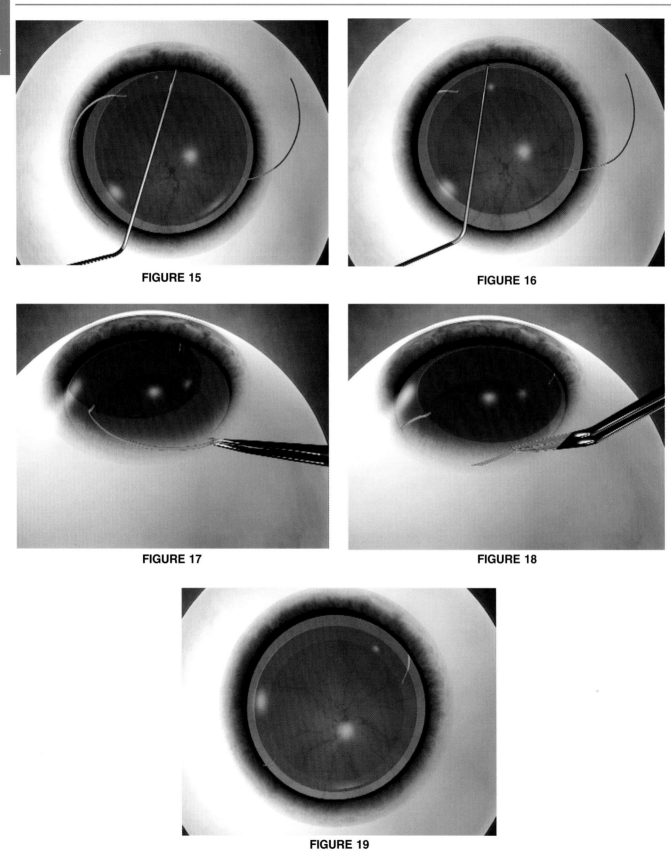

FIGURE 15

FIGURE 16

FIGURE 17

FIGURE 18

FIGURE 19

FIGURES 15 to 19: Illustrations depicting repositioning of the PC IOL into the sulcus

once again the wound has to be sutured back. Another technique one can use is Keiki Mehtas HEMA life boat. In this a contact lens is injected between the iris and the nucleus to prevent the nucleus from falling down. After the nucleus emulsification the contact lens is removed. The difference between this and the IOL scaffold is that in the IOL scaffold the IOL need not be removed. Also the fear of the IOL falling into the vitreous unlike the contact lens is not there as one haptic is still outside the eye. In the IOL scaffold technique, the wound remains clear corneal and there is no wound extension **(Figures 9 to 14)**. Since there is no wound extension, there is no need for suturing and thereby chance of induced astigmatism is also less. The foldable IOL acts as a barrier to nucleus pieces dropping into the vitreous and works like an artificial posterior capsule. The method is termed as "scaffold" since the IOL optic acts as a "temporary platform" over which the nucleus emulsification is performed. Since one haptic is kept out of the incision site the IOL position can be readily adjusted if the nucleus rotates in the anterior chamber and the chances of IOL drop are also decreased as the haptic is controlled from the incision **(Figure 12)**. The presence of the IOL also serves to compartmentalize the eye which in turn decreases hydration of the vitreous from the AC maintainer as well as prevents vitreous prolapse into the anterior chamber. Once the nucleus is removed the same PC IOL is repositioned into the sulcus **(Figures 15 to 19)**.

When compared to an open wound (after extension), PCR during phacoemulsification is associated with a relatively low incidence of vitreous loss because the self-sealing small clear corneal wound provides control of ocular integrity. This maintains the anterior chamber and intraocular pressure, discouraging forward movement of the vitreous, which would occur in the presence of an "open globe" as in ECCE.

Conclusion

Avoiding PCR is the goal of every cataract surgeon. If a tear occurs, management techniques and skills are required for preventing further complications. Early recognition of posterior capsular rupture combined with prevention of collapse of the anterior chamber may prevent extension of the tear, forward movement of the vitreous, and displacement of the lens posteriorly. Here in this technique, the anterior chamber is maintained by slow infusion, forward movement of the vitreous is prevented by the IOL scaffold and the nucleus fragment drop is stopped by the IOL which acts as a physical barrier. Thus we favor this new IOL scaffolding technique in PCR's with nonemulsified moderate to soft nucleus during phacoemulsification. However, in cases of hard cataract conversion to ECCE is ideal.

References

1. Vejarano LF, Tello A. Posterior capsular rupture. In Amar Agarwal: Phaco Nightmares; Conquering cataract catastrophes; Slack Inc, USA. 2006;253-64.
2. Vajpayee RB, Sharma N, Dada T, Gupta V, Kumar A, Dada VK. Management of posterior capsule tears. Surv Ophthalmol. 2001; 45(6):473-88.
3. Gimbel HV, Sun R, Ferensowicz M, Anderson Penno E, Kamal A. Intraoperative management of posterior capsule tears in phacoemulsification and intraocular lens implantation. Ophthalmology. 2001;108(12):2186-9; discussion 2190-2.
4. Dada T, Sharma N, Vajpayee RB, Dada VK. Conversion from phacoemulsification to extracapsular cataract extraction: incidence, risk factors, and visual outcome. J Cataract Refract Surg. 1998;24(11):1521-4.
5. Prasad S, Kamath GG. Converting from phacoemulsification to ECCE. J Cataract Refract Surg. 1999;25(4):462-3.
6. Thatte S, Raju VK. Phacosandwich technique. J Cataract Refract Surg. 1999;25(8):1039-40.
7. Chang DF, Packard RB. Posterior assisted levitation for nucleus rctricval using Viscoat after posterior capsule rupture. J Cataract Refract Surg. 2003;29(10):1860-5.
8. Michelson MA. Use of a Sheets' glide as a pseudo-posterior capsule in phacoemulsification complicated by posterior capsule rupture. Eur J Implant Refract Surg. 1993;5:70-2.
9. Hansson LJ, Larsson J. Vitrectomy for retained lens fragments in the vitreous after phacoemulsification. J Cataract Refract Surg. 2002;28(6):1007-11.
10. Monshizadeh R, Samiy N, Haimovici R. Management of retained intravitreal lens fragments after cataract surgery. Surv Ophthalmol. 1999;43(5):397-404.
11. Kumar DA, Agarwal A, et al. IOL Scaffold technique for posterior capsular rupture. J Refract Surg. 2012;28(5):314-5.

10
Creating an Artificial Posterior Capsule: Combining Glued IOL and IOL Scaffold in Cases of Posterior Capsular Rupture

Amar Agarwal, Soosan Jacob

Introduction

The first glued PC IOL implantation in an eye with a deficient capsule was done on 14th December 2007. Since 2007, a large number of cases have been done with this technique.[1-6] In 2011 we started a technique to prevent nuclear fragments from falling into the vitreous cavity called the IOL scaffold technique.[7] We wanted to combine the glued IOL with the IOL scaffold technique in certain cases thus creating an artificial posterior capsule in cases of posterior capsular rupture (PCR).

Concept and Indications

In the IOL scaffold technique, we implant a three piece foldable IOL above the iris or over the anterior capsule in cases of PCR. This prevents the nuclear pieces from descending into the vitreous, as the IOL acts as a scaffold or a temporary platform. Once the nucleus is emulsified the same IOL can then be placed into the sulcus or glued to the sclera depending on the availability of the anterior capsule.

The problem comes in cases in which the iris support is not sufficient and if with that there is no anterior capsular support to support the IOL scaffold technique. In such cases we cannot implant the IOL to support the nuclear pieces as then the IOL may sink. This can happen in cases like an iris coloboma **(Figure 1)** in which a PCR has occurred and there is no capsular support at all. Alternatively in cases like a floppy iris where the iris is not taut enough to support the IOL or cases in which the pupil is very dilated and not constricting due to trauma and once again there is no capsular support.

Surgical Technique

If there is a PCR **(Figure 2)** in a case one should stop phacoemuslfication. The remaining nuclear pieces are

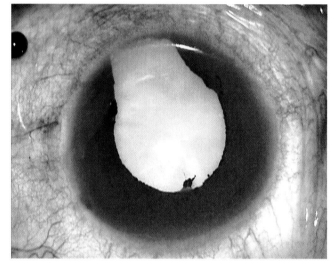

FIGURE 1: Iris coloboma with a mature cataract

brought to the anterior chamber **(Figure 3)**. One should now fix an infusion cannula **(Figure 4)** and create scleral flaps to prepare for glued IOL surgery **(Figure 4)**. A 20G needle then creates a sclerotomy 1 mm behind the limbus under the scleral flaps. A 23G vitrectomy is passed through the sclerotomy to perform vitrectomy so that there is no traction in the vitreous **(Figure 5)**. Vitrectomy is an essential step in the surgery as one can otherwise land up with a retinal detachment postoperatively.

The three piece foldable IOL is loaded onto the injector and the cartridge passed into the anterior chamber (AC) **(Figure 6)**. The haptic tip should be slightly out of the cartridge so that when one goes to grasp the haptic with the glued IOL forceps it is easy. The haptic tip is grasped with the glued IOL forceps and while the IOL is unfolding the haptic tip is still caught. The chances of the IOL falling down are not there as the haptic is caught with the forceps and the trailing haptic is still outside the clear corneal incision

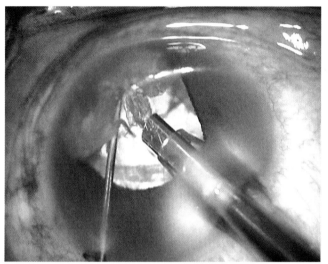

FIGURE 2: Phaco in mature cataract with iris coloboma. Note the posterior capsular rupture (PCR)

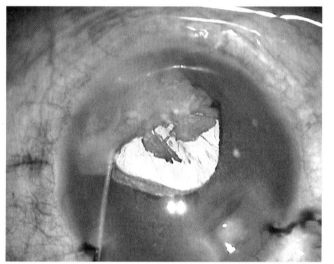

FIGURE 3: Posterior capsular rupture. Nuclear pieces brought to the anterior chamber

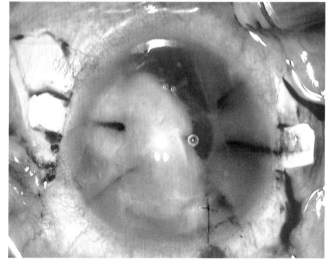

FIGURE 4: Preparation for glued IOL surgery. Scleral flaps created. Note the infusion cannula through a trocar cannula

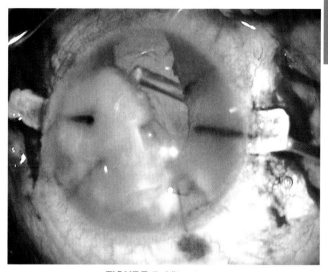

FIGURE 5: Vitrectomy

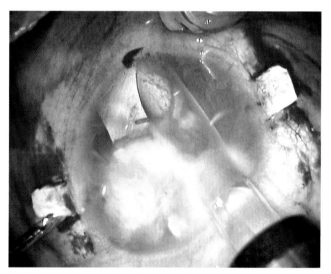

FIGURE 6: Three piece foldable IOL implantation. Note the cartridge in the AC. Also note the haptic is slightly out of the cartridge so that it is easy for the glued IOL forceps to grasp the tip of the haptic

(Figures 7 and 8). The haptic is subsequently externalized **(Figure 9)**. Using the handshake technique the trailing haptic is externalized **(Figures 10 and 11)**. If the nuclear pieces are occupying a lot of space in the AC this maneuver is sometimes difficult. One should use viscoelastic to dislodge the pieces to the side to gain visualization.

A 26G needle is used to create the Scharioth pocket **(Figure 12)** and the haptics tucked into the intrascleral pocket **(Figure 13)**. Phacoemulsification of the nuclear pieces is performed **(Figures 14 to 16)**. An artificial posterior capsule has been created using the combination of the glued IOL and the IOL scaffold technique. This prevents the nuclear fragments from

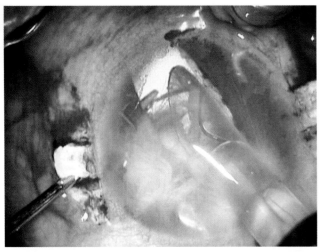

FIGURE 7: Haptic tip grasped with the glued IOL forceps (MST, USA)

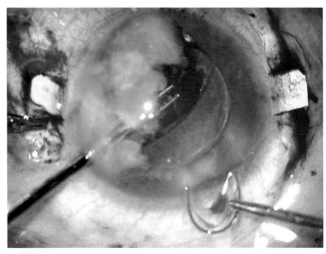

FIGURE 10: Trailing haptic flexed to pass it inside the AC. Note the glued IOL forceps passed through the side port incision to perform the handshake technique

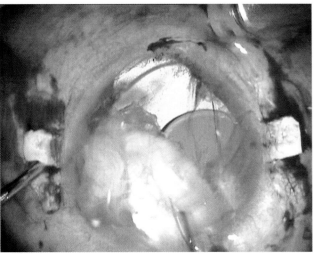

FIGURE 8: Three piece foldable IOL unfolded inside the eye. Note the haptic is not externalized till the IOL unfolds

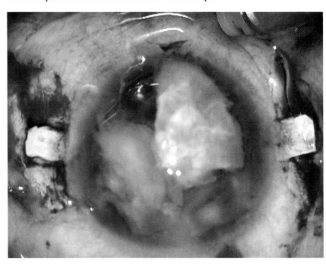

FIGURE 11: Both haptics externalized

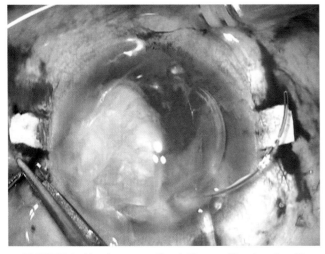

FIGURE 9: Haptic externalized. Note trailing haptic still outside the corneal incision

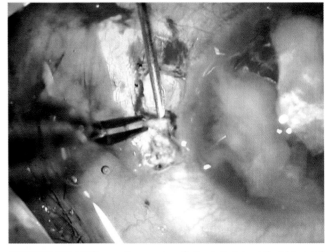

FIGURE 12: 26G needle creates Scharioth intrascleral tunnel

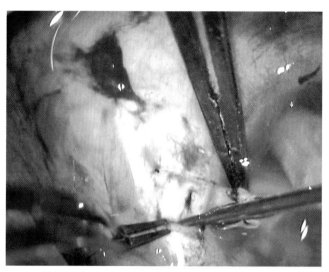

FIGURE 13: Haptic tucked in Scharioth pocket

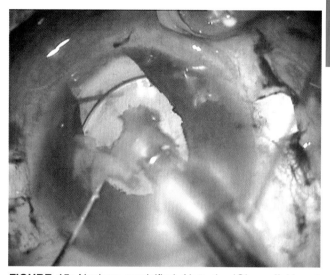

FIGURE 15: Nucleus emulsified. Note the IOL scaffold and the glued IOL procedure combined prevent the nucleus from falling down

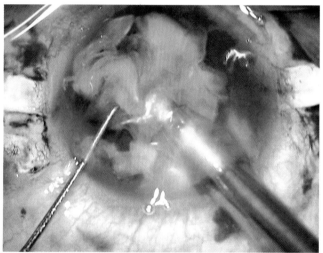

FIGURE 14: Phaco of the nuclear pieces. Artificial posterior capsule created by the IOL

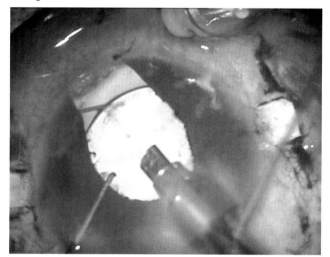

FIGURE 16: Nucleus totally emulsified

falling into the vitreous cavity. Finally air is injected into the AC and fibrin glue used to seal the haptics in the sclera **(Figure 17).**

Problems

The biggest problem is if the nuclear pieces are too big visualization of the haptic is difficult. Another problem is to be careful of endothelial damage. One should use viscoelastics to prevent endothelial damage.

Conclusion

Combining the glued IOL and the IOL scaffold techniques, one can create an artificial posterior capsule

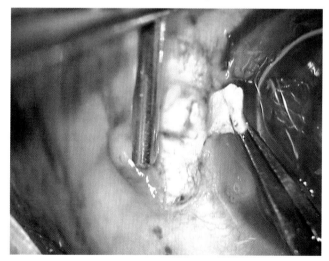

FIGURE 17: Fibrin glue application to seal the haptics to the scleral flap

80

in certain select cases of capsular deficiency where the iris is deficient or the pupil too large to support an IOL.

References

1. Agarwal A, Kumar DA, Jacob S, et al. Fibrin glue-assisted sutureless posterior chamber intraocular lens implantation in eyes with deficient posterior capsules. J Cataract Refract Surg. 2008;34:1433-38.

2. Prakash G, Kumar DA, Jacob S, et al. Anterior segment optical coherence tomography-aided diagnosis and primary posterior chamber intraocular lens implantation with fibrin glue in traumatic phacocele with scleral perforation. J Cataract Refract Surg. 2009;35:782-4.

3. Prakash G, Jacob S, Kumar DA, et al. Femtosecond assisted keratoplasty with fibrin glue-assisted sutureless posterior chamber lens implantation: a new triple procedure. J Cataract Refract Surg. In press (manuscript no 08-919).

4. Agarwal A, Kumar DA, Prakash G, et al. Fibrin glue-assisted sutureless posterior chamber intraocular lens implantation in eyes with deficient posterior capsules [Reply to letter]. J Cataract Refract Surg. 2009;35:795-6.

5. Nair V, Kumar DA, Prakash G, et al. Bilateral spontaneous in-the-bag anterior subluxation of PC IOL managed with glued IOL technique: A case report, Eye Contact Lens 2009. In Press (manuscript no ECL-07-281).

6. Gabor SGB, Pavilidis MM. Sutureless intrascleral posterior chamber intraocular lens fixation. J Cataract Refract Surg. 2007; 33:1851-4.

7. Kumar DA, Agarwal A, et al. IOL Scaffold technique for posterior capsular rupture. J Refract Surg. 2012;28(5):314-5.

11 | Sutureless Three Port Vitrectomy and Management of Dislocated IOLs

Dhivya Ashok Kumar, Amar Agarwal

Introduction

Dislocation of an intraocular lens (IOL) into the vitreous can occur as an early or late complication arising from posterior capsular rupture during phacoemulsification.[1,2] Management of such a situation with available instruments without compromising the visual outcome remains a challenge. Traditionally, dislocated IOLs have been managed either by repositioning the same or a different IOL with sutured scleral fixation[3-8] or replacing the lens with an anterior chamber IOL.[9,10] It is routinely combined with a conventional pars plana vitrectomy.[9-13]

We have described a new technique of sutureless vitrectomy using 20-gauge vitrectomy instrumentation and repositioning the dislocated IOL in the posterior chamber with transscleral fixation of haptics, intra-lamellar scleral tuck, and fibrin glue-assisted flap closure. This is an extension of the glued IOL technique.[14-18]

Sutureless 20G Vitrectomy

Two partial thickness limbal-based scleral flaps (**Figure 1A**; f1, f2), 2.5 × 2.5 mm, are created exactly 180° diagonally apart. A third scleral flap (**Figure 1A**; f3) is made 2 mm from the limbus in the inferotemporal quadrant. A pars plana sclerotomy (**Figure 1A**) 3 mm from the limbus is made with a 20-gauge needle under the scleral flap f3. A polyglactin 6-0 suture is placed (**Figure 1B**) and a 4 mm infusion cannula connected to a 500 ml bottle of balanced salt solution inserted through the sclerotomy. Infusion cannula with a halogen light source (Chandelier illumination) can also be used. The fluid flow is started after visualization of

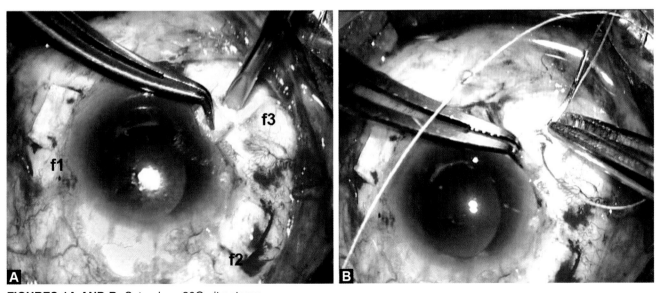

FIGURES 1A AND B: Sutureless 20G vitrectomy
A. Three scleral flaps made (f1, f2, f3). The scleral flaps f1 and f2 are 1.5 mm from the limbus and f3 is 2 mm from the limbus
B. Pars plana sclerotomy made and the infusion cannula attached with 6-0 polyglactin suture 3 mm from the limbus

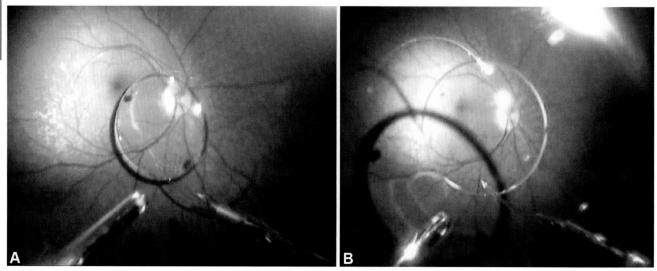

FIGURES 2A AND B: An intraoperative picture showing the IOL being lifted in a case of a dislocated IOL
A. An intraoperative picture showing the IOL caught with a forceps. Note the other hand has a vitrectomy probe to cut the vitreous
B. Internal illumination is from the halogen light source attached to the infusion cannula (Chandelier illumination) as seen in the upper right corner

the tip of the infusion cannula in the vitreous cavity. Two straight sclerotomies with a 20-gauge needle are then made 1.0 to 1.5 mm from the limbus under the existing scleral flaps (f1, f2). A vitrectomy system is used for posterior vitrectomy. Posterior vitreous detachment is induced mechanically using suction of the 20-gauge vitrectomy probe. A thorough vitrectomy to free all the vitreous attachments to the IOL is then done with a 20-gauge vitrectomy probe and endoilluminator. When the vitreous tractions are released, a diamond-coated 20-gauge intravitreal forceps (Grieshaber, Alcon Laboratories, Inc.) is used to hold the haptic tip **(Figures 2A and B)**. The IOL is gently lifted up to bring it to the level of the sclerotomy sites. The intravitreal forceps (holding the haptic) are then withdrawn from the sclerotomy site (f1), externalizing the haptic in the process. With the assistant holding the tip of the externalized haptic, the other haptic is pulled **(Figures 3A and B)** through the other sclerotomy (f2) using the intravitreal forceps. The tips of the haptic are then tucked through a Scharioth intralamellar scleral tunnel made with a 26-gauge needle at the point of externalization. The scleral flaps (f1, f2) are then closed with fibrin glue (Tisseel, Baxter, Deerfield, IL). The polyglactin suture and the infusion cannula are subsequently removed and the third scleral flap (f3) also sealed with the glue. The conjunctiva is also apposed at the peritomy sites with the tissue glue.

Chandelier Illumination

Visualization of the fundus during vitrectomy is done using a Chandelier illumination in which xenon light is fixed to a trocar cannula **(Figures 4A and B)**. This gives excellent illumination and one can perform a proper bimanual vitrectomy as an endoilluminator is not necessary for the surgeon to hold in the hand. An inverter has to be used if one is using a wide field lens. The supermacula lens helps give better steropsis so that one will not have any difficulty in holding the IOL with a diamond tipped forceps. One can also use a noncontact viewing system like a BIOM. When one is using the Chandelier illumination system one hand can hold the IOL with the forceps and the other hand can hold a vitrectomy **(Figures 2A and B)** probe to cut the adhesions of the vitreous thus doing a bimanual vitrectomy. One can also use two forceps to hold the lens thus performing a handshake technique.

Perfluorocarbon Liquids

Stanley Chang popularized the use of perfluorocarbon liquids for the surgical treatment of various vitreoretinal disorders. Due to their heavier-than-water properties, and their ease of intraocular injection and removal, perfluorocarbon liquids (PFCL) are highly effective for flattening detached retina, tamponading retinal tears,

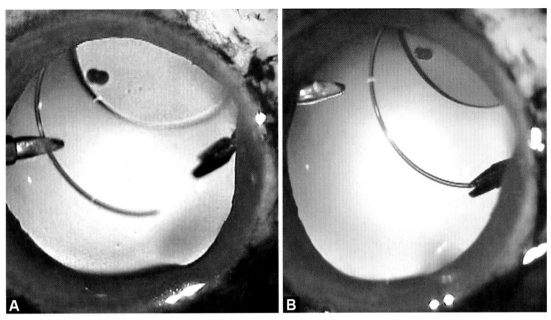

FIGURES 3A AND B: Handshake technique. Intravitreal forceps is used to hold the haptic while the IOL is brought to the pupillary plane

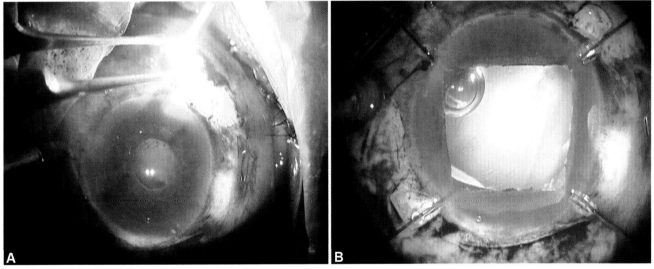

FIGURES 4A AND B: Chandelier illumination
A. Chandelier illumination being fixed onto the trocar and cannula
B. Note the bright vitreous cavity due to the Chandelier illumination

limiting intraocular hemorrhage, as well as floating dropped crystalline lens fragments and a dislocated IOL. We do not use PFCL for dislocated IOLs generally, but if one wants one can use them. One should remove the PFCL at the end of surgery.

Subluxated Three Piece IOL

The haptics of a subluxated three piece IOL are very comfortable to externalize through the sclerotomies without explanting the IOL **(Figures 2 and 3)**. The

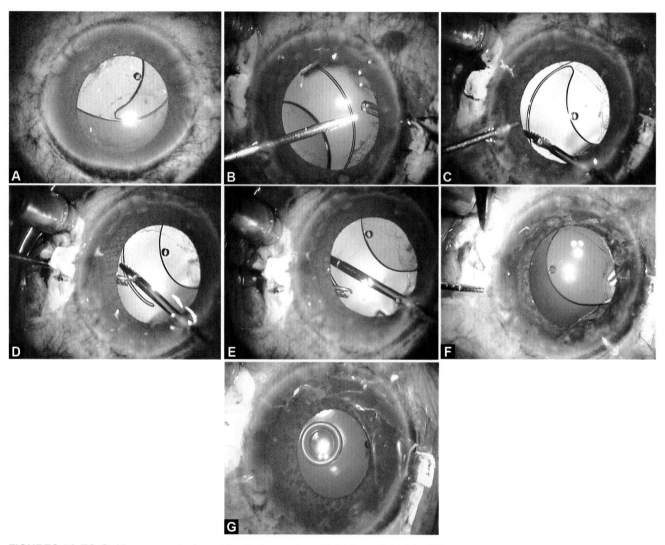

FIGURES 5A TO G: Management of a subluxated one piece PMMA non foldable IOL

A. Subluxated single piece polymethyl methacrylate (PMMA) IOL
B. Vitrectomy performed. Note one haptic held with the glued IOL forceps to prevent the IOL from falling down while vitrectomy is done
C. One haptic caught with the glued IOL forceps
D. Second forceps passed through the sclerotomy under the scleral flap to grab the haptic using the handshake technique
E. Haptic tip grasped to externalize the haptic
F. Haptic externalized. One should be careful when doing this in a single piece nonfoldable PMMA IOL as the haptic can break
G. Both haptics externalized and tucked. Glue will then be applied. Note the well centered IOL

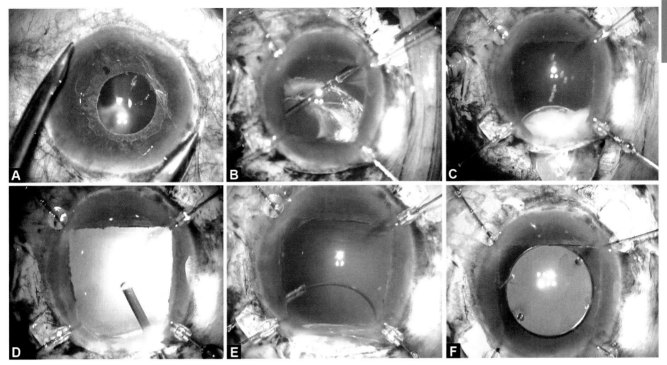

FIGURES 6A TO F: Management of a subluxated capsular bag-IOL complex. Note iris hooks used for better visualization as there is a miotic pupil

A. Subluxated capsular bag-IOL complex. Measure the white to white diameter of the cornea and if horizontal is more than 11 mm perform a vertical glued IOL

B. Scleral flaps made, infusion fixed and vitrectomy done. One hand holds the haptic with a glued IOL forceps to prevent the bag-IOL complex from falling down

C. Explantation of the bag-IOL complex through a sclera tunnel incision. One can perform a vitrectomy and chew up the bag but in some cases there are thick Sommering's rings which sometimes are difficult to chew and can fall down onto the retina. In such cases it might be more prudent to explant the entire complex

D. Vitrectomy

E. Glued IOL started with a three piece IOL

F. Haptics externalized and tucked. Finally glue to be applied

reason is that the haptics are quite malleable and so can be externalized easily. Issue is to hold the haptic with the glued IOL forceps while vitrectomy is being done with the other hand so that there is no vitreous traction. One should also remember to grab the tip of the haptic while externalizing so that the haptic is not deformed. The handshake technique helps in achieving this.

One Piece Nonfoldable PMMA Subluxated IOL

It is a bit tricky to reposition a single piece nonfoldable PMMA IOL using the glued IOL technique as one can break the haptic **(Figures 5A to G)**. One should create the scleral flaps and after fixing the infusion should perform vitrectomy. Using two glued IOL forceps and the handshake technique each haptic is then externalized

through the sclerotomies under the scleral flaps. They are then tucked and glued in the Scharioth tunnels.

Subluxated Capsular Bag-IOL Complex

The subluxated capsular bag-IOL complex are tricky to handle **(Figures 6A to F)**. In such cases there may be thick Sommering's rings. Vitrectomy of those can be done but sometimes they are quite thick and can fall down into the vitreous cavity. It might be better to explant the complex through a scleral tunnel incision. Once explanted and vitrectomy done a three piece IOL can then be glued into place.

One Piece Foldable IOL

The IOL which cannot be fixed and glued is the single

piece foldable IOL. The reason if that for the glued IOL technique we need a firm haptic to tuck and glue into the sclera. The haptics in a single piece foldable IOL are too flexible to tuck and glue. In such cases, one should explant the IOL and refixate a three piece IOL with the glued IOL technique. We do not suture these IOLs as the results of the glued IOL are much better. So though there is a slightly larger incision for explanting the IOL we still prefer it to suturing an existing foldable single piece IOL.

Discussion

The postoperative dislocated or luxated IOL remains an infrequent but significant complication of cataract surgery. The management options are observation, IOL exchange, or repositioning of the IOL. In all the procedures, combined pars plana vitrectomy has to be done, which requires multiple wounds of either sclerotomies[5,8-13] or clear corneal incisions.[4,5] This increases the risk of suture-induced astigmatism, postoperative inflammation, surgical time, and delayed visual rehabilitation. In this method of glued IOL repositioning, there is no IOL explantation; hence, chances of corneal wound astigmatism as seen in pars plana vitrectomy with IOL explantation and re-implantation are decreased. It can be performed with a dislocated rigid polymethyl methacrylate IOL, a three-piece foldable posterior capsule IOL, or IOLs with modified polymethyl methacrylate haptics. Unlike other methods, in this technique, we have used the same pars plicata sclerotomy port for vitrectomy and IOL haptic externalization.[8-13] If the IOL is on the retina one can lift the IOL through 23G sclerotomies through the pars plana and then externalize the haptics through the pars plicata incisions. This way it is very comfortable for the visualizing contact lens to be placed on the cornea.

Vitrectomy and IOL fixation through pars plicata have been reported in special situations. Although there is a possible risk of intraoperative hyphema because the sclerotomy is through the pars plicata, it was not observed in any of our patients. The probable reasons may be that the needle passes through the ciliary sulcus perpendicular to the sclera and continuous infusion flow is maintained to prevent decompression. Although it is known that a sclerotomy wound can cause prolapse and incarceration of uveal tissue and retinal fragments leading to vitreous traction and iatrogenic retinal breaks, the postoperative ultrasound biomicroscopy showed no vitreous traction or retinal incarceration in the pars plicata ports. We have done an intralamellar tucking of the IOL haptic followed by fibrin glue application after externalization.[14-18] We preferred this technique of glued IOL repositioning because the suture-related complications of scleral fixation IOL are reduced by this procedure. Because the IOL haptic is tucked in the scleral tunnel, it would prevent further movement of the haptic reducing pseudophakodonesis, minimizing slippage and late re-dislocation. Although complete scleral wound healing with collagen fibrils may take up to 3 months, because the haptic is snugly placed inside an intralamellar scleral tunnel, the IOL remains very stable from the early postoperative period. The risk of retinal photic injury that is known to occur in sutured scleral fixation IOLs would also be reduced in our technique because of the short surgical time. This method avoids additional corneal incisions or multiple sclerotomies, reduces surgical time, and intraocular pressure fluctuation by maintaining a closed system.

Conclusion

This method of glued IOL repositioning avoids additional corneal incisions or multiple sclerotomies, reduces surgical time, and intraocular pressure fluctuation by maintaining a closed system.

References

1. Gimbel HV, Condo GP, Kohen T, Olson RJ, Halkiadakis I. Late in-the-bag intraocular lens dislocation: incidence, prevention, and management. J Cataract Refract Surg. 2005;31:2193-2204.
2. Hayashi K, Hirata A, Hayashi H. Possible predisposing factors for in-the-bag and out-of-the-bag intraocular lens dislocation and outcomes of intraocular lens exchange surgery. Ophthalmology. 2007;114:969-75.
3. Mensiz E, Avtulner E, Ozerturk Y. Scleral fixation suture technique without lens removal for posteriorly dislocated intraocular lenses. Can J Ophthalmol. 2002;37:290-4.
4. Koh HJ, Kim CY, Lim SJ, Kwon OW. Scleral fixation technique using 2 corneal tunnels for a dislocated intraocular lens. J Cataract Refract Surg. 2000;26:1439-41.
5. Chan CK, Agarwal A, Agarwal S, Agarwal A. Management of dislocated intraocular implants. Ophthalmol Clin North Am. 2001;14:681-93.
6. Smiddy WE, Flynn HW Jr. Needle-assisted scleral fixation suture technique for relocating posteriorly dislocated IOLs. Arch Ophthalmol. 1993;111:161-2.
7. Kokame GT, Yamamoto I, Mandel H. Scleral fixation of dislocated posterior chamber intraocular lenses: temporary haptic externalization through a clear corneal incision. J Cataract Refract Surg. 2004;30:1049-56.

8. Kim SS, Smiddy WE, Feuer W, Shi W. Management of dislocated intraocular lenses. Ophthalmology. 2008;115:1699-1704.

9. Mitra RA, Connor B, Han DP, et al. Removal of dislocated intraocular lenses using pars plana vitrectomy with placement of an open-loop, flexible anterior chamber lens. Ophthalmology. 1998;105:1011-14.

10. Steinmetz RL, Brooks HL Jr, Newell CK. Management of posteriorly dislocated posterior chamber intraocular lenses by vitrectomy and pars plana removal. Retina. 2004;24:556-9.

11. Johnston RL, Charteris DG, Horgan SE, Cooling RJ. Combined pars plana vitrectomy and sutured posterior chamber implant. Arch Ophthalmol. 2000;118:905-10.

12. Campo RV, Chung KD, Oyakawa RT. Pars plana vitrectomy in the management of dislocated posterior chamber lenses. Am J Ophthalmol. 1989;108:529-34.

13. Flynn HW Jr, Buus D, Culbertson WW. Management of subluxated and posteriorly dislocated intraocular lenses using pars plana vitrectomy instrumentation. J Cataract Refract Surg. 1990;16:51-6.

14. Agarwal A, Kumar DA, Jacob S, Baid C, Agarwal A, Srinivasan S. Fibrin glue-assisted sutureless posterior chamber intraocular lens implantation in eyes with deficient posterior capsules. J Cataract Refract Surg. 2008;34:1433-8.

15. Prakash G, Ashokumar D, Jacob S, Kumar KS, Agarwal A, Agarwal A. Anterior segment optical coherence tomography-aided diagnosis and primary posterior chamber intraocular lens implantation with fibrin glue in traumatic phacocele with scleral perforation. J Cataract Refract Surg. 2009;35:782-4.

16. Prakash G, Jacob S, Kumar DA, et al. Femtosecond-assisted keratoplasty with fibrin glue-assisted sutureless posterior chamber lens implantation: new triple procedure. J Cataract Refract Surg. 2009;35:973-9.

17. Agarwal A, Kumar DA, Jacob S, Prakash G, Agarwal A. Reply to letter: Fibrin glue-assisted sutureless posterior chamber intraocular lens implantation in eyes with deficient posterior capsules. J Cataract Refract Surg. 2009;35:795-6.

18. Nair V, Kumar DA, Prakash G, Jacob S, Agarwal A, Agarwal A. Bilateral spontaneous in-the-bag anterior subluxation of PC IOL managed with glued IOL technique: a case report. Eye Contact Lens. 2009;35:215-7.

12 | Modifications in the Glued IOL Technique

Priya Narang, George Beiko
Toshihiko Ohta, Amar Agarwal

Introduction

Since its invention, the glued IOL technique[1-2] has continuously evolved and has now reached a stage where it is accepted worldwide. Various modifications have come up which have rectified and improvised each and every step of the surgery.

No Assistant Technique

No Assistant Technique is an effort to decrease the dependence on the assistant and make it more surgeon dependent. This technique is an attempt to make the process of 'Externalization of haptics' which is considered to be the most technically demanding part of the surgery; more easy and feasible. The concept of no assistant technique was conceptualized by one of us (PN).

Three Hands in Glued IOL Surgery

Normally in a glued IOL surgery, the assistant holds the leading haptic while the surgeon engages in the externalization of the trailing haptic. A definite part of surgical expertise is required for the assistant to hold the haptic properly. Undue pressure on the haptic causes it to flatten which is then difficult to tuck. Inability of the assistant to hold the leading haptic along the correct plane causes IOL torsion while externalization and renders the procedure difficult at times.

Physics

The entire technique works on the simple principle of physics—The vector forces. The mid-pupillary plane is the major contributor to the success of this technique.

Normal Scenario

After externalization of the leading haptic, there is a tendency of the haptic to slip back into the anterior chamber due to vector forces acting along the axis of the IOL (**Figure 1A**, Green arrows indicate the vector forces).

No Assistant Technique (Figure 1B)

When the trailing haptic crosses the mid-pupillary plane and is nearly at 6 o'clock position, the vector forces act in a way that causes further extrusion of the leading haptic from the sclerotomy site with virtually no chance of slippage of the leading haptic into the anterior chamber.

Surgical Technique

As usual, two partial scleral thickness flaps 2.5 × 2.5 mm are made 180° opposite followed by introduction of infusion into the eye by either an AC maintainer or a trocar cannula. A sclerotomy wound is created with a 20G needle approximately 1.0 mm from the limbus beneath the scleral flaps. Vitrectomy is then done from the same sclerotomy site with a 23G cutter.

Corneal tunnel is fashioned followed by a side port entry. The IOL is loaded and the tip of the haptic is slightly brought out from the cartridge. The loaded cartridge is then entered into the eye while the Glued IOL forceps is introduced from the sclerotomy site. The tip of the haptic is then grasped and the IOL is slowly unfolded (**Figures 2A to D**). When the entire IOL has unfolded, the leading haptic is pulled and externalized.

The trailing haptic is then grasped with the Glued IOL forceps while the left hand still holds onto the leading haptic. The trailing haptic is then moved inferiorly up to the 6 o'clock position. This ensures that no external forces are acting on the leading haptic which causes it to slip inside. The surgeon leaves the leading haptic and then introduces the Glued IOL forceps from the side port incision. The tip of the trailing haptic is then transferred to the second forceps (**Figures 3A to D**). Now the surgeon enters the eye

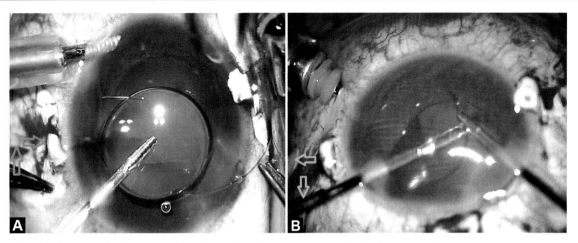

FIGURES 1A AND B: Physics in no assistant technique. Green arrows indicate the vector forces.
A. Normal Glued IOL surgery—At this stage, the assistant surgeon needs to hold the haptic because it tends to slip back into the eye as the vector forces are acting along the axis of the IOL (inwards)
B. No assistant technique—As the IOL crosses the mid-pupillary plane, the vector forces act in a way (outwards) which ensures that the haptic does not slip back into anterior chamber

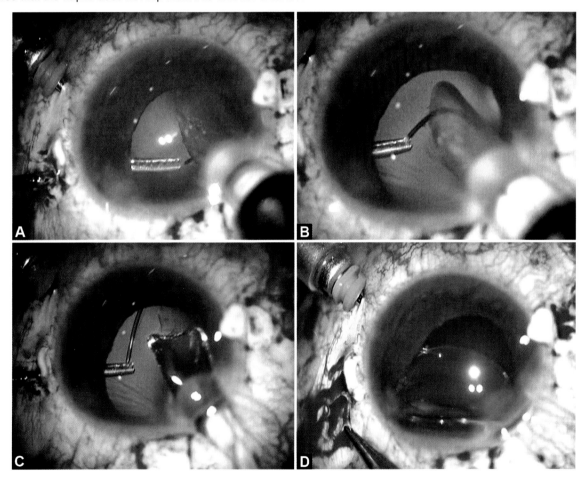

FIGURES 2A TO D: Leading haptic externalization in no assistant technique
A. Tip of the leading haptic about to be grasped with glued IOL forceps
B. Tip of the leading haptic caught with glued IOL forceps
C. Haptic still caught with the forceps while IOL is being injected. Note the haptic is not externalized
D. Leading haptic externalized after the entire IOL has unfolded. The trailing haptic is still outside the corneal incision. Once externalized the surgeon holds the haptic so that it does not slip back

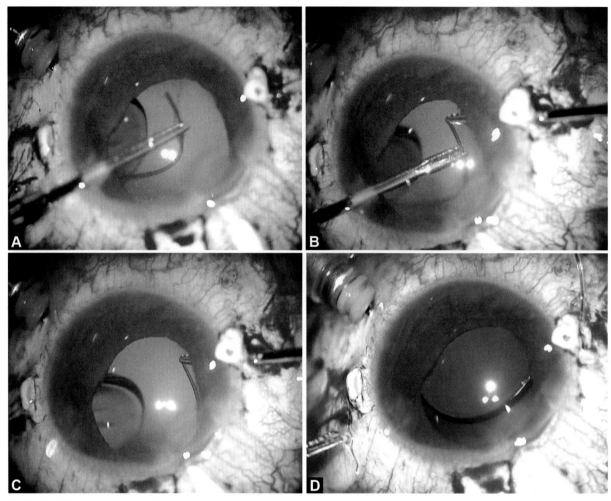

FIGURES 3A TO D: Trailing haptic externalization in no assistant technique
A. The trailing haptic is moved inferiorly up to the 6 o'clock position. This way the physics of vector forces come into play and the leading haptic now does not slip back into the eye. Surgeon leaves the leading haptic, and a glued IOL forceps introduced from the side port incision grasps the trailing haptic
B. The tip of the trailing haptic is transferred to the second forceps using the handshake technique
C. Tip of the trailing haptic is caught with the glued IOL forceps
D. Trailing haptic is externalized. Finally, both haptics are externalized without the help of an assistant

from the other sclerotomy site with the Glued IOL forceps and catches the tip of the trailing haptic using the handshake technique. The trailing haptic is then pulled out and externalized.

The haptics are then tucked in the scleral pockets and vitrectomy is done at the sclerotomy site. The infusion is stopped and the glue is applied beneath the scleral flaps and the corneal incision sites are also sealed with glue.

Advantages

1. Fast and easy.
2. Totally surgeon dependent. Manipulation and externalization of haptics becomes technically very handy.

Summary

'No Assistant Technique' is an armamentarium in the hands of the Glued IOL surgeon as it enables the surgeon to externalize the haptics without the need of any assistant to hold on to the leading haptic. It renders the surgery more 'surgeon' dependent rather than 'assistant' dependent.

Vertical Glued IOL

One should measure the horizontal white to white diameter of the cornea. If it is large more than 11 mm one can do a vertical glued IOL as the vertical diameter will always be shorter and one will have more haptic to tuck and glue. In vertical glued IOL which was started by Jeevan Ladi from India the idea is to make the scleral flaps at 12 and 6 o'clock. The surgeon sits temporally.

Needle-guided Intrascleral Fixation of Posterior Chamber Intraocular Lens for Aphakia Correction

Iñaki Rodríguez-Agirretxe and others from Instituto Clínico Quirúrgico de Oftalmología, Vizcaya, Spain came out with this concept. A 3-piece IOL is inserted into the anterior chamber and the IOL is then rotated so the tip of the haptic to be externalized faces the scleral flap. Using a 25-gauge needle, a straight sclerotomy is made 1.0 mm from the sclerocorneal limbus. The haptic is guided into the needle and the needle withdrawn. This ensures that the haptic is also withdrawn with the needle. Then intrascleral haptic fixation can be done.

Beiko's Modification

Choice of Tissue Glue

George Beiko has used both Tisseel (Baxter Corp.) and Evicel (Ethicon Inc.). The two tissue glues are similar; Tisseel contains aprotinin, an antifibrinolytic agent, while Evicel is manufactured without plasminogen and as such does not contain an antifibrinogen agent. There is a difference in the preparation of the agents. Evicel is stored frozen; once thawed, it has to be used within 24 hours if kept at room temperature or within 30 days if stored in a refrigerator. Tisseel is also stored frozen; it has to be thawed, then warmed to 33-37°C and has to be used within 4 hours of preparation.

Choice of Forceps Tips

23G instruments are recommended by Beiko. The tips can be either ridged or smooth. The problem with ridged tips is that they can result in crinkling of the haptics. Crinkling of haptics, especially prolene haptics, results in weakening and the haptics can easily break. Broken haptics can be a problem as the amount available for threading into the scleral tunnel will be limited.

Silicone Tires

The technique requires an assistant to hold the haptics of the IOL once they have been externalized through the sclerotomies. If an assistant is not available, it is likely that the externalized haptic will be pulled into the eye once the second haptic is externalized. In order to prevent the migration of the first haptic into the eye, it is possible to use a silicone tire **(Figures 4A to D)**. This silicone tire is readily available from a Mackool Capsular Support System (Impex Surgical) or MST Capsular Support (Microsurgical Technology Inc.). Placing the silicone tire on the haptic provides support for the haptic while other procedures are performed.

Toshihiko Ohta's Y-fixation Technique

Toshihiko Ohta from Japan started a simplified and safer method of sutureless intrascleral posterior chamber intraocular lens fixation. This is called the Y-fixation technique **(Figures 5A to G)**.

Technique

Under peribulbar anesthesia, a 5 mm conjunctival peritomy is done at the 2 o'clock and 8 o'clock positions **(Figures 6A to I)**. A reference marker and Y marker (Duckworth & Kent, England) are used for marking **(Figures 7 and 8)**. Then two Y-shaped incisions are made 2 mm from the limbus exactly 180 degrees apart diagonally. An infusion cannula or anterior chamber maintainer is inserted. To prevent interference with the creation of the Y-shaped incision, the infusion cannula should be positioned at 5 o'clock. Anterior vitrectomy is performed, if necessary. A 23-gauge MVR knife is used to perform a sclerotomy parallel to the iris at the Y-shaped incision, and a scleral tunnel is made parallel to the limbus at the end of the Y-shaped incision. Next, a 2.4 to 3.0 mm keratome is used to make a corneal incision at 10 o'clock for injector-assisted IOL implantation. A standard 3-piece IOL is implanted with an injector and the trailing haptic is left outside the corneal incision. The leading haptic is then grasped at its tip with a 25-gauge IOL haptic gripping forceps (Eye Technology, England), pulled through the sclerotomy, and externalized on the left side. After the trailing haptic is inserted into the anterior chamber with a forceps, a U-shaped hook (Duckworth & Kent, England) is used to guide it to the center of the pupil (U-shaped hook technique) **(Figures 9 and 10)**. Then the tip of the haptic is grasped with the 25-gauge forceps, pulled through the second sclerotomy, and externalized on the right side. The tip of the IOL

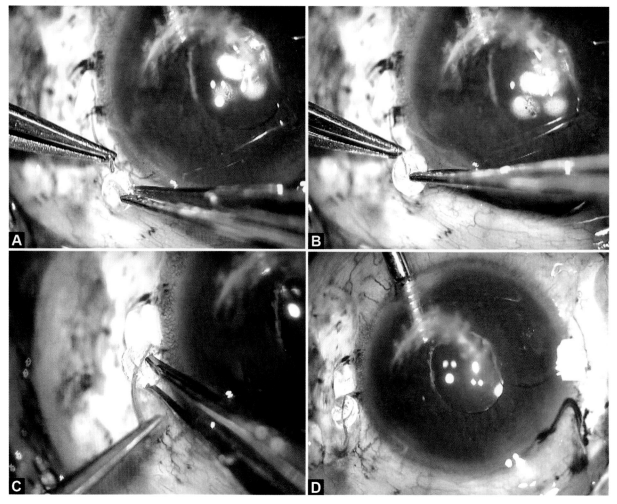

FIGURES 4A TO D: Beiko's modification
A and B. Haptic passed through the narrow opening in the silicone tire of an iris hook
C. Haptic passed fully
D. Silicone tire of iris hook prevents the haptic from slipping back into the vitreous cavity

haptic is subsequently inserted into the limbus-parallel scleral tunnel with a forceps, after which the IOL is positioned and centered. A single 8-0 nylon suture is used to fix the haptic to the scleral bed in order to prevent it shifting immediately after surgery and the incision is closed with 8-0 Vicryl. After the incision is closed completely and the haptic embedded into the sclera, the anterior chamber maintainer or infusion cannula is removed. Finally, the conjunctiva is closed with 8-0 Vicryl.

Results

This technique was used in 44 eyes of 42 patients. No intraoperative complications occurred. All IOLs were stable and centered at the end of surgery. Although

IOL decentration was subsequently observed in 2 eyes due to ocular contusion, correction was done without difficulty. There was no decline of best-corrected visual acuity (BCVA) except in one eye with postoperative retinal detachment. In 5 eyes with a dislocated IOL, the same IOL was used again. As for postoperative complications, compared with suture fixation, there was significantly less IOL decentration and tilt. Astigmatism of the IOL was also significantly less marked than with suture fixation, showing virtually no difference from intracapsular fixation.

Discussion

Gabor et al. described a technique for intrascleral fixation of both haptics in the ciliary sulcus by means of a parallel

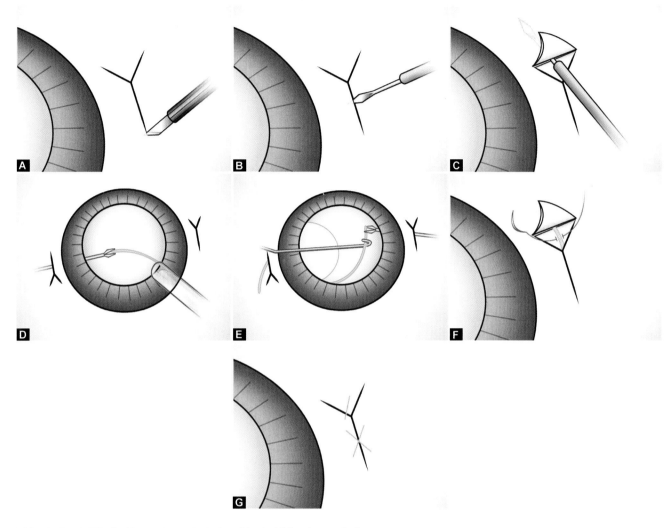

FIGURES 5A TO G: Illustrations depicting Ohta's Y-fixation technique
A. A Y-shaped incision is made 2 mm from the limbus
B. A 23-gauge MVR knife performs sclerotomy parallel to the iris
C. The 23-gauge MVR knife creates a scleral tunnel
D. Leading haptic caught with the 25 gauge forceps
E. A U-shaped hook is used to guide the IOL haptic to the center of the pupil. Then the tip of the IOL haptic is grasped with a 25-gauge forceps and pulled through the second sclerotomy
F. An 8-0 nylon suture is placed in the scleral bed to prevent shifting of IOL immediately after surgery
G. The sclera is sutured with 8-0 Vicryl, the incision is completely closed, and the haptic is embedded into the sclera

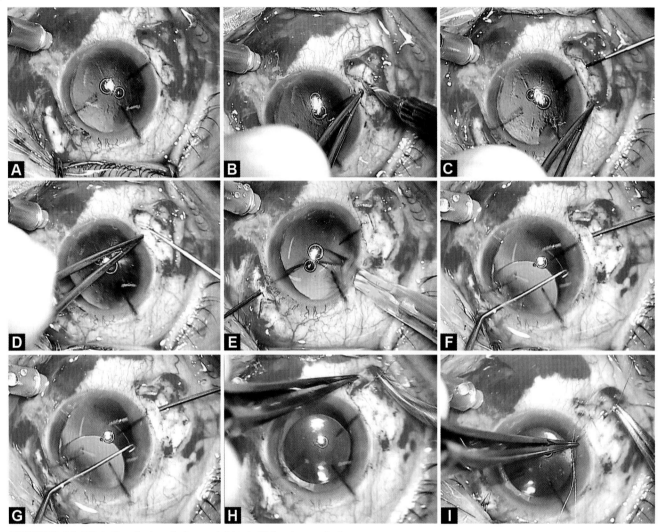

FIGURES 6A TO I: Surgical technique of Ohta's Y-fixation technique

A. A 5 mm conjunctival peritomy is done at 2 o'clock and 8 o'clock positions, a reference marker and Y-marker are used for marking
B. A Y-shaped incision is made 2 mm from the limbus
C. A 23-gauge MVR knife is used to perform a sclerotomy parallel to the iris
D. The 23-gauge MVR knife creates a scleral tunnel parallel to the limbus at the end of the Y-shaped incision
E. The leading haptic is grasped at the tip with a 25-gauge forceps and pulled through the sclerotomy
F. A U-shaped hook is used to guide the IOL haptic to the center of the pupil. Then the tip of the IOL haptic is grasped with a 25-gauge forceps and pulled through the second sclerotomy
G. The tip of the IOL haptic is inserted into the limbus-parallel scleral tunnel with a forceps
H. An 8-0 nylon suture is placed in the scleral bed to prevent the IOL shifting immediately after surgery
I. The sclera is sutured with 8-0 Vicryl, the incision is completely closed, and the haptic is embedded into the sclera

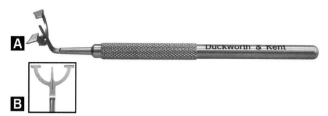

FIGURES 7A AND B: Ohta reference marker for the intrascleral IOL fixation technique (Duckworth & Kent, England)

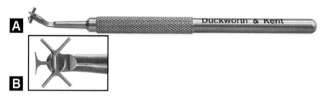

FIGURES 8A AND B: Ohta Y-marker for the intrascleral IOL fixation technique (Duckworth & Kent, England)

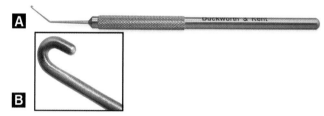

FIGURES 9A AND B: U-shaped hook for the intrascleral IOL fixation technique (Duckworth & Kent, England)

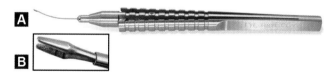

FIGURES 10A AND B: Ohta IOL haptic gripping forceps (25G) (Eye Technology, England)

scleral tunnel, with a 24-gauge needle being used to create a straight sclerotomy. However, extracting the haptic is difficult, it can only be done with a 3-piece IOL, and closure is problematic. Agarwal et al. used a 22-gauge needle to create a straight sclerotomy and bioadhesive to attach the haptics and to glue the scleral flaps and overlying conjunctiva. However, their technique has problems with regard to closure and postoperative hypotony, using fibrin glue, and the creation of a lamellar scleral flap. The Y-fixation technique is a new intrascleral IOL fixation method that does not involve complicated manipulation and achieves safer sutureless fixation. With the Y-fixation technique, a Y-shaped incision is made in the sclera and a 23-gauge MVR knife is used to create the sclerotomy instead of a needle. The Y-shaped incision eliminates the need to raise a lamellar scleral flap, while performing sclerotomy with the 23-gauge MVR knife simplifies extraction of the haptic and greatly improves wound closure.

Conclusion

The Y-fixation technique that Ohta devised is simpler and safer than the other intrascleral IOL fixation techniques. This technique is a new generation secondary IOL implantation method that achieves both anatomical and optical stability.

Problems with the Glued IOL Technique and their Solutions

Hypotony

Hypotony, sometimes severe (IOP 2-4 mm Hg) can be a common denominator in some cases. We need to learn how to solve this problem of hypotony.

A. Fill the AC with air. Do not over fill it too much as that pushes the iris way down. Just have enough air in the AC. Now inject some balanced salt solution (BSS) inside the eye if you feel the eye is hypotonic. The hypotony occurs not due to the sclerotomies or 26G tunnels. This can happen if you are not using glue but with glue hypotony will not occur due to these factors.

B. At the end of the case once you have stuck the flaps and conjunctiva with glue closed up the case, injected the subconjunctival injection and removed the speculum, check if the eye is hypotonic. If you feel the eye is soft inject immediately some BSS through the clear corneal incision till the eye becomes solid. What happens now is that air is in the AC and the fluid you inject will go through the pupil into the vitreous cavity and distend the eye.

C. The hypotony is due to the fact that we have removed vitreous and sometimes the fluid is not there. Point B will solve it.

D. Postoperatively if you see hypotony put the patient on systemic steroids and it will resolve. But with point B followed of BSS injected at the end of the case into the AC hypotony in your cases will generally not be there.

96

E. Do not leave an eye hypotonic at the end of the surgery. That is the key. Answer is not only an air bubble but fluid going from AC into the vitreous cavity.

Three Piece IOL Deformation

Any three piece IOL can be used. One main issue of deformation is if the tip of the haptic is not caught. Also if the haptic is slightly deformed you can straighten it outside the eye using two tying forceps once the haptic is externalized. The advantage is when we use a pushing injector then an assistant is not required. If you have externalized the haptics and got quite a bit of haptic out and the tip is deformed so tucking is difficult just take a scissor and cut the tip. It is like a thread being passed through a needle. Sometimes the thread tip gets deformed and does not pass through the eye of the needle. In such a case you just break the tip of the thread and then it passes through easily.

Too much Haptic Externalized so Haptics too Long to Tuck into the Tunnels

This is very easy to treat. Just chop the haptics if they are too long after externalization. Lets say you have 5 mm haptic externalized and it is too much just take a scissor and cut the extra portion and tuck the remaining haptic. Same will happen when you operate a microcornea eye with a coloboma. They may require a glued IOL.

Concerns of Late Redislocation

If the surgery is done well you will not get a dislocation after years even. If you get a dislocation you will get it within a month. This shows the haptics were not tucked well or the amount of haptic tucked was not enough, etc. If the surgery is done well you will not get a dislocation. Again scientifically if we see the haptic tucked and glued well there is no way that haptic can come out. The issue is not the same with sutures. A suture can break.

Conclusion

Various modifications have come out in the intrascleral haptic fixation of a PC IOL and Glued IOL techniques. Each technique has its own pros and cons. It is up to the surgeon to choose which technique is the best.

References

1. Agarwal A, Kumar DA, Jacob S, Baid C, Agarwal A, Srinivasan S. Fibrin glue-assisted sutureless posterior chamber intraocular lens implantation in eyes with deficient posterior capsules. J Cataract Refract Surg. 2008;34(9):1433-8.
2. Kumar DA, Agarwal A, Prakash G, Jacob S, Saravanan Y, Agarwal A. Glued posterior chamber IOL in eyes with deficient capsular support: a retrospective analysis of 1-year post-operative outcomes. Eye (Lond). 2010;24(7):1143-8.

3
Section

SPECIAL CONDITIONS

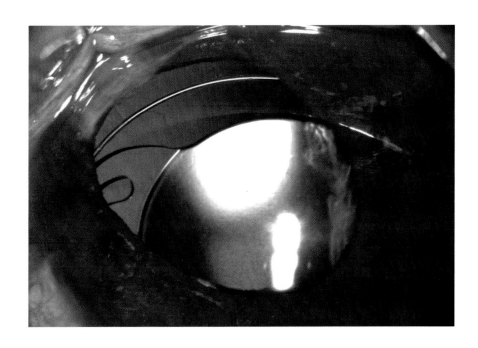

Gabor B Scharioth

Introduction

Due to the absence of sufficient capsular support for an IOL in subluxated/luxated lenses or aphakia, we developed a sutureless technique for posterior chamber IOL sulcus fixation using permanent incarceration of the haptics in a scleral tunnel parallel to the limbus, which combines the high degree of control in a closed-eye system with iris-independent good postoperative axial stability of the posterior chamber IOL.[1,2] The encouraging postoperative axial stability results prompted us to use the same technique for a multifocal posterior chamber IOL **(Figure 1)**.

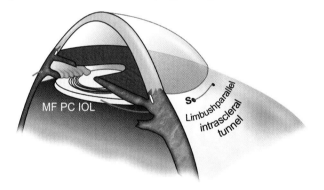

FIGURE 1: Schematic illustration of IOL position in intrascleral haptic fixation of a multifocal IOL (MIOL)

Multifocal IOL in Eyes with Deficient Capsules

The need for optimal centering and axial stability of a multifocal posterior chamber IOL for optimal refractive results is well documented. Any decentration and/or lens tilt would result in an untreatable insufficient refractive and visual outcome. In our technique an intraoperative "fine tuning" with intraoperative centration of the MIOL ab interno with a Sinskey hook is possible, and if the IOL remains decentered or tilted,

a new ciliary sulcus sclerotomy could be performed and the haptic reinserted. We have used IOL Master (Zeiss Meditec, Oberkochen, Germany) for biometry and IOL calculation. The SRK-T formula was used and the A-constant was similar to in-the-bag IOL placement. Any residual refractive error could be treated postoperatively with excimer laser treatment after the IOL implantation. This postoperative refractive treatment after cataract extraction and in-the-bag implantation of a PC IOL was first used by Zaldivar et al[3] in high myopic eyes and named bioptics. Later, bioptics became popular to minimize residual refractive errors after implantation of a multifocal IOL.

Results

We have used this technique in one myopic 24-year-old patient with bilateral subluxation of the crystalline lens of unknown etiology.[4] This was our first patient where we have used intrascleral haptic fixation technique for a multifocal IOL. In one eye postoperative refraction was emmetropia and the patient had uncorrected distance visual acuity of 0.8 and could read the newspaper. The second eye had a preexisting corneal astigmatism which was limiting the postoperative outcome. Preoperative corrected distance visual acuity of 0.4 improved to 0.63 with a manifest refraction of -0.50 D sphere and a cylinder of 6.00 D after IOL implantation. Customized LASEK using corneal wavefront ablation was performed 4 months after IOL implantation, as higher order aberrations were present—root-meansquare (RMS) at 6 mm was 0.45 μm with coma of 0.36 μm. Postoperative uncorrected distance visual acuity was 0.63 with RMS of 0.3 μm and coma of 0.3 μm. Postoperative refraction was -0.50 -0.50/155°. We advocate LASEK or PRK as the suction ring in LASIK is placed in the area where the IOL haptic is fixed intrasclerally. The IOL remained centered after LASEK

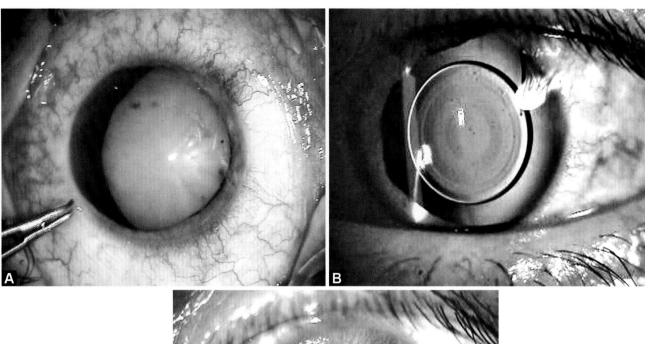

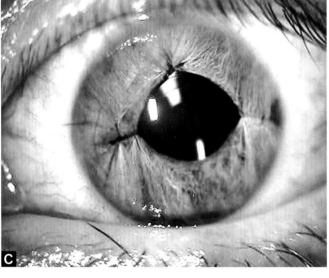

FIGURES 2A TO C

A. Traumatic subluxation of a crystalline lens after severe blunt trauma in a 34-year-old patient. Hypermature cataract developed 3 to 4 weeks after the trauma. Vitreous was present in the anterior chamber, pupil fixed in mydriasis (traumatic Urrets-Zavalia syndrome), visual acuity light perception. After pars plana lensectomy and vitrectomy peripheral retina showed a large retinal break, surgery was completed with shaving of the vitreous base, circular endolaser treatment and SF6 gas tamponade

B. Same patient after a second surgery with secondary implantation of a multifocal IOL with intrascleral haptic fixation. BUCVA for distance 0.8, reading newspaper was possible without additional reading glasses, but patient suffered from photophobia

C. Same patient after iris reconstruction, MIOL stable in place and well centered. BUCVA improved to 1.0 and patient was very satisfied, stereopsis was good (Lang test positive)

and in the three years follow-up remained uneventful. Since then we have used intrascleral haptic fixation of multifocal IOL in 8 patients with excellent results **(Figures 2A to C)**. All patients were under the age of 40 years and except the presented case all had unilateral implantation. Four eyes had spontaneous subluxation/luxation of the crystalline lens (Marfan syndrome and unknown etiology) and the other four eyes were trauma cases. We have used in seven eyes ReZoom (Abott Medical Optics, Santa Ana, USA) and in one eye the Tecnis Multifocal (Abott Medical Optics).

Conclusion

Multifocal IOLs can be implanted in eyes with deficient capsules.

References

1. Gabor SG, Pavlidis MM. Sutureless intrascleral posterior chamber intraocular lens fixation. J Cataract Refract Surg. 2007;33(11):1851-4.
2. Scharioth GB, Prasad S, Georgalas I, Tataru C, Pavlidis M. Intermediate results of sutureless intrascleral posterior chamber intraocular lens fixation. J Cataract Refract Surg. 2010;36(2):254-9.
3. Zaldivar R, Davidorf JM, Oscherow S, Ricur G, Piezzi V. Combined posterior chamber phakic intraocular lens and laser in situ keratomileusis: bioptics for extreme myopia. J Refract Surg. 1999;15(3):299-308.
4. Pavlidis M, de Ortueta D, Scharioth GB. Bioptics in sutureless intrascleral multifocal posterior chamber intraocular lens fixation. J Refract Surg. 2011;27(5):386-8.

14 Angle Kappa and Multifocal Glued IOL

Gaurav Prakash, Amar Agarwal

Introduction

Multifocal intraocular lens (IOL) implantation for the correction of ametropia aims for a good unaided visual acuity for both near and distance. This is done by creating multiple focal points, which focus for distance and near.[1-3]

Two inherent designs of multifocal optics have been used to develop these IOLs: refractive and diffractive. Refractive IOLs have multiple concentric rings in them with varying powers. Diffractive IOLs work on the Huygens-Fresnel principle.[4-6] Both the lens designs have improved significantly from their earlier prototypes. These include aspheric optics, change in the size of rings and making the IOL dominant for distance or near, and modifying the anterior or posterior surface of the IOLs.[3,5] Inspite of these modifications, the implantation of a multifocal IOL can have less than satisfactory visual acuity and quality, along with more photic phenomenon like haloes and glare compared to monofocal IOLs. Researchers have noted these factors and some studies have analyzed the governing factors for patient satisfaction after implantation of multifocal IOLs.[7, 9-22] Causes associated with photic phenomena noted in previous studies have included IOL decentration, retained lens fragments, posterior capsular opacification, dry-eye syndrome, uncorrected visual acuity, use of spectacles for distance purposes, postoperative astigmatism, and postoperative spherical equivalent.[10,22] However, none of the studies in published literature have evaluated the role of misalignment between the visual axis and the pupillary axis, or the angle kappa, as a specific predictor for patient symptoms.[23-28]

Angle Kappa

Angles of the eye have of late received a renewed interest secondary to the significant role they play in refractive surgery. Angle kappa is the angle between the visual axis and the pupillary axis (Figures 1A and B). It is clinically very important to the refractive surgeon as patients, especially hyperopes have a large angle kappa and the center of the pupil is thus no longer the point through which a fovea-centric ray of light passes. Thus any treatment that is performed centered on the pupil results in a decentered ablation. This effect is more pronounced with corrections for astigmatism and higher order aberrations if angle kappa is not compensated for.

Angle Kappa and Multifocal IOLs

But what role does angle kappa play for the cataract surgeon? We know that multifocal IOLs work by creating multiple focal points which focus for distance and near (Figures 2A and B). We also know that patients with monofocal IOLs have traditionally been more satisfied with their visual outcome with regard to postoperative blurry vision, haloes, glare and decreased contrast sensitivity. Multifocal IOLs have been associated with these symptoms despite uneventful surgery with the IOL well centered in the bag. Many factors have been proposed for these phenomena, the most important being a decrease in the intensity of light falling on the retina due to splitting up of incident light into multiple focal points and due to superimposition of the defocussed image onto the focussed image. But irrespective of these factors being common to all patients, not all patients are equally affected by the symptoms. One of the factors proposed to account for this difference in symptoms is varying degrees of neuro-adaptation. Other factors include IOL decentration, retained lens fragments, posterior capsular opacification, poor ocular surface and postoperative residual refractive error. The newer model multifocal IOLs have lesser symptoms associated with them.

A lesser studied entity is the angle kappa. Angle kappa is the distance between the center of the pupil

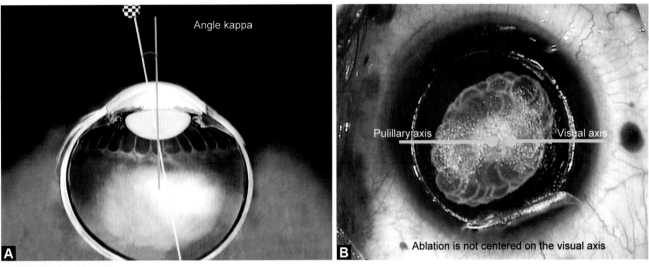

FIGURES 1A AND B
A. Angle kappa is the angle between the visual axis and the pupillary axis
B. Angle kappa in refractive surgery

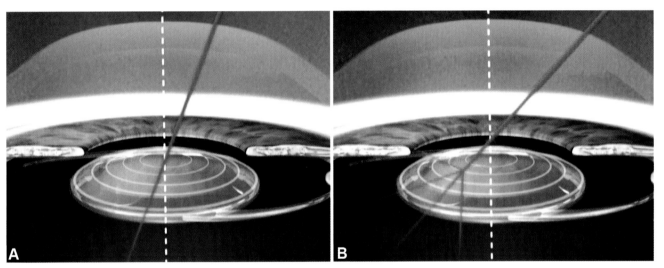

FIGURES 2A AND B
A. In eyes with small angle kappa, a fovea centric ray may pass through the central ring of the multifocal IOL
B. In eyes with large angle kappa, a fovea centric ray may hit on the edge of the ring causing edge glare effects and deterioration in quality of vision

and the light reflex. The vertex normal or the light reflex is near the visual axis at the corneal plane. Angle kappa can be measured with the synoptophore or using the Orbscan II. The average angle kappa is about ± 5 degrees. Effect of angle kappa on multifocal IOLs has been evaluated previously by attempting iridoplasty to make the pupil concentric to the center of the IOL. This could theoretically increase the effect of higher order aberrations because of an increase in the pupil size.

We also studied angle kappa in relation to visual satisfaction in multifocal patients and found photic phenomena to have an association with angle kappa. Multifocal IOLs work on either a refractive or a diffractive principle and have either multifocal zones or steps. In an eye with a small angle kappa, the ray of light would be able to pass through the IOL center without disturbance but in an eye with a large angle kappa, a fovea centric ray might hit on the edge of the ring, thus giving rise to edge glare effects, etc. **(Figures 3A and B)**. This might

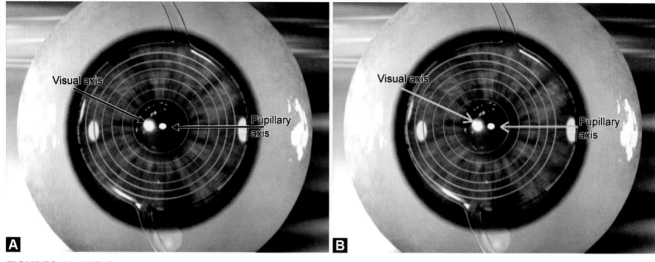

FIGURES 3A AND B
A. Figure shows a multifocal IOL which is centered on the pupillary axis but not on the visual axis in an eye with large angle kappa
B. Figure shows possible future customization of multifocal IOLs to allow centration of rings on the visual axis

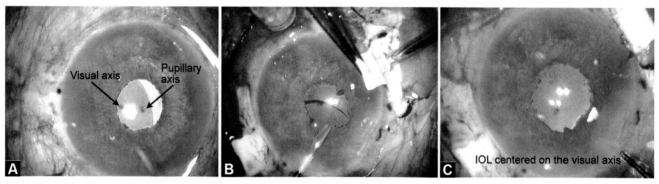

FIGURES 4A TO C: A glued multifocal IOL being done in an aphakic eye in an attempt to center the rings on the visual axis
A. Figure shows the pupillary axis and the visual axis marked preoperatively
B. Multifocal glued IOL
C. Figure shows the multifocal IOL rings centered on the pupillary axis after a glued IOL procedure which allows adjustment of the rings by adjusting the flaps, sclerotomies and the degree of tuck of individual haptics

be severe enough to result in having to explant such an IOL and replace it with a different IOL. A monofocal IOL in an eye with a large angle kappa would not cause as much visual disturbance as a decentered multifocal IOL because of the lack of steps or rings on its surface.

Multifocal Glued IOL

Just as the corneal intercept of the visual axis is used for centration of ablation in LASIK, we attempted to use the angle kappa measurement as an intraoperative guide to center a multifocal IOL. We marked the visual axis using the co-axially sighted light reflex. We then marked the pupillary center and centered a multifocal

IOL using the glued IOL technique **(Figures 4A to C)**. We marked the visual axis and the pupillary center on the cornea.

Despite the inability to ensure perfect accuracy, we did observe promising results with this technique.

There are certain situations where despite best attempts, a centered multifocal IOL in the bag may not be possible in a patient who is desirous of a multifocal. In such a patient, it is possible to perform a glued IOL and to adjust the centration by adjusting the location of the scleral flaps, sclerotomies and the degree of tuck of individual haptics. In other situations such as microspherophakia, our preferred practice is to do a lensectomy and implant a glued IOL, which if multifocal needs to be centered on its rings. It would also be ideal to combine this with ray optics and to be able to center the IOL ideally so that the light ray passes from fixation through the center of the rings to the fovea.

In the event of a posterior capsular rent, it is not advisable to place a multifocal IOL in the sulcus for fear of postoperative decentration. If in the bag multifocal IOL is not possible, a glued multifocal IOL may be preferable as the IOL is very stable with no postoperative decentration of the IOL occurring from its intraoperative positioning. In all these complicated situations as well as more importantly in the routine multifocal IOL patients, it is important to take the angle kappa into consideration for IOL centration. Future advances might also include IOL customization to match the angle kappa of the patients, though postoperative capsular contraction and IOL rotation would be challenges to be overcome.

Discussion

Multifocal IOL designs have come a long way since the earlier prototypes. At the cost of mild reduction in contrast sensitivity, many patients are satisfied with these newer models.[3,5,6,8] Neuroadaptation may also play a major role in some cases and hence enough time should be provided before drawing a conclusion on the severity of photic phenomenon.[6]

Improved patient compliance noticed with these newer IOLs was seen in our study too. The distance and near visual outcome was satisfactory with the multifocal IOL implantation in our study. We found that in cases having dissatisfaction, uncorrected postoperative visual acuity was the most important factor for patient satisfaction. This is intuitive because low intensity photic symptoms would happen in certain conditions, like around light sources or in night time driving, however, the effect of poor UCVA stays for the patient in all waking hours. Other than these factors, there was no effect of any other factor in the final resolution acuity satisfaction for distance or near. We did not find that cylindrical power had an effect independent of UCVA in patient dissatisfaction. Walcow and Klemen had similar findings with UCVA in a questionnaire based study on diffractive IOL, however they found cylindrical power to be an additionally important independent predictor of dissatisfaction.[22] The reason for this difference can be

in our exclusion of high cylinders from the preoperative data and the low postoperative cylinders. We do agree that both high cylinders and on same lines, induced higher order aberration (acquired aberropia) may have an impact on the final satisfaction of the patients.[23,24] We did not perform a wavefront analysis in our patients. A study correlating visual symptoms, angle kappa (and therefore coma aberration, which may be linked) and other higher order aberrations may provide further information on the same.[25-27]

Both the photic phenomenon evaluated in the study, i.e. haloes and glare, were found to have an association with angle kappa, which represents the angle between the visual axis and the pupillary axis. Even though many patients with high angle kappa were also asymptomatic, the strength of association was statistically significant, suggesting that angle kappa values may be considered in preoperative decision making in cases of multifocal IOL implantation. The reason for this association needs to be evaluated in detail, with simulation methods perhaps like ray tracing to confirm whether edge effect from the anterior IOL surface's rings may be responsible for the same. A higher angle kappa means that the actual misalignment between the anatomical center of the pupil-IOL complex (through which a foveo-centric ray should pass ideally) and the visual axis may be large enough to misalign the ray on to a ring edge **(Figures 5A and B)**. It may be noted that most self reporting questionnaires are biased by the expectation levels and the mindset of the patient itself, and therefore, in spite of a scale based on objective parameters, the subjective perception of a symptom may vary from one patient to another.

It needs to be seen if the lens can be customized to match the kappa angle of the patient. Due to multiple variable factors including capsular contraction and IOL rotation, it seems unlikely that a multifocal IOL intentionally decentered towards the visual axis would stay in the same position in the postoperative period. However, the situation can be different in a case of a glued IOL for aphakia.[28] In cases with glued multifocal IOL **(Figures 6A and B)** where the IOL is being placed without capsular support, one of the haptics may be pulled furthermore **(Figures 7A to C)** to position the central ring of IOL under the visual axis before tucking the haptic to fixate the IOL **(Figures 8A to E)**.

The externalized haptics tend to rub less against the ciliary body than a sutured SFIOL in which the haptic

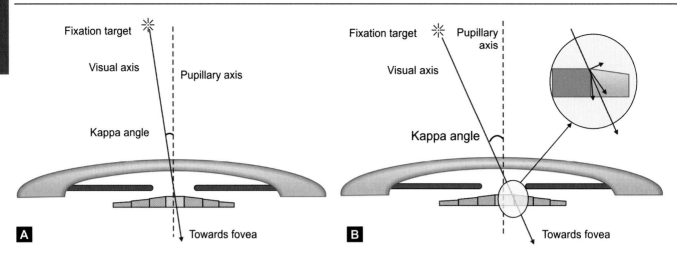

FIGURES 5A AND B
A. Schematic ray diagram showing the incident ray passing through the central area in an eye with small angle kappa
B. Schematic ray diagram showing the incident ray passing through the ring edge area in an eye with large angle kappa

lies curved within the eye close to the ciliary body. Potential to cause uveitis-glaucoma-hyphema (UGH) syndrome is also therefore less.

The perception of photic phenomenon is multifactorial as evaluated in previous studies.[10,22] Our study suggests that there may be an additional role of misalignment between the visual and pupillary axis in the occurrence of photic phenomenon after multifocal IOL implantation. Further studies will be required to analyze the effect of the same on induced higher order

aberrations and contrast sensitivity after multifocal IOL implantation.

Conclusion

To conclude, we propose that it is important to focus more research on the association between angle kappa and multifocal IOLs. It may be important to consider angle kappa for all prospective multifocal IOL patients and to avoid multifocal implantation in patients with

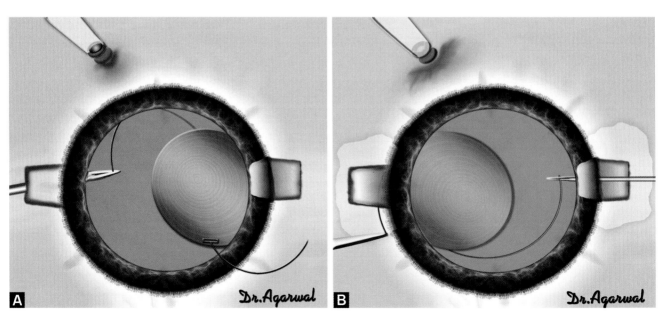

FIGURES 6A AND B: Illustration of multifocal glued IOL surgery

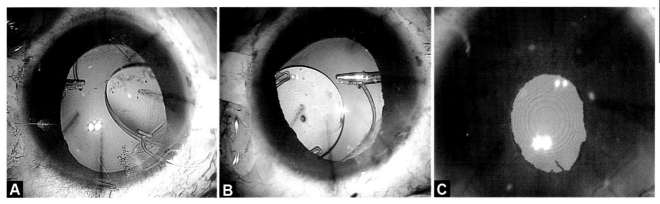

FIGURES 7A TO C: Multifocal glued IOL: Surgical steps

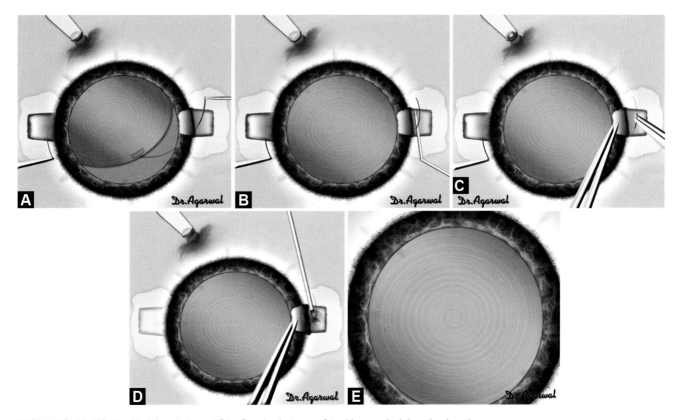

FIGURES 8A TO E: Multifocal glued IOL: Surgical steps of tucking and gluing the haptics

A. Haptic exteriorization: The second haptic is exteriorized by bringing the glued IOL forceps out through the sclerotomy. This brings both haptics out under the scleral flaps
B. Paralimbal scleral tunnel creation: A 26-gauge needle is used to create a scleral tunnel at the edge of the scleral flap. The needle is kept at the depth of the scleral flap and then advanced forwards to a sufficient degree parallel to the limbus to create a tunnel. The length of the tunnel should be sufficient enough to allow tuck of the haptics as well as to allow for intra-operative adjustment of the haptics.
C. Haptic tuck into scleral tunnel: Each haptic is tucked into its respective tunnel at the edge of the scleral flap. Centration of the IOL is then assessed intraoperatively and the degree of tuck of each individual haptic is then adjusted to allow for exquisite intraoperative centration of the IOL. This tuck of the haptic into a scleral tunnel prevents any movement of the haptic and makes the glued IOL very stable
D. Flap closure with fibrin glue: Fibrin glue is then applied under the scleral flap on either side and the flaps are sealed down
E. IOL centration: The lens is thus well centered by having adjusted the haptics. This can give perfect centration of the lens to any position desired. The lens can thus be made to center according to the surgeon's discretion either on the pupil or on the visual axis as determined by the angle kappa

large angle kappa till the time, advances make accurate centering of IOLs possible.

References

1. Bellucci R. Multifocal intraocular lenses. Curr Opin Ophthalmol. 2005;16:33-7.

2. Lane SS, Morris M, Nordan L, Packer M, Tarantino N, Wallace RB 3rd. Multifocal intraocular lenses. Ophthalmol Clin North Am. 2006;19:89-105.

3. Buznego C, Trattler WB. Presbyopia-correcting intraocular lenses. Curr Opin Ophthalmol. 2009;20:13-8

4. Jay JL, Chakrabarti HS, Morrison JD. Quality of vision through diffractive bifocal intraocular lens. Br J Ophthalmol. 1991;75: 359-66.

5. Cillino S, Casuccio A, Di Pace F, Morreale R, Pillitteri F, Cillino G, et al. One-year outcomes with new-generation multifocal intraocular lenses. Ophthalmology. 2008;115(9):1508-16.

6. Palomino Bautista C, Carmona González D, Castillo Gómez A, Bescos JA. Evolution of visual performance in 250 eyes implanted with the Tecnis ZM900 multifocal IOL. Eur J Ophthalmol. 2009;19(5):762-8.

7. Häring G, Dick HB, Krummenauer F, Weissmantel U, Kröncke W. Subjective photic phenomena with refractive multifocal and monofocal intraocular lenses. results of a multicenter questionnaire. J Cataract Refract Surg. 2001;27(2):245-9.

8. Leyland M, Zinicola E. Multifocal versus monofocal intraocular lenses in cataract surgery: a systematic review. Ophthalmology 2003;110:1789-98.

9. Dick HB, Krummenauer F, Schwenn O, Krist R, Pfeiffer N. Objective and subjective evaluation of photic phenomena after monofocal and multifocal intraocular lens implantation. Ophthalmology. 1999;106(10):1878-86.

10. Woodward MA, Randleman JB, Stulting RD. Dissatisfaction after multifocal intraocular lens implantation. J Cataract Refract Surg. 2009;35(6):992-7.

11. Pepose JS. Maximizing satisfaction with presbyopia-correcting intraocular lenses: the missing links. Am J Ophthalmol. 2008; 146(5):641-8.

12. Kohnen T, Kook D, Auffarth GU, Derhartunian V. Use of multifocal intraocular lenses and criteria for patient selection. Ophthalmologe. 2008;105(6):527-32.

13. Chang DF. Prospective functional and clinical comparison of bilateral ReZoom and ReSTOR intraocular lenses in patients 70 years or younger. J Cataract Refract Surg. 2008;34(6):934-41.

14. Blaylock JF, Si Z, Aitchison S, Prescott C. Visual function and change in quality of life after bilateral refractive lens exchange with the ReSTOR multifocal intraocular lens. J Refract Surg. 2008;24(3):265-73.

15. Chiam PJ, Chan JH, Haider SI, Karia N, Kasaby H, Aggarwal RK. Functional vision with bilateral ReZoom and ReSTOR intraocular lenses 6 months after cataract surgery. J Cataract Refract Surg. 2007;33(12):2057-61.

16. Alfonso JF, Fernández-Vega L, Baamonde MB, Montés-Micó R. Prospective visual evaluation of apodized diffractive intraocular lenses. J Cataract Refract Surg. 2007;33(7):1235-43.

17. Mester U, Hunold W, Wesendahl T, Kaymak H. Functional outcomes after implantation of Tecnis ZM900 and Array SA40 multifocal intraocular lenses. J Cataract Refract Surg. 2007; 33(6):1033-40.

18. Pepose JS, Qazi MA, Davies J, Doane JF, Loden JC, Sivalingham V, et al. Visual performance of patients with bilateral vs combination Crystalens, ReZoom, and ReSTOR intraocular lens implants. Am J Ophthalmol. 2007;144(3):347-57.

19. Chiam PJ, Chan JH, Aggarwal RK, Kasaby S. ReSTOR intraocular lens implantation in cataract surgery: quality of vision. J Cataract Refract Surg. 2006;32(9):1459-63.

20. Sen HN, Sarikkola AU, Uusitalo RJ, Laatikainen L. Quality of vision after AMO Array multifocal intraocular lens implantation. J Cataract Refract Surg. 2004;30(12):2483-93.

21. Hunkeler JD, Coffman TM, Paugh J, Lang A, Smith P, Tarantino N. Characterization of visual phenomena with the Array multifocal intraocular lens. J Cataract Refract Surg. 2002; 28(7):1195-204

22. Walkow L, Klemen UM. Patient satisfaction after implantation of diffractive designed multifocal intraocular lenses in dependence on objective parameters. Graefes Arch Clin Exp Ophthalmol. 2001;239(9):683-7

23. Agarwal A, Prakash G, Jacob S, Ashokkumar D, Agarwal A. Can uncompensated higher order aberration profile, or aberropia be responsible for subnormal best corrected vision and pseudo-amblyopia. Med Hypotheses. 2009;72(5):574-7.

24. Agarwal A, Jacob S, Agarwal A. Aberropia: a new refractive entity. J Cataract Refract Surg. 2007;33(11):1835-6.

25. Espinosa J, Mas D, Kasprzak HT. Corneal primary aberrations compensation by oblique light incidence. J Biomed Opt. 2009; 14(4):044003.

26. Lu F, Wu J, Shen Y, Qu J, Wang Q, Xu C, Chen S, Zhou X, He JC. On the compensation of horizontal coma aberrations in young human eyes. Ophthalmic Physiol Opt. 2008;28(3):277-82.

27. Tabernero J, Benito A, Alcón E, Artal P. Mechanism of compensation of aberrations in the human eye. J Opt Soc Am A Opt Image Sci Vis. 2007;24(10):3274-83.

28. Agarwal A, Kumar DA, Jacob S, Baid C, Agarwal A, Srinivasan S. Fibrin glue-assisted sutureless posterior chamber intraocular lens implantation in eyes with deficient posterior capsules. J Cataract Refract Surg. 2008;34(9):1433-8.

15

Glued IOL with Corneal Procedures

Rajesh Sinha, Himanshu Shekhar,
Namrata Sharma, Jeewan S Titiyal,
Rasik B Vajpayee

Introduction

The presence of corneal pathology in eyes with aphakia or malpositioned intraocular lens (IOL) is not infrequent. In most of these cases, penetrating keratoplasty (PKP) or Descemet's stripping automated endothelial keratoplasty (DSAEK) is an effective surgical modality for the treatment[1-5] of the corneal pathology. But some of these cases may require implantation or exchange of the intraocular lens (IOL) for full visual rehabilitation. Indications for intraocular lens exchange can be closed-loop IOLs, semiflexible anterior chamber (AC) IOLs, and iris-supported or malpositioned IOLs as these lenses may be associated with poor graft survival as well as suboptimal visual gain postoperatively.

IOL Implantation

Brunette et al[6] found that implanting a PC IOL at the time of PKP provides better results than an AC IOL; survival of the graft is longer, intraocular pressure is lower, and postoperative visual outcome is better even when the posterior capsule is damaged. Recent techniques for IOL exchange during keratoplasty, especially in cases with a deficient posterior capsule, are still evolving. Trans-sclerally sutured IOLs have been described in these situations[7,8] by some surgeons around the world. However, the technique is associated with a longer learning curve, prolonged intraoperative manipulation, postoperative pseudophacodonesis, and chances of postoperative decentration due to suture degradation or knot slippage.[9-15] Recently, fibrin glue assisted sutureless posterior chamber IOL implantation[16] has been described in cases of deficient posterior capsule. It involves trans-scleral exteriorization

and intrascleral tucking of both the haptics under diametrically opposite scleral flaps, which are then apposed with fibrin glue.

Indications

Pseudophakic bullous keratopathy (PBK) with an anterior chamber intraocular lens (AC IOL) is a leading indication for full-thickness penetrating keratoplasty (PKP) and IOL exchange.[1,2] Other indications may include PBK with decentred or subluxated IOL or corneal scar (post-traumatic or healed keratitis) with malpositioned IOL. These scenarios present as a surgical challenge because of a previous complicated surgery, compromised aqueous drainage, unhealthy wound configuration, and a deficient posterior capsule. Chen et al[17] have suggested reasons like limited AC space, a potential IOL-endothelium touch, difficult tissue handling, and air bubble management to conclude that exchanging a pre-implanted AC IOL with a posterior chamber IOL while undergoing DSAEK could be more beneficial. While performing full thickness keratoplasty, both corneal transplantation and IOL exchange should be optimized to achieve less "open sky" time to avoid the risk of expulsive hemorrhage or choroidal effusion and to ensure postoperative preservation of the donor endothelial cells. The tamponade effect of a securely fixated IOL can be helpful in maintaining the anterior chamber with the viscoelastic during suturing of the donor button (the open-sky period).

Aphakia with inadequate capsular support with endothelial decompensation is another condition where the surgical procedure may be challenging. Full visual rehabilitation requires implantation of an IOL apart from the corneal procedure. The possible options available are either an AC IOL or a transscleral fixated IOL (suture fixated, glued IOL, or iris fixated)[18,19] combined with a DSAEK procedure. However, an AC IOL requires an intact and healthy iris, which sometimes may not be the case in situations with complicated aphakia (distorted iris and loss of iris tissue), which along with other problems like decreased AC space may deter surgeons from using it as the first choice. As has been explained in a study, securely fixed haptics in the sclera instead of the sutured haptic attachment prevent a trampoline-like effect and provide a more stable configuration.[20] The glued IOL thus has potential advantages over both AC IOL and sutured SFIOL.

Preoperative Evaluation

The preoperative evaluation includes a complete ophthalmologic examination, tear film assessment, anterior segment measurements including corneal thickness, anterior chamber morphology evaluation by high-resolution noncontact anterior segment optical coherence tomography (AS-OCT) (Visante, Carl Zeiss Meditec AG), and ultrasonography of the posterior segment. Patients with significant stromal scarring are planned for PKP with glued IOL while DSAEK is performed in those with insignificant scarring.

DSAEK with Glued IOL

The donor corneoscleral tissue is mounted on an artificial anterior chamber (Moria ALTK, Moria). A 350 μm head is chosen for the microkeratome (Moria). The lamellar dissection is performed with the microkeratome. The posterior lamella with corneoscleral rim is placed on a teflon block with endothelial side up and an 8.0 mm donor lenticule is fashioned by a circular cutting trephine. The surgery can be performed under peribulbar anesthesia with 5 ml of 2% lignocaine hydrochloride and 5 ml of 0.5% bupivacaine hydrochloride. A temporal or superior approach can be selected. Here we are describing DSAEK performed through the superior approach with IOL haptics fixed nasally and temporally.

A localized peritomy is done nasally and temporally. The sclera is marked 1.5 mm and 3.0 mm from the limbus (Figure 1). Two partial thickness radial scleral incisions are made parallel to each other between

1.5 mm and 3 mm points from the limbus (Figure 2). A crescent blade is used to perform the lamellar dissection between the two incisions (Figure 3). The lamellar dissection is extended beyond the radial incisions on the temporal aspect on one side and nasally on the other side. Partial thickness scleral flaps are raised by cutting the roof of the tunnel at the forniceal side so as to create a limbus based scleral flap (Figure 4). The cornea is marked with an 8-mm circular cutting disposable corneal trephine. Two paracentesis are made at the limbus at 10 and 2 o'clock positions. An AC maintainer is placed through the 2 o'clock paracentesis. The scoring of Descemet's membrane along with endothelium is performed with a reverse Sinskey hook through the paracentesis made at 10 o'clock position (Figure 5) and the membrane is taken out. Limited anterior vitrectomy is performed to clear any vitreous strands from the anterior chamber. Two sclerotomies are made, one each in the bed of the scleral flap 1.5 mm from the limbus.

A superior limbal tunnel is made with a 2.75 mm keratome. The limbal tunnel is enlarged to 6.0 mm. A posterior chamber multipiece IOL is introduced into the anterior chamber with a McPherson forceps. The haptic is then held at the tip with a 23 gauge vitreoretinal or lens fixing forceps introduced through the sclerotomy site (Figure 6) and exteriorized through one sclerotomy site. The second haptic is managed similarly, exteriorized with the help of a forceps inserted through the other sclerotomy (Figure 7) and guided into the scleral pocket dissected adjacent to the scleral flap (Figure 8). The tip of the other haptic is then tucked into the adjacent scleral pocket. The reconstituted fibrin glue (Baxter AG, Vienna, Austria) is then injected into the pockets and over the beds of the scleral flap (Figure 9). The scleral flap is replaced and gentle pressure is applied locally over the flap for 20-30 seconds to promote the action of the glue to adhere the scleral flaps. The conjunctival flaps are also replaced by sticking it to the sclera with the application of fibrin glue (Figure 10). The donor lenticule is then placed into the Busin glide (Figure 11) and inserted into the anterior chamber by pulling with a forceps introduced through a limbal paracentesis made at the 6 o'clock position (Figure 12). The donor lenticule is unfolded and brought into position by gently stroking the cornea. The corneal tunnel is closed with 10-0 monofilament nylon suture. Air is injected to fill the AC and achieve tamponade for 10 minutes (Figure 13). At the end of

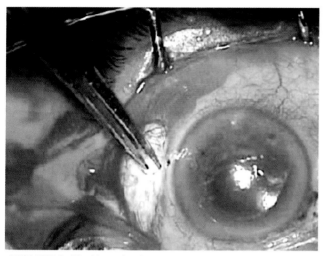

FIGURE 1: Marking of sclera 1.5 mm and 3.0 mm from the limbus

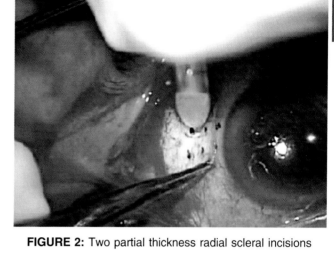

FIGURE 2: Two partial thickness radial scleral incisions

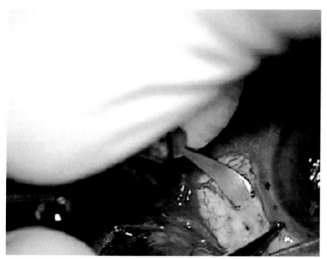

FIGURE 3: Lamellar dissection performed between the two incisions with a crescent blade

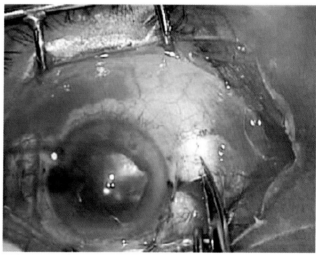

FIGURE 4: Creation of partial thickness scleral flaps by cutting the roof of the tunnel at the forniceal side with a curved Vannas' scissors

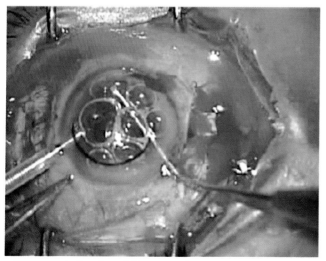

FIGURE 5: Scoring of Descemet's membrane performed with a reverse Sinskey hook

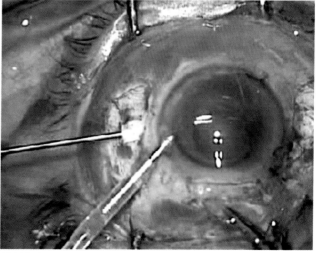

FIGURE 6: The haptic of a posterior chamber multipiece IOL held with a 23-gauge vitreoretinal forceps and exteriorized

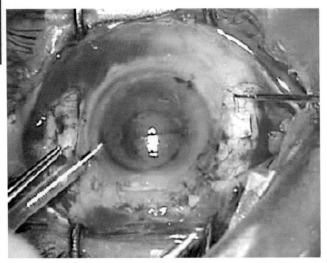

FIGURE 7: The second haptic is also exteriorized through the sclerotomy site

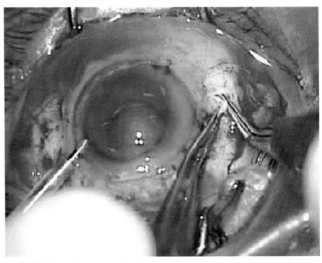

FIGURE 8: The exteriorized haptic tucked into the scleral pocket dissected adjacent to the scleral flap

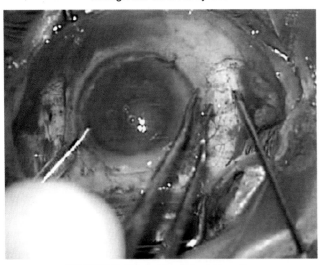

FIGURE 9: Fibrin glue injected on the scleral bed and flap replaced

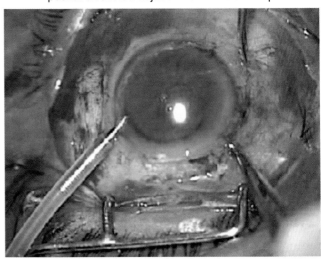

FIGURE 10: Conjunctival flap being replaced after injecting fibrin glue under it

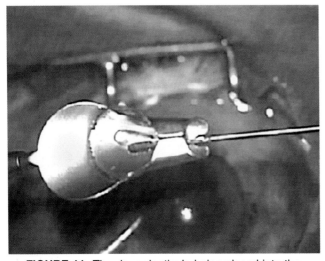

FIGURE 11: The donor lenticule being placed into the Busin glide

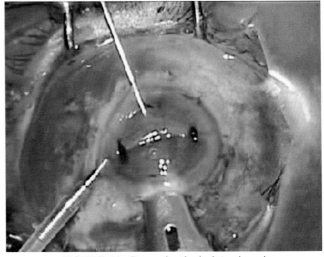

FIGURE 12: Donor lenticule introduced into the anterior chamber

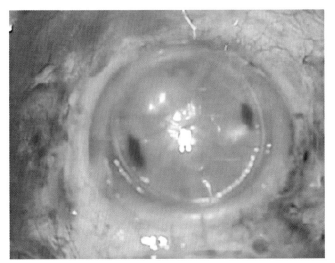

FIGURE 13: Air injected into the AC to achieve tamponade for donor lenticule

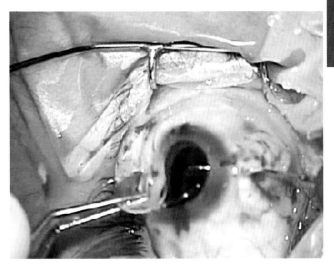

FIGURE 14: Tip of a multipiece IOL is held and exteriorized through the sclerotomy

10 minutes, half the air in the chamber is exchanged with saline. Postoperatively, the patient is asked to lie in a strict supine position with face towards the ceiling for 8-10 hours.

Penetrating Keratoplasty (PKP) with Glued IOL

The donor tissue is prepared using a manual trephine from a freshly prepared corneoscleral button by punching on a Teflon block. The scleral flaps and the adjacent groove are created in a similar fashion as described earlier. One should make the 20G sclerotomy under the scleral flaps before opening the eye, as otherwise the eye is too soft. It is better to create the scleral pockets also beforehand. The host cornea is trephined using a 7.2 mm circular cutting disposable trephine. A multipiece IOL is held with a McPherson forceps at the pupillary plane with one hand and then exteriorized through the sclerotomy on one side followed by the other with a vitreoretinal or lens fixing forceps inserted through the sclerotomy sites as described earlier **(Figure 14)**. The tips of the haptics are then tucked into the scleral pocket dissected on both sides. The graft is then placed and cardinal sutures applied using 10-0 monofilament nylon sutures in an interrupted fashion **(Figure 15)**. Similarly, other 12 sutures are applied to appose the graft host junction. The reconstituted fibrin glue is injected through the cannula of the double syringe delivery system under the scleral flaps **(Figure 16)**. Local pressure is applied over the flaps for 30 seconds to allow formation of adhesion

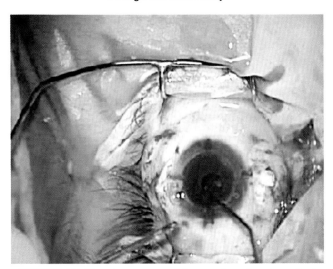

FIGURE 15: The donor corneal tissue placed and cardinal sutures applied

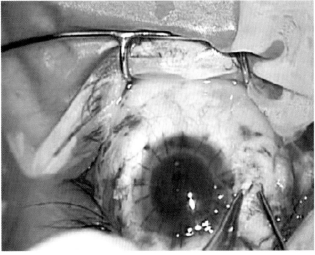

FIGURE 16: Fibrin glue injected under the scleral flaps

114

of the flap with bed. The conjunctiva is also apposed to the sclera using fibrin glue.

Postoperative Regime, Evaluation and Follow-up

Postoperative treatment, follow-up and evaluation after the procedure is similar to that followed after any corneal transplantation procedure. Postoperatively the patients are prescribed topical antibiotic drops such as topical moxifloxacin 0.5% 3 times a day, topical corticosteroid drops in the form of prednisolone acetate 1% eye drops 6 times a day, tropicamide 1% eye drops twice a day, and preservative-free lubricating drops 6 times a day. The corticosteroid drops are subsequently tapered. Follow-up visits are scheduled at 1, 7 and 14 days after the surgery and then monthly till the end of one year **(Figures 17 and 18)** and yearly thereafter. Additional visits are scheduled in cases of complications or problems. During the follow-up, a complete ophthalmological examination is performed which includes parameters like corneal transparency, corneal thickness, endothelial counts, visual outcome, and complications (keratoplasty related and IOL related).

Advantages

The intrascleral glue fixation of IOL has potential benefits as a combined procedure with DSAEK in comparison to anterior chamber IOL because it does not reduce the

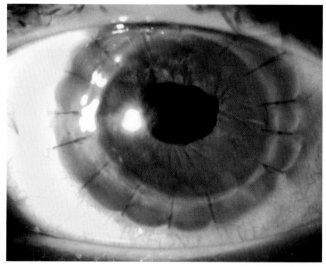

FIGURE 18: Postoperative picture of intrasclerally glue-fixed IOL with PKP at 1 year

anterior chamber volume, does not require intact iris tissue, and unlike suture-fixated IOL, does not have knot slippage or pseudophakodonesis.[20] In PKP also, intrascleral fixation of IOL with fibrin glue can be used as a safe and effective alternative. This technique reduces the surgical time[20,21] and the time of IOL fixation in an open globe after host trephination as the additional time required for the procedure is only in externalization and tucking of the haptic; thereby reducing the risk of expulsive hemorrhage or choroidal effusion.

Intraocular lens exchange is arguably the more challenging step in this surgery. The safety and long-term efficacy of a trans-sclerally sutured PC IOL are less than satisfactory.[10-12] The trans-sclerally sutured IOL is associated with a steep learning curve and requires special steps that an anterior segment surgeon may not use routinely. Study has shown that ultrasound biomicroscopy showed that trans-scleral suturing of an IOL had problems related to accurate suturing at the ciliary sulcus.[10] In addition, there are issues with IOL iris contact, pigment dispersion, high aqueous flare, and vitreous incarceration. In PKP, the conventional wisdom is to reduce the "open-sky" duration to as short a time as possible as there is an associated risk for expulsive hemorrhage or choroidal effusion. Transscleral suture fixation requires adjustment of the sutures and knots to maintain the IOL in position, leading to requirement of a specially designed IOL. An open-sky procedure is often associated with anterior vitrectomy. The resultant hypotony makes suture placement and adjustment difficult. In an open sky procedure with a deficient posterior capsule, there is no

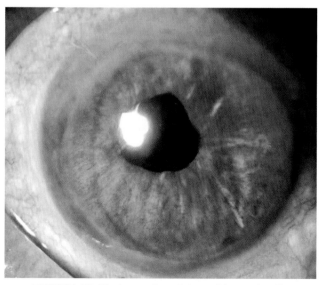

FIGURE 17: Postoperative picture of intrasclerally glue-fixed IOL with DSAEK at 1 year

tamponade effect and the results can be disastrous if the patient strains or coughs. The aim of the surgeon in this scenario should be to reduce the surgical time. Most of the time consumption in these cases is in passing the straight needle and tying and adjusting the sutures. A glued IOL can be used as a safe and effective alternative. Most steps, except externalization and tucking, are part of routine anterior segment procedures.[16] There is no requirement for an extra set of sutures and a straight needle, which can be difficult to pass in a hypotonous open globe. While doing scleral fixation with sutures, the surgeon must readjust the knots to maintain the central position of the IOL. While in cases of glued IOL, simply manipulating the amount of externalization can cause proper centration of the IOL. The final tucking of the haptic provides further stabilization. The pseudophacodonesis associated with sutured IOL may result in progressive endothelial loss. However, in glued IOL, rigid haptics are used for fixation on the scleral side and the stable optic-haptic junction prevents torsional and anteroposterior instability. Therefore, there is much less pseudophacodonesis. The haptics are covered in the scleral flap and tucked well inside the scleral pocket. There is an additional well-apposed layer of conjunctiva over the sclera. This further reduces the chances of haptic extrusion.

Complications

Although PKP or DSAEK combined with the replacement of an anterior chamber IOL for a scleral-fixated posterior chamber IOL has a high anatomic success rate, visual acuity may be low due to many postoperative complications and fundus comorbidities. There is not much information in literature stating the postoperative complications of this combined procedure. Some of these problems result from the PKP procedure itself that include surgically induced astigmatism, suture-related complications, delayed stromal wound healing, graft rejection, graft infection and decompensation. Other complications may be IOL related and include bleeding, dislocation, subluxation and decentration, glaucoma, vitreous incarceration, endophthalmitis, and haptic extrusion.[22-25]

Conclusion

In summary, the intrascleral fixation of an IOL assisted by fibrin glue in combination with DSAEK or PKP appears to be a safe and effective method for the management of pseudophakic corneal edema with aphakia or malpositioned IOLs. However, the more this technique is used by different surgeons, the greater will be the information regarding its benefits as well as limitations.

References

1. Lyle WA, Jin J-C. An analysis of intraocular lens exchange. Ophthalmic Surg. 1992;23:453-8.
2. Lois N, Kowal VO, Cohen EJ, Rapuano CJ, Gault JA, Raber IM, et al. Indications for penetrating keratoplasty and associated procedures, 1989-1995. Cornea. 1997;16:623-9.
3. Forster W, Atzler U, Ratkay I, Buss H. Therapeutic use of the 193-nm excimer laser in corneal pathologies. Graefes Arch Clin Exp Ophthalmol. 1997;235:296-305.
4. Chen ES, Terry MA, Shamie N, Hoar KL, Friend DJ. Descemet-stripping automated endothelial keratoplasty: six-month results in a prospective study of 100 eyes. Cornea. 2008;27(5):514-20.
5. Balazs E, Balazs K, Modis L Jr, Berta A. Penetrating keratoplasty for pseudophakic bullous keratopathy. Acta Chir Hung. 1997;36:11-3.
6. Brunette I, Stulting RD, Rinnie JR, Waring GO 3rd, Gemmil M. Penetrating keratoplasty with anterior or posterior chamber intraocular lens implantation. Arch Ophthalmol. 1994;112: 1311-9.
7. Soong HK, Meyer RF, Sugar A. Techniques of posterior chamber lens implantation without capsular support during penetrating keratoplasty: A review. Refract Corneal Surg. 1989;5:249-55.
8. Kocak Altintas AG, Kocak Midillioglu I, Dengisik F, Duman S. Implantation of scleral-sutured posterior chamber intraocular lenses during penetrating keratoplasty. J Refract Surg. 2000;16:456-8.
9. Busin M, Brauweiler P, Boker T, Spitznas M. Complications of sulcus-supported intraocular lenses with iris sutures, implanted during penetrating keratoplasty after intracapsular cataract extraction. Ophthalmology. 1990;97:401-5.
10. Manabe S, Oh H, Amino K, Hata N, Yamakawa R. Ultrasound biomicroscopic analysis of posterior chamber intraocular lenses with transscleral sulcus suture. Ophthalmology. 2000;107: 2172-8.
11. Buckley EG. Safety of transscleral-sutured intraocular lenses in children. J AAPOS. 2008;12:431-9.
12. Asadi R, Kheirkhah A. Long-term results of scleral fixation of posterior chamber intraocular lenses in children. Ophthalmology. 2008;115:67-72.
13. Vote BJ, Tranos P, Bunce C, Charteris DG, Da Cruz L. Long term outcome of combined pars plana vitrectomy and scleral fixated sutured posterior chamber intraocular lens implantation. Am J Ophthalmol. 2006;141:308-12.
14. Guell JL, Barrera A, Manero F. A review of suturing techniques for posterior chamber lenses. Curr Opin Ophthalmol. 2004;15: 44-50.
15. Hannush SB. Sutured posterior chamber intraocular lenses: indications and procedure. Curr Opin Ophthalmol. 2000;11: 233-40.

16. Agarwal A, Kumar DA, Jacob S, Baid C, Agarwal A, Srinivasan S. Fibrin glue-assisted sutureless posterior chamber intraocular lens implantation in eyes with deficient posterior capsules. J Cataract Refract Surg. 2008;34:1433-8.

17. Chen ES, Terry MA, Shamie N, et al. Retention of an anterior chamber IOL versus IOL exchange in endothelial keratoplasty. J Cataract Refract Surg. 2009;35:613.

18. Baykara M, Ozcetin H, Yilmaz S, et al. Posterior iris fixation of the iris claw intraocular lens implantation through a scleral tunnel incision. Am J Ophthalmol. 2007;144:586-91.

19. Menezo JL, Martinez MC, Cisneros AL. Iris-fixated Worst claw versus sulcus-fixated posterior chamber lenses in the absence of capsular support. J Cataract Refract Surg. 1996;22:1476-84.

20. Prakash G, Agarwal A, Jacob S, Kumar DA, Chaudhary P, Agarwal A. Femtosecond-assisted descemet stripping automated endothelial keratoplasty with fibrin glue-assisted sutureless posterior chamber lens implantation. Cornea. 2010;29(11):1315-9.

21. Prakash G, Jacob S, Ashok Kumar D, Narsimhan S, Agarwal A, Agarwal A. Femtosecond-assisted keratoplasty with fibrin glue-assisted sutureless posterior chamber lens implantation: new triple procedure. J Cataract Refract Surg. 2009;35(6):973-9.

22. Chang JH, Lee JH. Long-term results of implantation of posteriorchamber intraocular lens by suture fixation. Korean J Ophthalmol. 1991;5:42-46.

23. Holland EJ, Daya SM, Evangelista A, Ketcham JM, Lubniewski AJ, Doughman DJ, et al. Penetrating keratoplasty and trans-scleral fixation of posterior chamber lens. Am J Ophthalmol. 1992;114:182-7.

24. Djalilian AR, Anderson SO, Fang-Zen M, Lane SS, Holland EJ. Long-term results of trans-sclerally sutured posterior chamber lenses in penetrating keratoplasty. Cornea. 1998;17:359-64.

25. van der Schaft TL, van Rij G, Renardel de Lavalette JG, Beekhuis WH. Results of penetrating keratoplasty for pseudophakic-bullous keratopathy with the exchange of an intraocular lens. Br J Ophthalmol. 1989;73:704-8.

16 | Penetrating Keratoplasty with Glued IOL

Gaurav Prakash, Amar Agarwal

Introduction

Pseudophakic bullous keratopathy (PBK) with an anterior chamber intraocular lens (AC IOL) is a leading indication for full-thickness penetrating keratoplasty (PKP) and IOL exchange.[1,2] It presents a unique surgical challenge because of a previous complicated surgery, compromised aqueous drainage, unhealthy wound configuration, and a deficient posterior capsule. Both the corneal transplantation and the IOL exchange should be optimized to achieve less "opensky" time, easier intraoperative procedures, faster wound healing, and maximum provision and postoperative preservation of the donor endothelial cells.

A paradigm shift has occurred in keratoplasty with the use of the femtosecond laser for sculpting the donor and host corneas. The top-hat configuration has resulted in a more stable wound configuration, faster healing, and more endothelial cells (compared with those in a standard manual procedure with a comparable epithelial side diameter).[3-8] In contrast, current techniques for IOL exchange during keratoplasty, especially in cases with a deficient posterior capsule, are less than satisfactory. Transsclerally sutured IOLs have been used in this situation.[9,10] Unfortunately, this technique is associated with a longer learning curve, prolonged intraoperative manipulation, postoperative pseudophacodonesis, and chances of postoperative decentration due to suture degradation or knot slippage.[10-17]

We have successfully performed fibrin glue-assisted sutureless posterior chamber IOL (PC IOL) implantation in eyes with deficient posterior capsule support.[18] It involves trans-scleral exteriorization and intrascleral tuck of both the haptics under diametrically opposite scleral flaps, which are then apposed with scleral glue. This sutureless technique can be performed with routinely available three piece PCIOLs and has a short learning curve.

Penetrating Keratoplasty with Glued IOL

When one is performing a keratoplasty with a glued IOL, it is better to create the scleral flaps first and also the sclerotomy with a 20G needle under the scleral flap 1 mm behind the limbus. The reason is that it is difficult to do these maneuvers once the eye is opened. One can then use a manual trephine perform the open-sky vitrectomy externalize the haptics and then suture the new graft. Once air is injected at the end one can use the glue to seal the scleral flaps.

Femto-assisted Keratoplasty with Glued IOL

The initial part of the surgery is done at the femtosecond laser facility. Donor buttons are prepared from whole globes. The patient is prepared (Figure 1A). After the suction ring is applied and adequate vacuum and centration are achieved, a top-hat configuration is created using a femtosecond laser [IntraLase FS (IntraLase Corp.)] (Figures 1B and C). For the host cut, the patient is given topical anesthesia. After the suction ring is applied and adequate vacuum and centration are achieved, a top-hat configuration is created. The donor cornea and patient are then moved to the keratoplasty operating room.

The rest of the surgery is performed under peribulbar anesthesia. A limited peritomy is done in the inferotemporal and superonasal areas 180 degrees apart, and a 3.0-3.0 mm area is marked on the sclera. Two partial-thickness limbal-based scleral flaps of

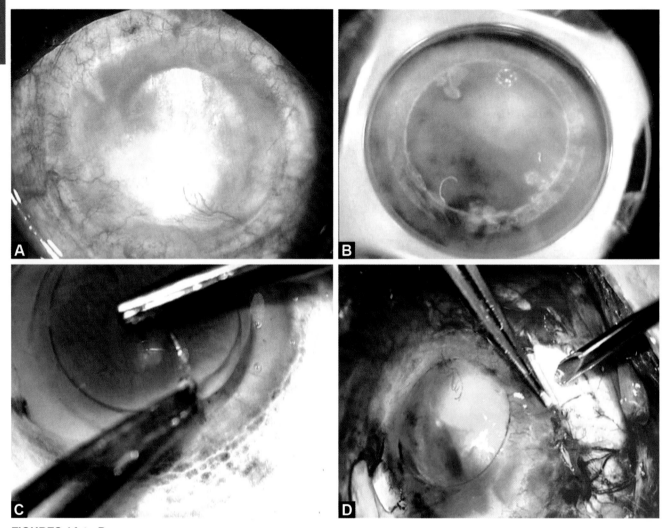

FIGURES 1A to D
A. Preoperative photograph showing pseudophakic bullous keratopathy (PBK) with an AC IOL *in situ*
B. Femtosecond laser-created top-hat configuration
C. Femtosecond-assisted top-hat configuration showing the predictable and uniform wound formation
D. Inferior straight sclerotomy made with a 20-gauge needle 1.5 mm from the limbus under the existing scleral flaps. Note the diametrically opposite scleral flaps

3.0 mm are created. Two straight sclerotomies, one slightly inferior to the other are made with a 20-gauge needle 1.0 to 1.5 mm from the limbus under the existing scleral flaps **(Figure 1D)**. The top hat is inspected for completeness. The diseased cornea is removed **(Figures 2A and B)**. After the host button is removed, the AC IOL is explanted **(Figure 2C)**. Limited open sky anterior vitrectomy is then performed.

A posterior chamber 6.5 mm IOL is held with a McPherson forceps at the pupillary plane with one hand. It is better to use a three piece IOL as the optic haptic junction would not easily break on externalization of the haptics. An end-gripping 25-gauge microcapsulorhexis forceps (Micro Surgical Technology) is passed through the inferior sclerotomy with the other hand. The tip of the leading haptic is grasped with the microcapsulorhexis forceps and pulled through the inferior sclerotomy following the haptic curve **(Figure 2D)**. The haptic is then externalized under the inferior scleral flap **(Figure 3A)**. The trailing haptic is also externalized through the superior sclerotomy under the scleral flap **(Figure 3B)**. After both haptics have been externalized, the graft is placed and cardinal sutures are applied **(Figure 3C)**. With a 26-gauge needle, a scleral tunnel is created along the curve of the externalized haptic at the edge of the scleral bed of the flap **(Figure 3D)**. The haptic is tucked

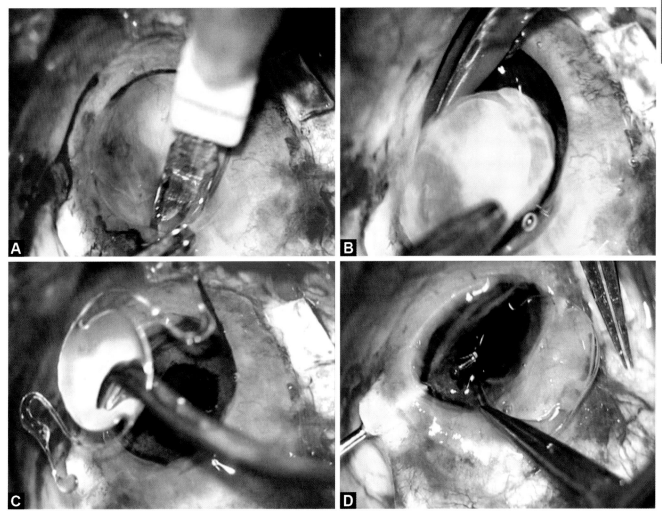

FIGURES 2A TO D

A. Augmentation of the top-hat configuration in areas that had poor laser penetration because of overlying opacity

B. Posterior uncut tissue dissected with a Vannas scissors

C. Explantation of the AC IOL after removal of the host button

D. Leading haptic grasped with the microcapsulorhexis forceps for being pulled through the inferior sclerotomy following the haptic curve

into this tunnel **(Figures 4A and B)**. A similar tunnel is created in the complementary area on the other side, and tucking is performed. Fibrin glue (Tisseel, Baxter) is reconstituted from a pack containing freeze-dried human fibrinogen, freeze-dried human thrombin, and aprotinin solution. The reconstituted fibrin glue is injected through the cannula of the syringe delivery system under the superior and inferior scleral flaps **(Figure 4C)**. Local pressure is applied to the flaps for 30 seconds to allow polypeptide formation. The same glue is applied in the area between the sutures at the entire graft-host junction **(Figure 4D)**. The conjunctiva is also apposed with the glue.

Discussion

In penetrating keratoplasty (PKP) cases, all attempts should be made to minimize endothelial cell loss in the intraoperative and postoperative periods. To provide the maximum number of endothelial cells to the host, there may be a tendency toward larger grafts in conventional keratoplasty for bullous keratopathy. However, this is associated with an increased epithelial cell load, which is probably associated with a higher risk for graft rejection. Since a top-hat configuration is larger at the inner end, it provides a greater number of endothelial cells for the same number of epithelial cells. In

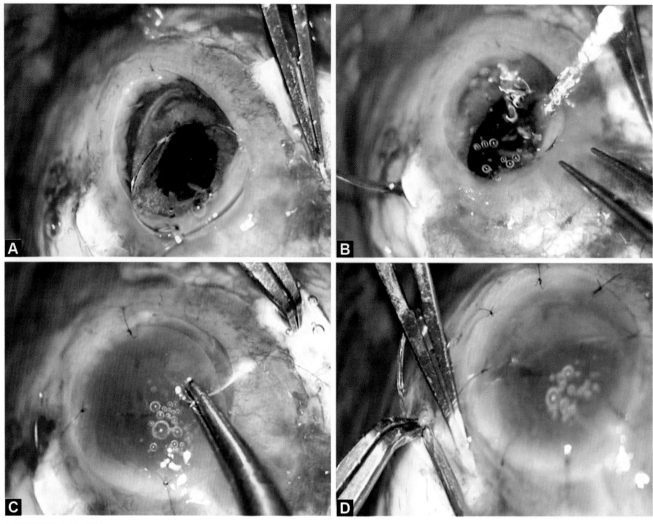

FIGURES 3A TO D
A. Leading haptic externalized completely under the inferior scleral flap
B. The trailing haptic externalized through the superior sclerotomy under the scleral flap
C. The graft button placed and cardinal sutures applied
D. Scleral tunnel created along the curve of the externalized haptic in the superonasal area at the edge of the scleral bed of the flap

addition, with the top-hat configuration, smaller outer sizes can be prepared and the graft-host junction can be farther from the limbus centripetally, reducing chances of neovascularization. These two unique advantages of the top-hat configuration may enhance graft survival by reducing chances of graft rejection and promoting endothelial survival.

Intraocular lens exchange is arguably the more challenging step in this surgery. The safety and long-term efficacy of a transsclerally sutured PC IOL are less than satisfactory.[12-14] The transsclerally sutured IOL is associated with a steep learning curve and requires special steps that an anterior segment surgeon may not

use routinely. In a previous study,[12] ultrasound biomicroscopy showed that transscleral suturing of an IOL had problems related to accurate suturing at the ciliary sulcus. In addition, there are issues with IOL iris contact, pigment dispersion, high aqueous flare and vitreous incarceration.

In PKP, the conventional wisdom is to reduce the "open-sky" duration to as short a time as possible as there is an associated risk for expulsive hemorrhage or choroidal effusion. The tamponade effect of a securely fixated IOL can be helpful in the duration between completion of host dissection and suturing of the donor button (the open-sky period). Transscleral

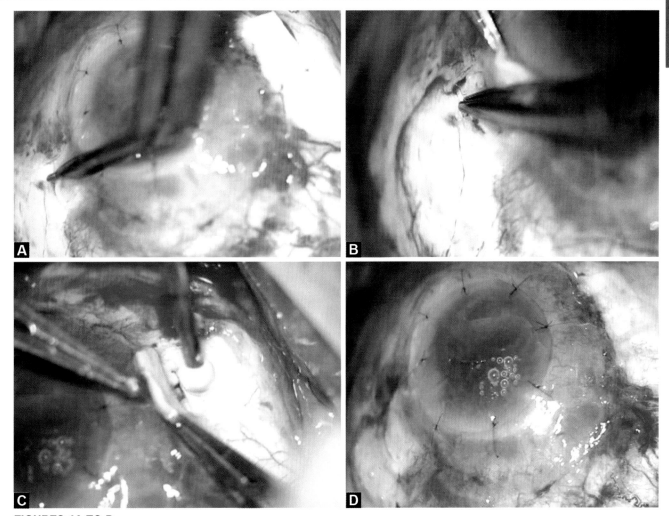

FIGURES 4A TO D
A. The superior haptic tucked into the superonasal tunnel
B. The tucking shown at higher magnification
C. Reconstituted fibrin glue injected through the cannula of the syringe delivery system under the inferior scleral flap
D. The glue applied at the graft-host junction

suture fixation requires adjustment of the sutures and knots to maintain the IOL in position, leading to a delay in placement of the donor button. It also requires a special IOL with eye haptics and may not be readily available.

An open-sky procedure is often associated with anterior vitrectomy. The resultant hypotony makes suture placement and adjustment difficult. In an open-sky procedure with a deficient posterior capsule, there is no tamponade effect and the results can be disastrous if the patient strains or coughs. The aim of the surgeon in this scenario should be to reduce the surgical time. Most of the time consumption in these cases is in passing the straight needle and tying and adjusting the

sutures. A glued IOL can be used as a safe and effective alternative. The new technique has a short learning curve. Most steps, except externalization and tucking, are part of routine anterior segment procedures.[18] There is no requirement for an extra set of sutures and a straight needle, which can be difficult to pass in a hypotonous open globe.

While doing scleral fixation with sutures, the surgeon must readjust the knots to maintain the central position of the IOL. In our procedure, simply manipulating the amount of externalization can cause proper centration of the IOL. The final tucking of the haptic provides further stabilization. A sutured scleral-fixated IOL hangs in the posterior chamber, with the sutures passing through the haptic eyes, similar to a hammock, causing dynamic torsional and antero-posterior oscillation. This pseudophacodonesis may result in progressive endothelial loss. However, in this technique, haptics are used for fixation on the scleral side and the stable optic-haptic junction prevents torsional and anteroposterior instability. Therefore, there is much less pseudophacodonesis **(Figure 5)**. The haptics are covered in the scleral flap and tucked well inside the scleral pocket. There is an additional well-apposed layer of conjunctiva over the sclera. This further reduces the chances of haptic extrusion.

Femtosecond laser-assisted keratoplasty with top-hat configuration and a glued IOL provides a unique solution in cases with bullous keratopathy and AC IOLs. This is an improvement over the traditional technique of manual trephination and transscleral suture fixation of the IOL **(Figure 5)**. The femtosecond laser's top-hat configuration provides a greater number

of endothelial cells in the donor lenticule and a more stable wound configuration. Better dynamic stability of the glued IOL prevents pseudophacodonesis and may reduce endothelial cell loss or repositioning surgery. Combining, these two surgical modalities may improve results.

Conclusion

The unique benefits of femtosecond laser and a "glued IOL" could be adjunctive and provide enhanced results in cases having PKP and IOL implantation.

References

1. Lyle WA, Jin J-C. An analysis of intraocular lens exchange. Ophthalmic Surg. 1992;23:453-8.
2. Lois N, Kowal VO, Cohen EJ, Rapuano CJ, Gault JA, Raber IM, et al. Indications for penetrating keratoplasty and associated procedures, 1989-1995. Cornea. 1997;16:623-9.
3. Cheng YYY, Tahzib NG, van Rij G, van Cleynenbreugel H, Pels E, Hendrikse F, Nuijts RMMA. Femtosecond laser-assisted inverted mushroom keratoplasty. Cornea. 2008;27:679-85.
4. McAllum P, Kaiserman I, Bahar I, Rootman D. Femtosecond laser top hat penetrating keratoplasty: wound burst pressures of incomplete cuts. Arch Ophthalmol. 2008;126:822-5.
5. Bahar I, Kaiserman I, McAllum P, Rootman D. Femtosecond laser-assisted penetrating keratoplasty;stability evaluation of different wound configurations. Cornea. 2008;27:209-1.
6. Price FW Jr, Price MO. Femtosecond laser shaped penetrating keratoplasty: one-year results utilizing a top-hat configuration. Am J Ophthalmol. 2008;145:210-4.
7. Steinert RF, Ignacio TS, Sarayba MA. "Top hat"-shaped penetrating keratoplasty using the femtosecond laser. Am J Ophthalmol. 2007;143:689-91.
8. Ignacio TS, Nguyen TB, Chuck RS, Kurtz RM, Sarayba MA. Top hat wound configuration for penetrating keratoplasty using the femtosecond laser; a laboratory model. Cornea. 2006;25: 336-40.
9. Soong HK, Meyer RF, Sugar A. Techniques of posterior chamber lens implantation without capsular support during penetrating keratoplasty: a review. Refract Corneal Surg. 1989;5: 249-55.
10. Koçak-Altintas AG, Koçak-Midillioglu I, Dengisik F, Duman S. Implantation of scleral-sutured posterior chamber intraocular lenses during penetrating keratoplasty. J Refract Surg. 2000;16: 456-8.
11. Busin M, Brauweiler P, Böker T, Spitznas M. Complications of sulcus-supported intraocular lenses with iris sutures, implanted during penetrating keratoplasty after intracapsular cataract extraction. Ophthalmology. 1990;97:401-5; discussion by RF Meyer, 405-6.
12. Manabe S-I, Oh H, Amino K, Hata N, Yamakawa R. Ultrasound biomicroscopic analysis of posterior chamber intraocular lenses with transscleral sulcus suture. Ophthalmology. 2000;107: 2172-8.

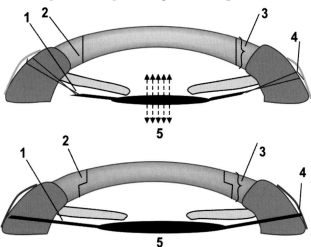

FIGURE 5: Diagram showing biomechanical and kinetic properties of manual keratoplasty with transscleral suture-fixated PC-IOL (TSF IOL) (top) and femtosecond-assisted keratoplasty (FAK) with glued IOL (bottom). Differences between the 2 approaches are indicated by the points. Point 1, top: Haptic-suture junction in the TSF IOL, with the IOL hanging like a hammock. Point 1, bottom: Rigid PMMA haptic in glued IOL fixated with the sclera. Point 2, top: Transverse graft-host junction. Point 2, bottom: More stable top-hat configuration. Point 3, top: Size of epithelial side (outer cut) same as that of endothelial side (inner cut). Point 3, bottom: Size of epithelial side (outer cut) less than that of endothelial side (inner cut), leading to greater number of endothelial cells for smaller epithelial load and placement of sutures farther from limbus. Point 4, top: Knots in TSF IOL may degrade and slip. Point 4, bottom: Haptic is securely tucked and sealed with fibrin glue in glued IOL. Point 5, top: More pseudophacodonesis with TSF IOL. Point 5, bottom: Less pseudophacodonesis with glued IOL

13. Buckley EG. Safety of transscleral-sutured intraocular lenses in children. J AAPOS. 2008;12:431-9.

14. Asadi R, Kheirkhah A. Long-term results of scleral fixation of posterior chamber intraocular lenses in children. Ophthalmology. 2008;115:67-72.

15. Vote BJ, Tranos P, Bunce C, Charteris DG, Da Cruz L. Longterm outcome of combined pars plana vitrectomy and scleral fixated sutured posterior chamber intraocular lens implantation. Am J Ophthalmol. 2006;141:308-12.

16. Güell JL, Barrera A, Manero F. A review of suturing techniques for posterior chamber lenses. Curr Opin Ophthalmol. 2004;15: 44-50.

17. Hannush SB. Sutured posterior chamber intraocular lenses: indications and procedure. Curr Opin Ophthalmol. 2000; 11:233-40.

18. Agarwal A, Kumar DA, Jacob S, Baid C, Agarwal A, Srinivasan S. Fibrin glue-assisted sutureless posterior chamber intraocular lens implantation in eyes with deficient posterior capsules. J Cataract Refract Surg. 2008;34:1433-8.

Endothelial Keratoplasty with Glued IOL

Soosan Jacob, Gaurav Prakash, Amar Agarwal

Introduction

Suture fixated IOLs tend to simulate the crystalline lens-bag-zonule complex, which due to its 360 degree attachment to the ciliary area, is a trampoline like structure **(Figures 1A to D).** However, the prolene sutures (2 or 4, depending on the technique) rather act as a hammock, which provides lesser torsional stability than the natural state. We used the glued IOL technique with DSAEK[1] in cases with aphakic corneal decompensation with good results.[2] The same technique has also been used in cases of aphakia (as a secondary

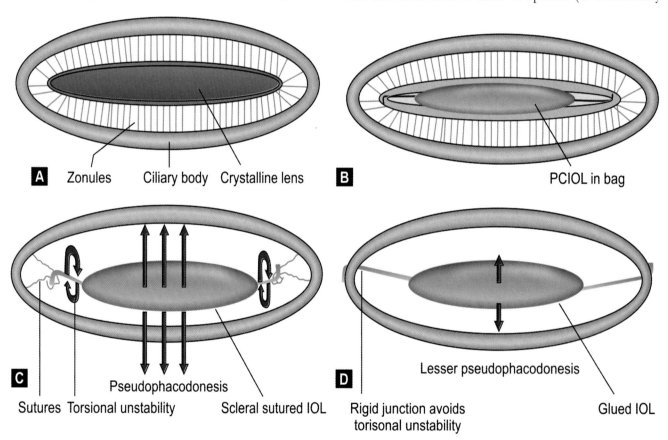

A Zonules Ciliary body Crystalline lens **B** PCIOL in bag

C Pseudophacodonesis **D** Lesser pseudophacodonesis

Sutures Torsional unstability Scleral sutured IOL Rigid junction avoids torisonal unstability Glued IOL

FIGURES 1A TO D: Schematic diagrams showing:
A. Normal trampoline line arrangement of ciliary body, zonules and crystalline lens in a normal eye
B. The change in the case of a pseudophakic eye with an in-the-bag IOL
C. The situation in the case of a pseudophakic eye with an sutured scleral fixated IOL: increased torsional unstability and increased pseudophacodonesis due to ciliary body-suture-haptic attachment
D. The situation in the case of a pseudophakic eye with an glued IOL: reduced torsional unstability and lesser pseudophacodonesis due to rigid ciliary body-haptic-optic attachment

IOL) as well as in cases requiring full thickness keratoplasty. In our experience of DSAEK with glued IOL, there has been no incidence of donor dislocation into the posterior segment. We feel the difference from sutured secondary posterior chamber IOL lies in the rigid, non-elastic attachment of the IOL to the ciliary area with the glued IOL technique. This reduces the torsional and oscillatory freedom of the implant because the resultant IOL-haptic-ciliary body complex is more stable than the IOL-haptic-suture-ciliary body complex of the suture fixated IOLs **(Figures 1A to D)**. This same biomechanical model is the reason for lesser pseudophacodonesis seen after glued IOL in comparison to suture fixated IOLs.[3,4] The learning curve for the glued IOL procedure is fairly simple for most anterior segment surgeons and the detailed steps for the combination surgery have been provided in literature.[2] Other authors have also noted the disastrous complications of the donor lenticule falling into the vitreous in aphakic eyes.[5,6] The placement of glued IOL *in situ* before placement of the lenticule compartmentalizes the aphakic eye from a unicameral to bicameral environment. This will produce lesser instability in the anterior segment and will also act as a rigid barrier preventing the donor lenticule from falling into the vitreous.

DSAEK with AC IOL vs Glued IOL

Descemet stripping automated endothelial keratoplasty (DSAEK) has emerged as the surgical treatment of choice for endothelial decompensation in the recent years since Gerrit Melles started endothelial keratoplasty. The advantages include early rehabilitation, lesser number of sutures, and decreased-risk of graft rejection compared with fullthickness penetrating keratoplasty. Performing DSAEK along with intraocular lens (IOL) implantation in a case of aphakic corneal decompensation can be challenging. An essential prerequisite for DSAEK is a normal anterior chamber (AC) volume and minimal anterior synechia for better surgical manipulation, which is often not the case with an anterior chamber IOL (AC IOL). Limited AC space, a potential IOL-endothelium touch, difficult tissue handling, and air bubble management are reasons to conclude that exchanging a pre-implanted AC IOL with a posterior chamber IOL while undergoing DSAEK could be more beneficial. This also makes an AC IOL unsuitable for a primary combined endothelial keratoplasty—IOL implant procedure.

A posterior chamber-fixated lens, like a transscleral fixated IOL, may be the solution in such a scenario, ensuring that the AC volume is not compromised, leading to easier surgical maneuverability with the donor lenticule inside the chamber and chances of better postoperative anatomical results. "Glued IOL" is a new sutureless technique of transscleral haptic-fixated posterior chamber IOL implantation. It involves exteriorization of the haptics under partial thickness scleral flaps. The haptics are intrasclerally tucked for additional stability. These flaps are later sealed with fibrin glue, which holds the flap till they adhere by fibrosis (2-3 weeks). Therefore, unlike a suture-fixated IOL (SFIOL), there are no sutures, and the haptics act as points of attachment with the sclera. Glued IOL has been used previously in multiple situations including surgical aphakia, traumatic phacocele, dislocated IOL in bag, and in combination with femtosecond-assisted keratoplasty.

Surgical Technique of DSAEK with Glued IOL

An infusion cannula is placed via a sclerotomy in the inferonasal area. Limited conjunctival peritomy is done. Two 2.5 × 2.5 mm areas are marked on the sclera at the temporal and nasal areas 180 degrees apart. Two partial-thickness limbal based scleral flaps are created **(Figure 2A)**. Center of the cornea and limits of Descemet stripping are marked with a marking pen and an 8.5 mm blunt trephine, respectively, to facilitate the Descemet stripping and donor placement **(Figure 2B)**. A 5.5 mm long partial-thickness scleral incision is made 1 mm from the limbus, and lamellar dissection is done to stop short of entry into the AC. Two straight sclerotomies, one slightly inferior to the other, are made with a 20-gauge needle 1.0 mm from the limbus under the existing scleral flaps. The positions of the flaps are chosen to facilitate the exteriorization and tucking process. AC entry is done from the superior limbal incision, and trypan blue dye is injected to stain the endothelium. Descemet membrane is scored and stripped using a bent 26G needle and a reverse Sinskey hook, respectively **(Figure 2C)**. Limited anterior vitrectomy is performed to clear any vitreous strands.

A posterior chamber 3-piece IOL is used. They have an optic diameter of 6 mm and overall length of 13 mm. It is held with a McPherson forceps at the scleral entry with one haptic into the AC. An end-gripping 23-gauge microcapsulorhexis forceps (Micro

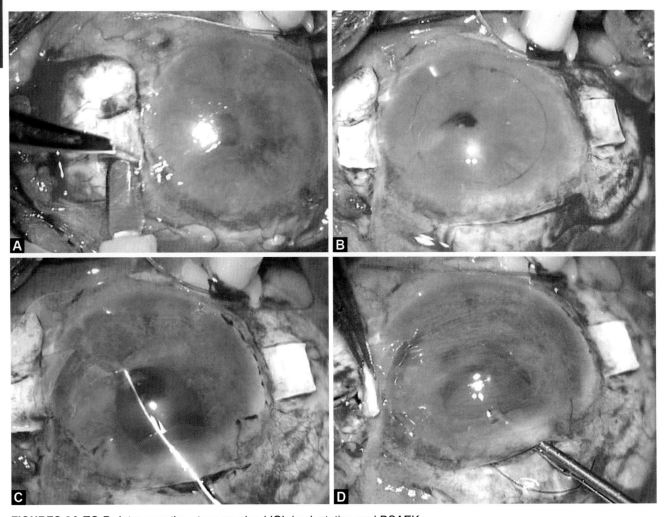

FIGURES 2A TO D: Intraoperative steps on glued IOL implantation and DSAEK

A. Partial-thickness limbal-based scleral flap of 2.5 mm × 2.5 mm is created after limited peritomy and placement of infusion cannula. A similar flap is created on the complementary side

B. After both the flaps are made, the cornea is marked with a marking pen at the center of the corneal dome and an 8.5 mm blunt trephine is used to mark the area concentric to this mark to facilitate in Descemet scoring and stripping

C. After Descemet scoring, the Descemet is being stripped with a reverse Sinskey hook

D. The IOL is held with McPherson forceps and inserted through the scleral incision. The leading haptic is grasped with a microcapsulorhexis forceps

Surgical Technology, Redmond, WA) is passed through the sclerotomy with the other hand. The tip of the leading haptic is grasped with the microcapsulorhexis forceps **(Figure 2D)**. The haptic is then pulled by the microcapsulorhexis forceps through the inferior sclerotomy following the haptic curve. The haptic is then externalized under the inferior scleral flap. The trailing haptic is also externalized through the superior sclerotomy under the scleral flap **(Figure 3A)**. After both haptics have been externalized, a 26-gauge needle is used to make a scleral pocket along the curve of the externalized haptic at the edge of the scleral bed of the

flap. The haptic is tucked into this pocket **(Figure 3B)**. A similar pocket is created in the complementary area on the other side, and tucking is performed.

The donor lenticule is gently lifted from the corneal button. A drop of viscoelastic is placed on the endothelial side, and the donor lenticule is folded in a 40-60 fashion. It is held gently with a noncrushing forceps and is inserted into the AC **(Figure 3C)**. The donor lenticule is unfolded by injecting saline **(Figure 3D)**. Air is injected to fill the AC and achieve tamponade for 10 minutes. Meanwhile, the scleral incision is sutured with 10-0 monofilament nylon

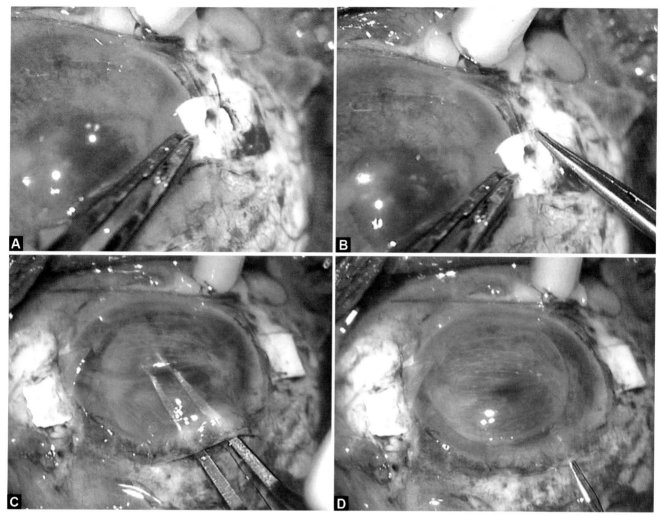

FIGURES 3A TO D: Intraoperative steps on glued IOL implantation and DSAEK
A. The trailing haptic is exteriorized via the sclerotomy
B. The trailing haptic is tucked into the intrascleral lamellar pocket
C. The donor lenticule is inserted into the eye
D. The donor lenticule is unfolded with saline injection and adjusted

(MFN), and the lamellar scleral flaps for the haptics are apposed with fibrin glue **(Figure 4).** The conjunctiva is also closed with the fibrin glue. Donor lenticule stability is confirmed before patching the eye.

DMEK with Glued IOL

Descemet's membrane is a vital layer of the cornea and any damage to the endothelial cells can lead to endothelial decompensation. This can occur primarily as part of Fuch's syndrome or secondary to surgical trauma. The most common cause of surgical trauma is cataract surgery and consequent aphakic or pseudophakic bullous keratopathy. Though many of the patients with

pseudophakic bullous keratopathy do have the IOL well placed in the bag or sulcus, one often also comes across a number of patients who have had complicated eye surgery resulting in insufficient capsular support and inability to place an in-the-bag or sulcus supported IOL. These patients are most commonly variably implanted with an anterior chamber intraocular lens (AC IOL), a sutured scleral fixated IOL (SFIOL) or are left aphakic. Another rarer presentation is when the Posterior Chamber IOL (PC IOL) has been placed in the anterior chamber (AC) either accidentally or intentionally resulting in consequent corneal decompensation. Patients with an AC IOL or a PC IOL in the AC or aphakic patients with bullous keratopathy need secondary IOL

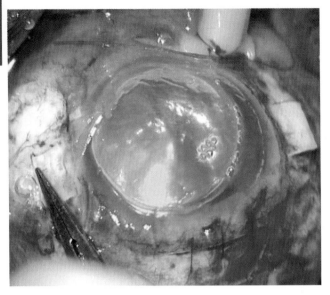

FIGURE 4: Air is injected into the AC to fix the donor lenticule. Fibrin glue is used to seal the scleral flaps

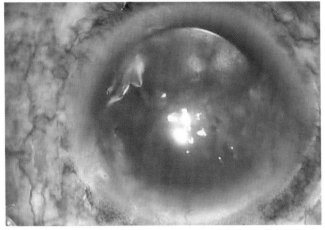

FIGURE 5: Preoperative pseudophakic bullous keratopathy. Note: PC IOL implanted in the AC

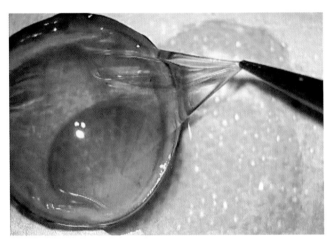

FIGURE 6: Descemet's membrane endothelial keratoplasty (DMEK) graft being prepared

implantation combined with corneal transplantation in the form of penetrating or lamellar keratoplasty. DMEK was first described by Gerrit Melles. We described Glued IOL first in 2007. We also now perform Descemet's membrane endothelial keratoplasty (DMEK) combined with secondary IOL implantation using the Glued IOL technique.

Surgical Technique of DMEK with Glued IOL

Patients are there with pseudophakic bullous keratopathy who require DMEK **(Figure 5)**. The basic technique consists of preparing the donor graft by partially trephining it and then using the Sinskey hook to lift up the edge of the cut Descemet's membrane. Once an adequate edge is lifted, a non-toothed forceps is used to gently grab the Descemet's membrane at its very edge and the graft is separated from the underlying stroma in a capsulorhexis-like circumferential manner **(Figure 6)**. It is then stained with trypan blue and replaced in the sterile corneal storage medium while the recipient eye is prepared.

An anterior chamber maintainer is inserted and two points are marked on the sclera exactly 180 degrees apart. Two 2.5 mm × 2.5 mm lamellar scleral flaps are created on either side centered on the marks. Trypan blue is used to stain the patient's Descemet's membrane before scoring and stripping it from approximately 8.5 mm diameter (as marked from above the corneal

surface) using a reverse Sinskey hook. A 20-gauge needle is used to create a sclerotomy about 1 to 1.5 mm from the limbus under each scleral flap and a 23-gauge vitrector introduced through the sclerotomy to perform anterior vitrectomy. In case of PC IOL in the AC **(Figure 5)**, it is repositioned in a closed globe manner by exteriorizing its haptics through the sclerotomies **(Figures 7A and B)**. In case of AC IOL, it is explanted and a new IOL is implanted by performing the conventional glued IOL technique. In aphakic eyes, a foldable IOL is injected into the AC and its haptics are exteriorized through the sclerotomy. In all situations, once both haptics are exteriorized, the Scharioth tuck is employed to tuck them into scleral tunnels made at the edge of the scleral flaps using a 26-gauge needle. Intracameral pilocarpine is then used to constrict the pupil and, if necessary, a pupilloplasty is performed.

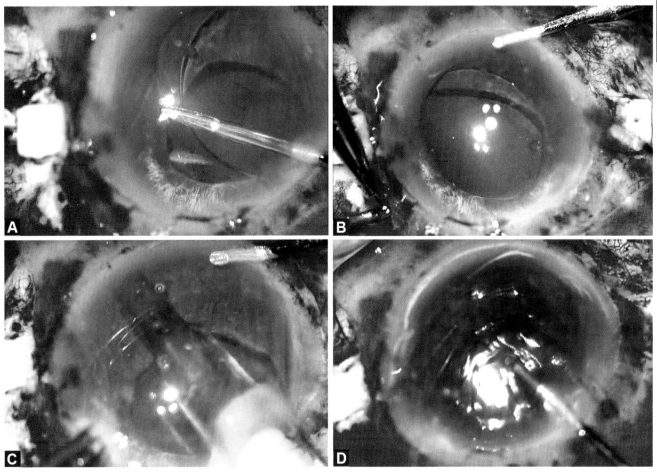

FIGURES 7A TO D: DMEK with glued IOL

A. PCIOL implanted in AC leading to corneal decompensation. The same PCIOL is being relocated into the posterior chamber using a closed globe glued IOL technique. The haptic is grabbed from over the iris using an end gripping MST forceps (Microsurgical Technology, USA) and using a handshake technique is transferred between the two hands till the tip of the haptic is held

B. The haptic is exteriorized through the sclerotomy made under the scleral flap. The same procedure is followed for the second haptic too which is exteriorized through a sclerotomy under a second scleral flap created 180 degrees away from the first. Each haptic is then tucked into a scleral tunnel created at the edge of the scleral flap

C. The DMEK graft loaded in a Staar ICL injector is injected into the anterior chamber

D. The DMEK graft is unrolled and an air bubble is used to appose it against the overlying stroma

The graft is then carefully loaded into a Staar ICL injector with the cartridge tip held occluded with a finger. It is then injected gently into the anterior chamber by plunging the soft tipped injector, taking care not to fold the graft **(Figure 7C)**. Wound-assisted implantation is avoided and the ACM flow is titrated carefully to prevent backflow and extrusion of the graft through the incision. The graft orientation is then checked and it is unfolded gently using a small air bubble as described by Melles. Once unfolded, an adequately tight air bubble is injected under the graft to float it up against the stroma **(Figure 7D)**. Fibrin glue (Tiessel, Baxter, USA) is finally used to seal the lamellar scleral flaps, conjunctiva and the clear corneal incisions.

Discussion

In cases with aphakia, loss of bicamerality of the eye because of absence of an iris-lens diaphragm is seen. This leads to poor tamponade effect and posterior migration of the injected air. A disastrous complication of the same can be dislocation of the lenticule into the vitreous cavity.[1] These problems are solved when combining endothelial keratoplasty with a glued IOL.

This technique (Endothelial keratoplasty with glued IOL) combines the advantages of stable fixation of the IOL as well as the advantages of lamellar keratoplasty. In contrast, an AC IOL has the disadvantage of decreased IOL-endothelial distance which can cause a long term graft failure when combined with PK. It becomes especially disadvantageous when combined with Descemet's stripping endothelial keratoplasty (DSEK) where the endothelium with donor stroma also occupies space within the anterior chamber, thereby bringing the anterior surface of the AC IOL very close to the DSEK lenticule. Hence, the need for these patients is explantation of the AC IOL with secondary IOL fixation and corneal transplantation.

Sutured scleral fixated IOLs can be combined with endothelial keratoplasty but they have the disadvantage of a longer open-sky period making it more vulnerable to potential complications such as expulsive hemorrhage. There is also more pseudophakodonesis associated with sutured IOLs as the fixation to the sclera is via sutures at two points whereas in the Glued IOL technique, the haptic of the IOL itself is anchored to the sclera along a significant portion of its length. This stability of the glued IOL can, in our opinion, lead to a decreased rate of graft dislocation as compared to a sutured scleral fixated IOL which has more intraocular mobility. The glued IOL also offers the ability to adjust the centration of the IOL at any time during surgery by simply adjusting the degree of tuck of the haptics into the scleral tunnel unlike the longer and more tedious procedure that would be required to recenter a decentered sutured scleral fixated IOL. All suture related complications such as erosion, degradation, and exposure are also done away with. The fibrin glue seals the flaps hermetically over the haptics and makes the procedure safe. Another problem in endothelial keratoplasty in aphakic eyes with deficient capsules is the chance of the graft falling into the vitreous. This is avoided with the combination of DMEK with the glued IOL technique.

Conclusion

A rigid compartmentalization of an aphakic eye by glued IOL can reduce donor lenticule dislocation into the vitreous after endothelial keratoplasty.

References

1. Afshari NA, Gorovoy MS, Yoo SH, Kim T, Carlson AN, Rosenwasser GO, et al. Dislocation of the Donor Graft to the Posterior Segment in Descemet Stripping Automated Endothelial Keratoplasty. Am J Ophthalmol. 2011 Nov 19. [Epub ahead of print].
2. Prakash G, Agarwal A, Jacob S, Kumar DA, Chaudhary P, Agarwal A. Femtosecond-assisted Descemet stripping automated endothelial keratoplasty with fibrin glue-assisted sutureless posterior chamber lens implantation. Cornea. 2010;29(11):1315-9.
3. Prakash G, Jacob S, Ashok Kumar D, Narsimhan S, Agarwal A, Agarwal A. Femtosecond-assisted keratoplasty with fibrin glue-assisted sutureless posterior chamber lens implantation: new triple procedure. J Cataract Refract Surg. 2009;35(6):973-9.
4. Kumar DA, Agarwal A, Prakash G, Jacob S, Saravanan Y, Agarwal A. Glued posterior chamber IOL in eyes with deficient capsular support: a retrospective analysis of 1-year post-operative outcomes. Eye (Lond). 2010;24(7):1143-8.
5. Singh A, Gupta A, Stewart JM. Posterior dislocation of descemet stripping automated endothelial keratoplasty graft can lead to retinal detachment. Cornea. 2010 ;29(11):1284-6.
6. Grueterich M, Messmer E, Kampik A. Posterior lamellar disc dislocation into the vitreous cavity during descemet stripping automated endothelial keratoplasty. Cornea. 2009;28(1): 93-6.

18 | Anterior Segment Transplantation

Soosan Jacob, Amar Agarwal

Introduction

Extensive anterior segment pathologies such as anterior staphyloma are challenging entities. An anterior staphyloma is characterized by diffuse corneal involvement and cicatrization of the uveal tissue along with high intraocular pressures resulting in a large ectatic area. Multiple causative factors have been noted in literature, the common ones being keratitis and congenital malformations, with sporadic reports of disorders like neurofibromatosis and sarcoidosis.[1-12]

The surgical options for anterior staphyloma and similar diffuse corneal lesions include conventional keratoplasty, overlay grafts, and partial or full thickness sclerokeratoplasty.[1,2,7,13-17] However, anterior staphyloma is often associated with additional problems other than corneal ectasia. The lens may be cataractous with compromised zonules that has to be addressed at the time of surgery. In addition, staphylectomy invariably leads to loss of iris tissue creating an iatrogenic aniridia. Therefore, an ideal transplant for an anterior staphyloma or similar diffuse anterior pathology should also resolve these issues.

Anterior Segment Transplantation

Biosynthetic implants hold a niche in ophthalmology, and are used in special circumstances with unique indications. A Boston keratoprosthesis, for example, is implanted in cases with very poor prognosis for conventional keratoplasty and combines the biointegration of corneal tissue and the optical clarity of the polymethyl methacrylate cylinder.[18-21] Another commonly used biosynthetic implant is the glaucoma valve with a scleral/fascia lata patch which reduces extrusion rates.[22-24] The biosynthetic graft described in this report in the treatment of anterior staphyloma, transplants a cornea and scleral rim as the biologic tissue, and

simulates the iris and lens with the help of an aniridia IOL. The surgical technique described herein combines sclerokeratoplasty, aniridia implant, and fibrin glue-assisted transscleral intraocular lens fixation, all three of which have their unique advantages and complement each other.[1,13,15,25-40]

This concept of anterior segment transplantation was conceptualized by one of us (SJ).[41]

Surgical Technique

Under general anesthesia, the maximum horizontal and vertical diameters of the staphyloma at its base were measured **(Figures 1A and B)**. This served as a measure of the intended size of the graft.

Assembly of the Graft

It consisted of two parts. The biological part was fashioned out of a cadaveric whole globe and the synthetic part consisted of an aniridia intraocular lens (IOL). We used the IOL style ANI5 (Intraocular Care, Gujarat, India) aniridia implant. It had an overall diameter of 12.75 mm, an optic diameter of 5 mm (clear optic zone)/9.5 mm (opaque annulus) and power of + 24.5 diopter.

A 3 mm by 2.5 mm area on the sclera was marked 180 degrees apart in the horizontal axis. A partial thickness limbal-based scleral flap was created up to the limbus **(Figures 2A to C)**. A similar flap was made 180 degrees apart. Two straight sclerotomies were created with a 20-gauge needle 1.5 mm from the limbus under the existing scleral flaps. After this, a scleral incision was made at the premarked area, and it was extended gradually along the preplaced marks with a corneoscleral scissor. The dissection was carried out so as to create a plane between the uveal tissue and the sclera. Once, the entire 360-degree dissection was

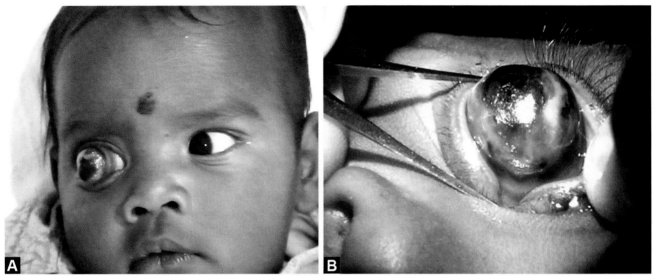

FIGURES 1A AND B: 5-month-old child with anterior staphyloma
A. Side profile view of the anterior staphyloma of the right eye
B. Measurement of the horizontal extent of the staphyloma

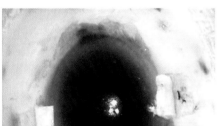 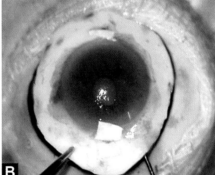 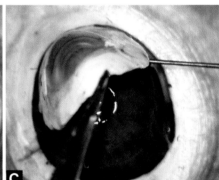

FIGURES 2A TO C: Donor preparation
A. Partial thickness scleral flaps made
B. A small incision extended from the premarked area
C. The dissection completed to create a plane between the uvea and the sclera. Cyclodialysis induced by a blunt rod to complete the separation. The corneoscleral button removed from the donor

completed, a cyclodialysis was induced to separate the uveal tissue from the dissected corneoscleral button. After completion of cyclodialysis, the corneoscleral button was removed from the globe. The corneoscleral graft was placed concave side up (endothelial side up), and the endothelial surface was coated with viscoelastic.

The aniridia IOL was held with the McPherson's forceps in one hand **(Figures 3A to C)**. An end-gripping 25-gauge microrhexis forceps (Micro Surgical Technology, Redmond, WA) was passed through the sclerotomy incision of the right side with the other hand. The tip of the leading haptic was grasped with the microrhexis forceps and externalized by pulling out through the sclerotomy after the curve of the haptic. The other haptic was also externalized through the diametrically opposite sclerotomy under the scleral flap. The biosynthetic assembly was thus completed and gently flipped to convex side up position and kept in a bowl of McCarey-Kaufman medium. The externalized haptics were directly visible now, and they were adjusted slightly to maintain IOL centration. The biosynthetic assembly thus consisted of donor cornea and sclera and a simulated iris and lens (Aniridia IOL).

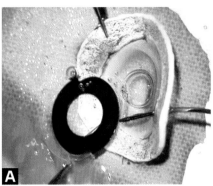 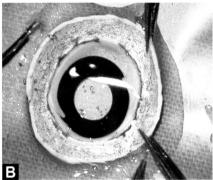 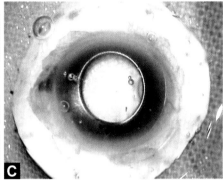

FIGURES 3A TO C: Preparation of the biosynthetic graft

A. The Aniridia IOL held near the concave side. Note that the endothelium has been coated with viscoelastic to prevent any inadvertent damage. One haptic externalized via the sclerotomies in the scleral flap
B. Similar externalization done for the other haptic
C. The complete assembly simulating an anterior segment: corneoscleral button with a transsclerally externalized haptics of Aniridia IOL

Host Dissection

A Flieringa scleral fixation ring was sutured to the recipient eye. A small incision was created in the staphylomatous cornea and the globe was decompressed by controlled aqueous drainage. The incision was enlarged using a Vannas' scissors **(Figures 4A and B)** and extended 360 degrees with a corneoscleral scissors ensuring that the dissection removed the entire staphylomatous area. A cataractous lens with compromised zonules was found. It was removed by open-sky lensectomy, leaving behind an intact posterior capsule.

Donor-Host Suturing

The graft was now placed on the host and one cardinal 8 '0' monofilament nylon (MFN) suture was placed to secure it at the graft-host junction. The donor scleral rim was now trimmed by free hand dissection to match the host size **(Figures 5A and B)**. The graft-host junction was secured with interrupted 8 '0' MFN sutures. Vitrector-assisted posterior capsulectomy and anterior vitrectomy were performed to clear the visual axis of any potential future obscuration because of posterior capsular opacity. The remaining 8 '0' MFN sutures were applied.

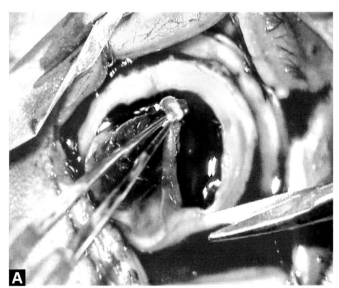 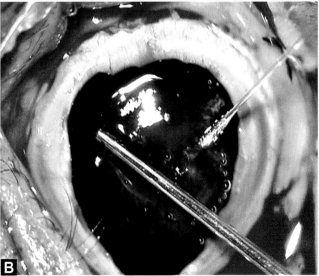

FIGURES 4A AND B: Host preparation

A. A small incision extended from the initial area of decompression. Staphylomatous area completely dissected
B. Open-sky lensectomy performed. An intact posterior capsule left behind

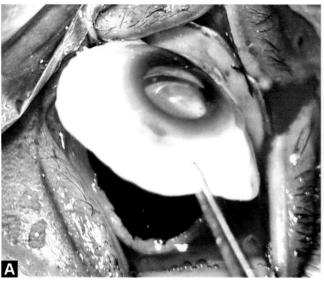 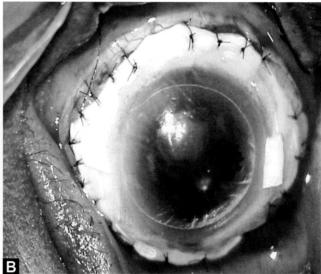

FIGURES 5A AND B: Graft-host suturing
A. Free hand dissection to trim the donor graft
B. 8-0 Monofilament nylon sutures to appose the graft. Note the well exposed scleral bed and externalized haptic under the everted flap. Then vitrector assisted capsulectomy and limited anterior vitrectomy to remove any possible vitreous strands is done

Haptic Tuck and Glue

IOL centration was reconfirmed by adjusting the amount of exteriorization of the haptics on both sides. Then, a scleral tunnel was created in the host along the curve of the exteriorized haptic at the edge of the scleral bed of the flap with a curved 26-gauge needle. The haptic was grasped with McPherson's forceps and nudged into the scleral tunnel **(Figures 6A to D)**. The haptic was tucked into this tunnel. A similar tunnel was created in the complementary area on the other side and tucking of the haptic was performed. Fibrin glue (Tisseel, Baxter, IL) was reconstituted from a pack containing freeze-dried human fibrinogen, freeze-dried human thrombin and aprotinin solution. The reconstituted fibrin glue was injected through the cannula of the syringe delivery system under the medial and lateral scleral flaps. Local pressure was applied to the flaps of the graft for 30 sec to allow for polypeptide formation and flap adhesion. The IOL was found to be well centered, and the flaps were well apposed. The host conjunctiva was advanced to cover the suture line and was apposed near the donor cornea with fibrin glue.

Postoperative Follow-up

On the first postoperative day, the child was following light with the operated eye and lid closure and cosmesis were markedly improved **(Figures 7A and B)** compared with the preoperative status. Previously, the child was unable to close the eyes because of the obstructive effect of the staphyloma. After the surgery, the lid closure was complete and the intrapalpebral aperture was 8 mm (fellow eye 7 mm). On examination under anesthesia, the cornea was clear with the conjunctiva apposed, and the IOL was well centered. The child was given ocular occlusion therapy in a 1:1 protocol.

Between first and fourth month follow-up, the child was following light and reaching out for objects with the normal eye occluded. The corneal area was clear with no evidence of rejection or failure. The aniridia IOL was stable and well centered. As the aniridia IOL blocked view of the peripheral fundus, an ultrasound B scan of the posterior segment was performed and found to be within normal limits. The intraocular pressure was 12 mm Hg. Indirect ophthalmoscopy revealed a normal posterior pole with a good view. The child was asymptomatic and was performing lid and extraocular movements comfortably. At fifth month follow-up, the child was noted to have an epithelial defect, which did not respond to conservative measures. This subsequently resulted in localized graft edema. At 6 months, a nebulomacular opacity had developed in the area of the epithelial defect, which was partially obscuring the visual axis.

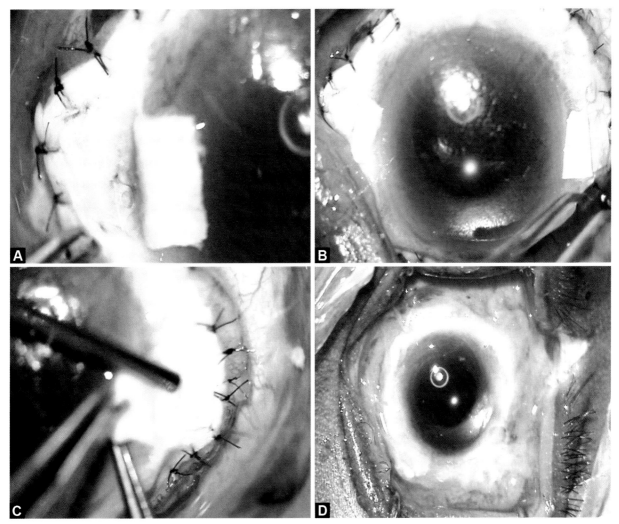

FIGURES 6A TO D: Intralamellar scleral tuck and fibrin glue assisted closure
A. The haptic grasped to tuck into the intrascleral lamellar pocket
B. The haptic in situ after intralamellar scleral tuck
C. Fibrin glue applied to the scleral bed
D. Conjunctiva closed with fibrin glue. The IOL is well centered

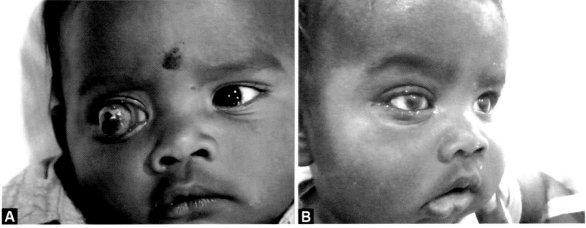

FIGURES 7A AND B
A. Preoperative face photograph.
B. Postoperative day 1 face photograph

The child subsequently had stem cell deficiency and the graft did not survive.

Conclusion

To conclude, this technique demonstrates the surgical feasibility and early postoperative outcome of this biosynthetic graft in cases with diffuse corneoscleral pathology.We did not succeed in a good result in the long term follow-up but perhaps this could be a precursor of things to come.

References

1. Panda A, Sharma N, Angra SK, Singh R. Sclerokeratoplasty versus penetrating keratoplasty in anterior staphyloma. Ophthalmic Surg Lasers. 1999;30:31-6.
2. Grieser EJ, Tuli SS, Chabi A, Schultz S, Downer D. Blueberry eye: Acquired total anterior staphyloma after a fungal corneal ulcer. Cornea. 2009;28:231-2.
3. Mullaney PB, Risco JM, Heinz GW. Congenital corneal staphyloma. Arch Ophthalmol. 1995;113:1206-7.
4. Loeffler KU. Unilateral congenital corneal staphyloma with retinal neovascularization. A case report. Graefes Arch Clin Exp Ophthalmol. 1992;230:318-23.
5. Rohrbach JM, Süsskind D, Szurman P, Siepmann K. Corneal staphyloma anterior chamber agenesia-microphakia syndrome. Klin Monatsbl Augenheilkd. 2006;223:168-75.
6. Ozdek S, Bahçeci UA, Onol M, Ezgü FS, Hasanreisoglu B. Postoperative secondary glaucoma and anterior staphyloma in a patient with homocystinuria. J Pediatr Ophthalmol Strabismus. 2005;42:243-6.
7. Miller MM, Butrus S, Hidayat A, Wei LL, Pontigo M. Corneoscleral transplantation in congenital corneal staphyloma and Peters' anomaly. Ophthalmic Genet. 2003;24:59-63.
8. Matsubara A, Ozeki H, Matsunaga N, Nozaki M, Ashikari M, Shirai S, et al. Histopathological examination of two cases of anterior staphyloma associated with Peters' anomaly and persistent hyperplastic primary vitreous. Br J Ophthalmol. 2001;85:1421-5.
9. Zaidman GW, Juechter K. Peters' anomaly associated with protruding corneal pseudo staphyloma. Cornea. 1998;17:163-8.
10. Kremer I, Gaton DD. Anterior scleral staphyloma associated with neurofibromatosis. Ann Ophthalmol. 1991;23:356-8.
11. Zeiter JH, Bhavsar A, McDermott ML, Siegel MJ. Ocular sarcoidosis manifesting as an anterior staphyloma. Am J Ophthalmol. 1991;112:345-7.
12. Bernuy A, Contreras F, Maumenee AE, O'Donnell FE Jr. Bilateral, congenital, dermis-like choristomas overlying corneal staphylomas. Arch Ophthalmol. 1981;99:1995-7.
13. Jonas JB, Rank RM, Budde WM. Tectonic sclerokeratoplasty and tectonic penetrating keratoplasty as treatment for perforated or predescemetal corneal ulcers. Am J Ophthalmol. 2001;132:14-8.
14. Esquenazi S, Shihadeh WA, Abderkader A, Kaufman HE. A new surgical technique for anterior segment ectasia: Tectonic lamellar sclerokeratoplasty. Ophthalmic Surg Lasers Imaging. 2006;37:434-6.
15. Panda A, Sharma N, Angra SK, Singh R. Therapeutic sclerokeratoplasty versus therapeutic penetrating keratoplasty in refractory corneal ulcers. Aust N Z J Ophthalmol. 1999;27: 15-9.
16. Panda A. Lamellolamellar sclerokeratoplasty. Where do we stand today? Eye. 1999;13:221-5.
17. Yalçindag FN, Celik S, Ozdemir O. Repair of anterior staphyloma with dehydrated dura mater patch graft. Ophthalmic Surg Lasers Imaging. 2008;39:3467.
18. Khan BF, Harissi-Dagher M, Khan DM, Dohlman CH. Advances in Boston keratoprosthesis: Enhancing retention and prevention of infection and inflammation. Int Ophthalmol Clin. 2007;47:61-71.
19. Ma JJ, Graney JM, Dohlman CH. Repeat penetrating keratoplasty versus the Boston keratoprosthesis in graft failure. Int Ophthalmol Clin. 2005;45:49-59.
20. Khan B, Dudenhoefer EJ, Dohlman CH. Keratoprosthesis: An update. Curr Opin Ophthalmol. 2001;12:282-7.
21. Yaghouti F, Dohlman CH. Innovations in keratoprosthesis: Proved and unproved. Int Ophthalmol Clin. 1999;39:27-36.
22. Egrilmez S, Yagci A, Ates H, Azarsiz SS, Andac K. Glaucoma implant surgery with autogenous fascia lata in scleromalacia perforans. Ophthalmic Surg Lasers Imaging. 2004;35:338-42.
23. Lam DS, Cheuk W, Lai JS. Short-term results of using Lamellar Corneoscleral patch graft for the Ahmed glaucoma valve implant surgery. Yan Ke Xue Bao. 1997;13:109-12.
24. Tanji TM, Lundy DC, Minckler DS, Heuer DK, Varma R. Fascia lata patch graft in glaucoma tube surgery. Ophthalmology. 1996;103:1309-12.
25. Schmitz K, Viestenz A, Meller D, Behrens-Baumann W, Steuhl KP. Aniridia intraocular lenses in eyes with traumatic iris defects. Ophthalmologe. 2008;105:744-52.
26. Karatza EC, Burk SE, Snyder ME, Osher RH. Outcomes of prosthetic iris implantation in patients with albinism. J Cataract Refract Surg. 2007;33:1763-9.
27. Menezo JL, Martínez-Costa R, Cisneros A, Desco MC. Implantation of iris devices in congenital and traumatic aniridias: surgery solutions and complications. Eur J Ophthalmol. 2005; 15:451-7.
28. Brown MJ, Hardten DR, Knish K. Use of the artificial iris implant in patients with aniridia. Optometry. 2005;76:157-64.
29. Mavrikakis I, Mavrikakis E, Syam PP, Bell J, Casey JH, Casswell AG, Brittain GP, Liu C. Surgical management of iris defects with prosthetic iris devices. Eye. 2005;19:205-9.
30. Hanumanthu S, Webb LA. Management of traumatic aniridia and aphakia with an iris reconstruction implant. J Cataract Refract Surg. 2003; 29:1236-8.
31. Agarwal A, Kumar DA, Jacob S, Baid C, Agarwal A, Srinivasan S. Fibrin glue-assisted sutureless posterior chamber intraocular lens implantation in eyes with deficient posterior capsules. J Cataract Refract Surg. 2008;34:1433-8.
32. Agarwal A, Kumar DA, Jacob S, Prakash G, Agarwal A. Reply: Fibrin glue assisted sutureless posterior chamber IOL implantation in eyes with deficient posterior capsules. J Cataract Refract Surg. 2009;35:795-6.
33. Prakash G, Kumar DA, Jacob S, Kumar KA, Agarwal A, Agarwal A. Anterior Segment Optical Coherence Tomography aided diagnosis and primary posterior chamber IOL implantation with fibrin glue in traumatic phacocele with scleral perforation. J Cataract Refract Surg. 2009;35:782-4.

34. Prakash G, Jacob S, Kumar DA, Narsimhan S, Agarwal A, Agarwal A. Femtosecond assisted keratoplasty with fibrin glue-assisted sutureless posterior chamber lens implantation: a new triple procedure. J Cataract Refract Surg. 2009;35: 973-9.

35. Phillips PM, Shamie N, Chen ES, Terry MA. Transscleral sulcus fixation of a small-diameter iris-diaphragm intraocular lens in combined penetrating keratoplasty and cataract extraction for correction of traumatic cataract, aniridia, and corneal scarring. J Cataract Refract Surg. 2008;34:2170-3.

36. Beltrame G, Salvetat ML, Chizzolini M, Driussi GB, Busatto P, Di Giorgio G, et al. Implantation of a black diaphragm intraocular lens in ten cases of post-traumatic aniridia. Eur J Ophthalmol. 2003;13:62-8.

37. Thompson CG, Fawzy K, Bryce IG, Noble BA. Implantation of a black diaphragm intraocular lens for traumatic aniridia. J Cataract Refract Surg. 1999;25:808-13.

38. Williams KA, Esterman AJ, Bartlett C, Holland H, Hornsby NB, Coster DJ. How effective is penetrating corneal transplantation? Factors influencing long-term outcome in multivariate analysis. Transplantation. 2006;81: 896-901.

39. Cosar CB, Laibson PR, Cohen EJ, Rapuano CJ. Topical cyclosporine in pediatric keratoplasty. Eye Contact Lens. 2003;29: 103-7.

40. Zetterstrom C, Kugelberg M. Paediatric cataract surgery. Acta Ophthalmol Scand. 2007;85:698-710.

41. Soosan J, Agarwal A, et al. Anterior Segment Transplatation Eye & Contact Lens. 2010;36:1.

19

Combined Surgical Management of Capsular and Iris Deficiency with Glued IOL: Glued Iris Prosthesis and Glued IOL with Pupilloplasty

Dhivya Ashok Kumar, Amar Agarwal

Introduction

Traumatic aniridia with combined lens injuries leading to aphakia is one of the sequelae after severe blunt trauma. Congenital aniridia with badly subluxated cataract is also not uncommon. Such conditions with iris and lens abnormalities leads to both cosmetic and an optical defect. An intact iris diaphragm is essential as it reduces the optical aberrations arising from the crystalline lens and thereby increases the depth of focus.[1,2] Thus, total aniridia is known to cause incapacitating glare and photophobia. Moreover, associated aphakia induce additional refractive problems to the existing defect. Managing both (aniridia and aphakia) together is always challenging for a cataract surgeon. Iris reconstructive implants have been implanted intracapsularly in some cases of aniridia with a capsular bag.[3] In eyes with partial aniridia, iris enclavation has been tried.[4] However, in eyes with total aniridia and aphakia, transscleral fixation was the option.[3] We managed total aniridia and aphakia with an aniridia IOL implanted with the Glued IOL technique.[5,6] We also managed partial iris defects and aphakia with Glued IOL and pupilloplasty.

Aniridia

Aniridia is an ocular condition characterized by total or partial absence of iris. It can be congenital or acquired. The exact pathogenesis of aniridia is unknown. It has been reported to be caused by a mutation in the *PAX6* gene on chromosome 11 **(Figure 1)**. Aniridia may be familial or sporadic. Acquired aniridia is due to trauma or post-surgery. Cataracts are known to occur in 50-85% of patients with congenital aniridia, usually

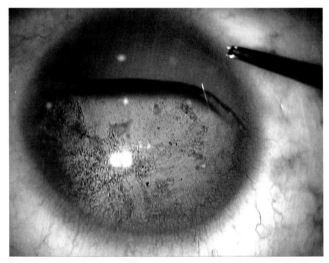

FIGURE 1: Congenital aniridia. Note the anirida, subluxated colobomatous cataract and stem cell deficiency. Patient had glaucoma also

acquired during the first 2 decades of life. Ectopia lentis, corneal defects, strabismus, nystagmus, foveal or optic nerve hypoplasia are some of the associations. Patients with aniridia typically complain of glare and photophobia. Iris prosthesis has been used as one of the surgical treatment options in these eyes to reduce the symptoms. However, in eyes with deficient posterior capsule, this is not possible. Hence, we have used our glued IOL technique in these eyes with absent or hypoplastic iris to give better cosmetic and functional outcome.[7]

Iris Prosthesis

Use of colored lens diaphragm has been reported way back in 1964. An anterior chamber lens with an optic surrounded by a colored diaphragm was initially designed by Choyce.[8] Later Reinhard et al and Sundmacher et al[9] reported implantation of a single-piece black iris diaphragm intraocular lens (IOL) for the correction of aniridia. They also showed that implantation of the black diaphragm aniridia IOL improved visual acuity in the majority of patients with a variety of endogenous problems in addition to aniridia.[10-12] Subsequently, Rosenthal reported the first use of a smaller incision artificial iris implant in the United States in 1996 in a case of iris dysgenesis. Osher and Burk[13] placed multiple/single fin Morcher (Morcher GmBH, Stuttgart, Germany) endocapsular ring type prosthesis within the capsular bag for iris reconstruction along with cataract removal. Dr Schmidt's (Intraocularlinsen GmbH, St. Augustin, Germany) foldable, biocompatible silicone artificial iris is custom-made with hand-crafted adjustment of the color, structure, and diameter of the implant. This has also been tried in eyes with iris defects. B Tanzer et al[14] implanted a black iris diaphragm in eyes with aniridia and aphakia. However, the aniridia IOL was transsclerally fixated with sutures in eyes with lens capsular deficiency. Pozdeyeva et al[15] placed the iris lens diaphragm in the ciliary sulcus and showed good results. Dong et al[16] reported transscleral suture fixation of iris prosthesis in vitrectomized eyes. Endocapsular iris prosthesis for iris defects and small incision iris prosthesis for functional and traumatic iris deficiency have also been reported.[17] In all the previous reports[14,16,18-20] of iris prosthesis implantation in eyes with deficient capsules, the iris prosthesis is transsclerally fixated with sutures.

Glued Iris Prosthesis

The glued iris prosthesis is a PMMA aniridia IOL implanted by the glued IOL technique (Figure 2). We used the OV lens Style ANI5 (Intra Ocular Care, Gujarat, India) aniridia implant. The overall diameter of the implant is about 12.75 mm. The optic has a central clear zone about 5 mm (clear optic zone) with a peripheral opaque or pigmented annulus about 9.5 mm. The haptics are also made of PMMA with acute angulations and has an eye on both haptics for prolene suture placement during transscleral fixation.

Surgical Technique of Glued Iris Prosthesis

Two partial thickness scleral flaps about 2.5 × 2.5 mm are created exactly 180 degrees diagonally apart (Figures

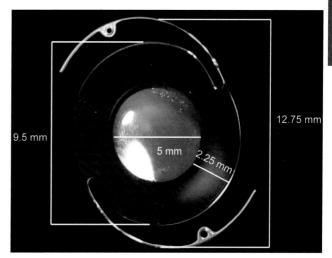

FIGURE 2: Aniridia IOL

3A to E). Infusion cannula or anterior chamber (AC) maintainer is fixed. Superior 2.8 mm entry with keratome is made and lensectomy is performed to remove the subluxated cataractous lens with a vitrectomy cutter. Anterior vitrectomy is completed to remove any vitreous traction. Two straight sclerotomies with a 20G needle are made under the existing scleral flaps. The limbal incision is enlarged with a sharp keratome or corneoscleral scissors. The PMMA aniridia implant is then introduced through the limbal incision using a McPherson forceps. An end gripping 25/23G micro-rhexis forceps (Micro Surgical Technology, Redmond, WA, USA) is passed through one of the sclerotomies to hold the tip of the haptic. The haptics are then externalized under the scleral flap. Precaution is taken during externalization as the angulation of the haptic with optic in the implant is different from the routine in-the-bag or scleral fixated IOLs. A scleral tunnel is made with a 26G needle at the point of externalization of the haptic and the haptic is tucked into the intralamellar scleral tunnel. The scleral flaps are then closed with fibrin glue (Tisseel, Baxter, USA). The infusion cannula or AC maintainer are then removed. The procedure can be performed with 23G trocar cannula infusion also. The limbal wound is closed with 10-0 monofilament nylon sutures. The conjunctiva is also apposed with the fibrin glue (Figures 4A to F). The same technique can be done in cases of acquired aniridia (Figures 5A to E).

Sutured Aniridia IOL vs Aniridia Glued IOL

Intrascleral sutureless PCIOL implantation in eyes with

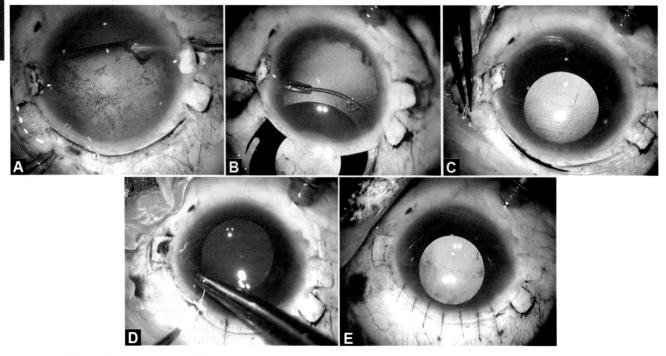

FIGURES 3A TO E: Aniridia glued IOL
A. Congenital aniridia. Note the two scleral flaps and a third flap for trabeculectomy. Lensectomy started
B. Aniridia IOL implantation and the haptic tip caught with the glued IOL forceps. Note the trocar cannula in the upper right corner for fluid infusion
C. One haptic externalized
D. Both haptics externalized and suturing of scleral tunnel being performed
E. Both haptics tucked in Scharioth pockets. Fibrin glue to be applied. One should be careful not to apply the fibrin glue in the trabeculectomy area

deficient capsule was introduced by Gabor et al.[21] We use scleral flaps to cover the haptics in the scleral tunnel and fibrin glue to create a hermetic seal unlike Gabor et al where the haptics are introduced directly into the scleral tunnel. As compared to sutured iris prosthesis, 10-0 or 9-0 prolene which is used for transcleral fixation of the prosthesis to the sclera is not used. Instead scleral tuck and fibrin glue are used for good surgical adhesion. Our earlier reports on glued IOL method[4,22,23] have shown good results with IOL centration. The limitation with aniridia IOL implantation with this method is the need for large incisions which can lead to postoperative astigmatism. Nevertheless, the technique can be performed with ease in any available aniridia IOL which has rigid haptics. Hanumanthu et al[24] reported retinal detachment after iris prosthesis. According to their report, eyes that have undergone surgery for traumatically disorganized anterior segment are likely to have an increased tendency towards proliferative postoperative inflammation. There was no sight threatening complications observed in any of the operated eyes in our case series. None of the eyes developed retinal detachment or endophthalmitis. Elevated IOP was the most common postoperative complication reported after implantation of the full sized black aniridia IOL.[12,20,25-27] However, there was only one patient with congenital aniridia who had increased IOP postoperatively and that was managed medically. Another important advantage of this technique is the prevention of suture-related complications like suture erosion, suture knot exposure or dislocation of IOL after suture disintegration or broken suture reported with sutured scleral fixated IOL. Dong[26] et al reported bullous keratopathy on a long-term in eyes with black diaphragm aniridia IOL. Posterior capsule opacification (PCO) has also been reported[27] in eyes with sulcus inserted aniridia IOL after phacoemulsification cataract surgery. However, PCO chance is absent in eyes which has undergone glued iris prosthesis since the lens is removed with the capsular bag.

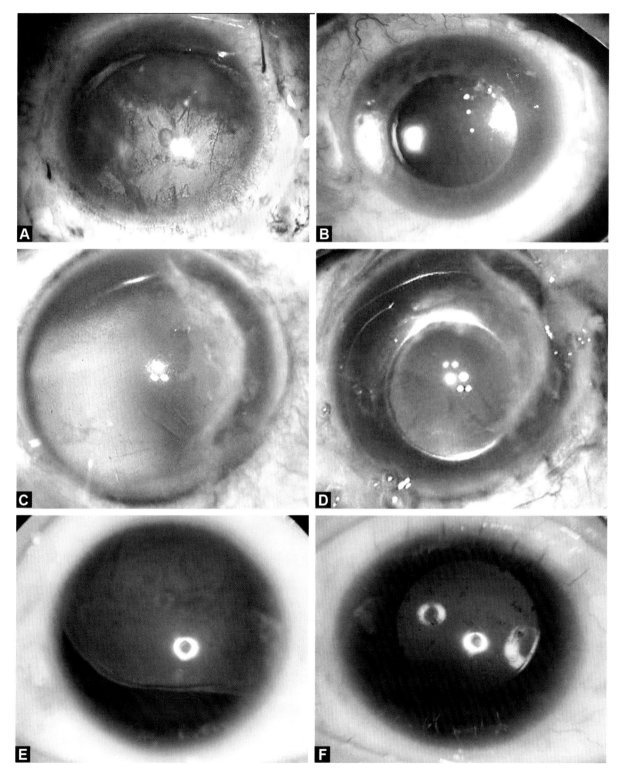

FIGURES 4A TO F: Postoperative outcome in glued iris prosthesis
A. Preoperative image of congenital aniridia with subluxated cataract
B. Postoperative outcome
C. Traumatic aniridia with aphakia
D. Postoperative image
E. Congenital aniridia with subluxated lens
F. Postoperative image of the same patient

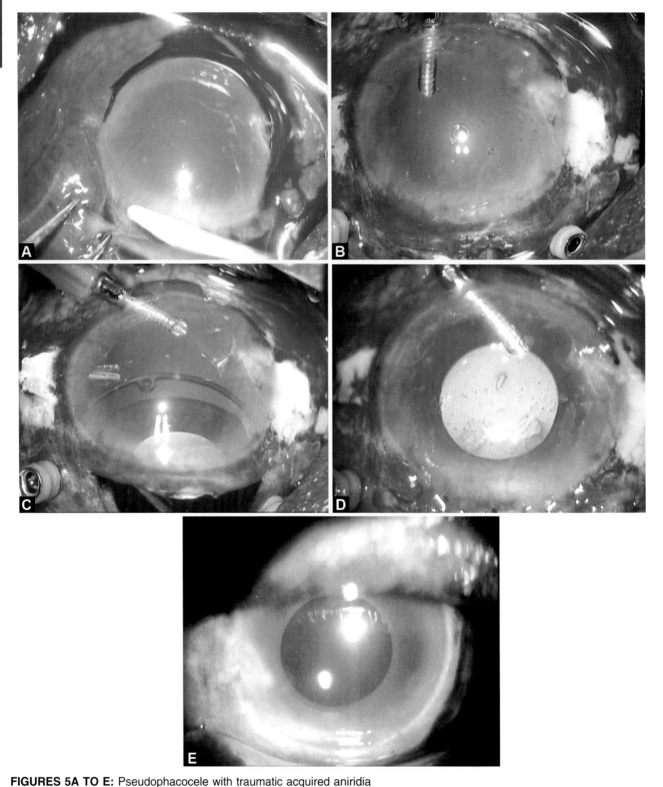

FIGURES 5A TO E: Pseudophacocele with traumatic acquired aniridia
A. Pseudophacocele. Note the PC IOL lying in the subconjunctival space on the left. Media is hazy due to the injury and vitreous hemorrhage. Vision PL +
B. PC IOL removed from the subconjunctival space. Vitreous hemorrhage cleared. Note the acquired aniridia
C. Aniridia IOL implantation
D. Both haptics tucked and glued
E. One month postoperative photo. Vision 20/30

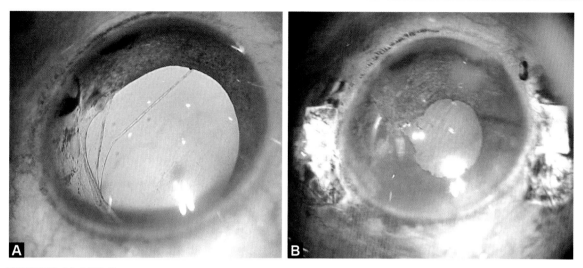

FIGURES 6A AND B

A. Clinical picture showing post-surgical aphakia with partial iris defect
B. Iridoplasty with glued IOL implantation

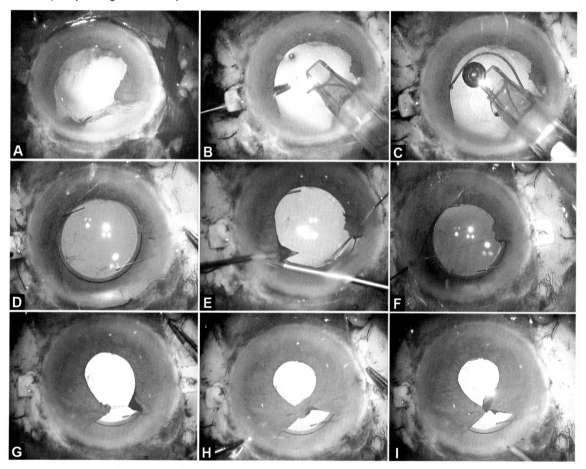

FIGURES 7A TO I: Glued IOL with iridoplasty

A. Aphakia with iris defect
C. Glued IOL forceps grasps the haptic tip
   while the IOL is injected
E. Iridoplasty started using 10 '0' prolene sutures
F. Sutures passed and knot made
H. Suture tied

B. Foldable three piece IOL in cartridge. Glued IOL
   forceps ready to grasp the haptic tip
D. Both haptics externalized then tucked in Scharioth pockets
G. Suture tying
I. Suture ends cut. Then haptics can be
   glued at the end of surgery

IOL Power Calculation

IOL power calculation is another important factor affecting visual outcome in the postoperative period. By definition, the anterior segment is malformed in aniridia, but the SRK/T formula predicts the postoperative effective lens position using constants derived from standard eyes. It is also difficult to gain accurate axial length measurements from patients who have a congenital absence of the fovea. Pre-existing nystagmus can also prevent accurate power calculation. However, Aslam et al[27] showed that biometry was reasonably accurate while implanting black iris diaphragm IOL for aniridia. Improvement in Snellen's visual acuity can be attributed to the removal of the cataract and correction of aphakia. However, patients consistently noted improvement in their quality of vision and glare disability after surgery.

Glued IOL with Pupilloplasty

In cases of glued IOL with iridoplasty **(Figures 6A and B)**, the scleral flaps are created, followed by implantation of the 3 piece foldable IOL (Sofport, Bausch & Lomb, Rochester, NY) and intrascleral tuck of haptics **(Figures 7A to D)**. The iridoplasty was then performed **(Figures 7E to I)** and finally the scleral flaps were closed with fibrin glue. All patients are prescribed topical 1% prednisolone acetate and 0.3% gatifloxacin in the postoperative period for 4 weeks. For iridoplasty, McCannel suture with Siepser slip knot technique can be used. A 10-0 polypropylene (Prolene) suture on a CIF-4 needle is passed through the iris adjacent to the edge of the pupil through limbal paracentesis incisions.

Conclusion

Operating on a traumatized or congenitally aniridic eye presents special challenges. From our results we believe that in cases with deficient capsule, implantation of glued iris prosthesis for total aniridia and glued IOL with iridoplasty for partial iris defects is a safe and effective method. We think the combined method has a useful role in anterior segment reconstruction procedures.

References

1. Thompson CG, Fawzy K, Bryce IG, Noble BA. Implantation of a black diaphragm intraocular lens for traumatic aniridia. J Cataract Refract Surg. 1999;25:808-13.
2. Shaw MW, Falls HF, Neel JV. Congenital aniridia. Am J Hum Genet. 1960;12:389-15.
3. Pozdeyeva NA, Pashtayev NP, Lukin VP, Batkov YN. Artificial iris-lens diaphragm in reconstructive surgery for aniridia and aphakia. J Cataract Refract Surg. 2005;31(9):1750-9.
4. Hanumanthu S, Webb LA. Management of traumatic aniridia and aphakia with an iris reconstruction implant. J Cataract Refract Surg. 2003;29(6):1236-8.
5. Agarwal A, Kumar DA, Jacob S, et al. Fibrin glue-assisted sutureless posterior chamber intraocular lens implantation in eyes with deficient posterior capsules. J Cataract Refract Surg. 2008;34:1433-8.
6. Prakash G, Kumar DA, Jacob S, et al. Anterior segment optical coherence tomography-aided diagnosis and primary posterior chamber intraocular lens implantation with fibrin glue in traumatic phacocele with scleral perforation. J Cataract Refract Surg. 2009;35:782-4.
7. Kumar DA, Agarwal A, Prakash G, Jacob S. Managing total aniridia with aphakia using a glued iris prosthesis. J Cataract Refract Surg. 2010;36(5):864-5.
8. Choyce P. Intraocular Lenses and Implants. London, England, HK Lewis, 1964;21.
9. Reinhard T, Sundmacher R, Althaus C. Irisblenden-IOL bei Traumatischer Aniridie. Klin Monatsbl Augenheilkd. 1994;205:196-200.
10. R Sundmacher R, Reinhard T, Althaus C. Black diaphragm intraocular lens for correction of aniridia. Ophthalmic Surg. 1994;25:180-5.
11. Sundmacher R, Reinhard T, Althaus C. Black diaphragm intraocular lens in congenital aniridia. Ger J Ophthalmol. 1994;3:197-201.
12. Reinhard T, Engelhardt S, Sundmacher R. Black diaphragm aniridia intraocular lens for congenital aniridia: long-term follow-up. J Cataract Refract Surg. 2000;26:375-81.
13. Osher RH, Burk SE. Cataract surgery combined with implantation of an artificial iris. J Cataract Refract Surg. 1999;25:1540-7.
14. Tanzer DJ, Smith RE. Black iris-diaphragm intraocular lens for aniridia and aphakia. J Cataract Refract Surg. 1999;25:1548-51.
15. Pozdeyeva NA, Pashtayev NP, Lukin VP, Batkov YN. Artificial iris-lens diaphragm in reconstructive surgery for aniridia and aphakia. J Cataract Refract Surg. 2005;31:1750-9.
16. Dong X, Yu B, Xie L. Black diaphragm intraocular lens implantation in aphakic eyes with traumatic aniridia and previous pars plana vitrectomy. J Cataract Refract Surg. 2003;29:2168-73.
17. Burk SE, Da Mata AP, Snyder ME, et al. Prosthetic iris implantation for congenital, traumatic, or functional iris deficiencies. J Cataract Refract Surg. 2001;27:1732-40.
18. Ozbek Z, Kaynak S, Zengin O. Transscleral fixation of a black diaphragm intraocular lens in severely traumatized eyes requiring vitreoretinal surgery. J Cataract Refract Surg. 2007;33:1494-8.
19. Omulecki W, Synder A. Pars plana vitrectomy and transscleral fixation of black diaphragm intraocular lens for the management of traumatic aniridia. Ophthalmic Surg Lasers. 2002;33:357-61.
20. Thompson CG, Fawzy K, Bryce IG, Noble BA. Implantation of a black diaphragm intraocular lens for traumatic aniridia. J Cataract Refract Surg. 1999;25:808-13.
21. Gabor SG, Pavlidis MM. Sutureless intrascleral posterior chamber intraocular lens fixation. J Cataract Refract Surg. 2007;33:1851-4.

22. Kumar DA, Agarwal A, Prakash G, Jacob S, Saravanan Y, Agarwal A. Glued posterior chamber IOL in eyes with deficient capsular support: a retrospective analysis of 1-year postoperative outcomes. Eye (Lond). 2010;24:1143-8.

23. Kumar DA, Agarwal A, Prakash D, Prakash G, Jacob S, Agarwal A. Glued intrascleral fixation of posterior chamber IOL in children. Am J Ophthalmol. 2011. Accepted. In press.

24. Hanumanthu S, Webb LA. Management of traumatic aniridia and aphakia with an iris reconstruction implant. J Cataract Refract Surg, 2003;29:1236-8.

25. Menezo JL, Martínez-Costa R, Cisneros A, Desco MC. Implantation of iris devices in congenital and traumatic aniridias: surgery solutions and complications. Eur J Ophthalmol. 2005; 15:451-7.

26. Dong XG, Cheng J, Xie LX. Long-term complications of black diaphragm aniridia intraocular lens implant in traumatic aniridia. Zhonghua Yan Ke Za Zhi. 2009;45:982-6.

27. Aslam SA, Wong SC, Ficker LA, MacLaren RE. Implantation of the black diaphragm intraocular lens in congenital and traumatic aniridia. Ophthalmology. 2008;115:1705-12.

20

Pediatric Glued IOL

Dhivya Ashok Kumar, Amar Agarwal

Introduction

Pediatric eyes differ from adults due to their rapid growth and significant refractive changes in early childhood. Hence, intraocular lens (IOL) implantation after cataract surgery in these eyes should be matched to the growing and changing refraction. IOL implantation in eyes with large posterior capsular rent or ectopia lentis becomes further complicated due to lack of normal capsular support. Anterior chamber (AC) IOLs or sutured scleral fixated IOLs have been performed in such cases.[1-3] Scleral fixated IOLs, by virtue of their anatomic location, offer numerous advantages over the AC IOL. Glued intrascleral fixation places a posterior chamber (PC) IOL in eyes with deficient capsules using a quick-acting surgical fibrin sealant derived from human blood plasma, with both hemostatic and adhesive properties **(Figures 1A to F).** We have performed intrascleral IOL fixation with fibrin glue (glued IOL) in adult eyes with deficient capsules in the recent past and have had encouraging results.[4-11]

IOL Implantation

The choice of IOL implantation in eyes with deficient capsules is challenging, especially in children. Childhood aphakia attributable to cataract surgery treated by contact lens or spectacle correction shows poor compliance. Hence, IOL implantation is nowadays recommended in children.[12] Anterior chamber IOL,[13,14] scleral sutured IOL,[15,16] or iris-fixated lenses[17,18] have been tried in these eyes, with variable results.

AC IOL

Anterior chamber IOL can induce recurrent uveitis, especially in a growing anterior chamber, and can cause endothelial decompensation. However, recent advances in AC IOL design have yielded lenses that provide a safe, effective alternative to sutured PC IOLs. In a study by Morrison and associates, no patients experienced corneal decompensation, increased intraocular pressure, persistent inflammation, IOL displacement, or explantation after 1 year of follow-up.[13] However, Epley and associates[19] reported corectopia, haptic migration, and pigment deposits on the lens. In eyes with pre-existing aniridia where AC IOLs cannot be implanted, glued IOL can be performed using the glued iris prosthesis.[11]

Sutured Scleral Fixated IOL

Another alternative in these eyes is the sutured scleral-fixated IOL. Transscleral suture-fixated IOL have been reported by Bardorf and associates to be safe over a 3-year period.[19] However, they claim that the surgery is more difficult to perform than capsular bag or sulcus implantation and potentially carries greater risks. Scleral fixation of PC IOL with 10-0 prolene sutures has shown long-term side effects attributable to suture degradation.[20-23] Suture inflammation, loose suture, or a broken suture can lead to malposition of the IOL. It has been shown in an ultrasound biomicroscopy study that trans-scleral suture-fixated IOL haptics are not exactly positioned in the ciliary sulcus where they are supposed to be.[24] Though short-term postoperative results after sutured scleral-fixated IOLs in pediatric eyes were encouraging, long-term risks are not totally eliminated.[1,15,16,19,25]

Glued IOL

Gabor and Pavilidis[26] introduced the intrascleral haptic fixation of a standard 3-piece PC IOL without sutures and showed good intermediate results in adults.[27] Our

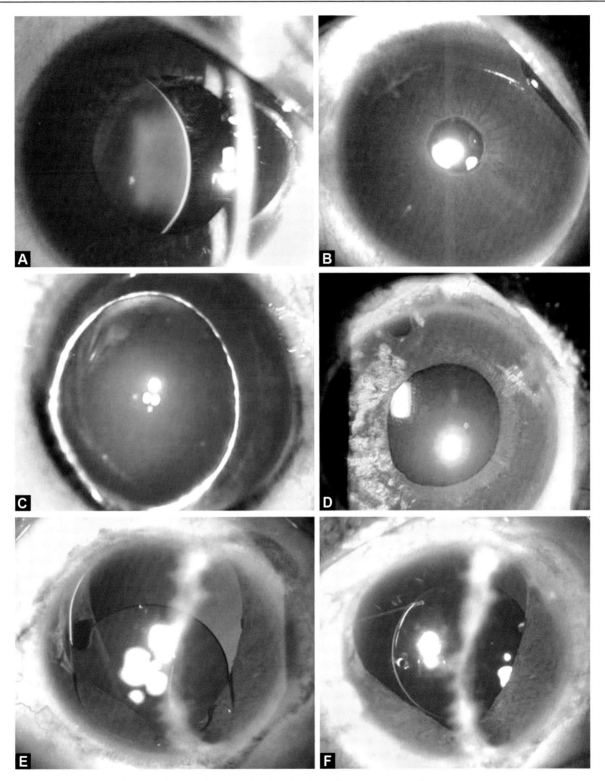

FIGURES 1A TO F: Intraocular lens (IOL) status in glued IOL follow-up in children
A. Preoperative picture of subluxated crystalline lens
B. 2-year postoperative picture
C. Preoperative clinical photograph of total subluxated lens with spherophakia
D. 3-year postoperative picture
E. Preoperative clinical photograph of decentered posterior chamber IOL
F. 2-year postoperative picture after glued IOL

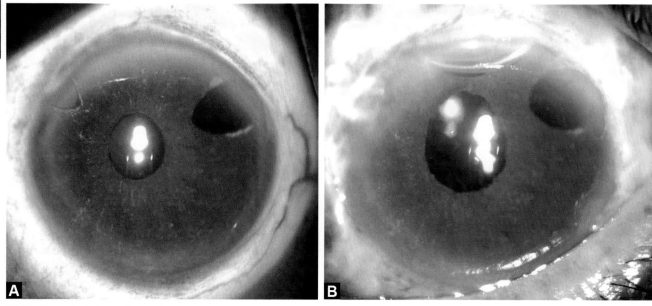

FIGURES 2A AND B: Secondary glued intraocular lens (IOL) in aphakic eye
A. Preoperative image showing aphakia with clear cornea
B. Postoperative day 1 image showing clear cornea; an air bubble is noted

technique differed from other sutureless methods by the use of fibrin glue, which enhances the rate of adhesion with hemostasis **(Figures 2A and B)**, and also by the use of available IOLs, unlike other techniques[28] that may require a new-design IOL. Needle-guided intrascleral fixation of PC IOL has also been tried in aphakia.[29] The glued IOL technique **(Figure 3)** is devoid of suture-related complications associated with sutured scleral-fixated IOLs.[30] Moreover, with foldable IOLs the chances of suture induced astigmatism are less and there is early visual rehabilitation. It also has less pseudophakodonesis as compared to IOLs sutured to the sclera with 10-0 prolene. There is no need for a new design IOL as the standard PC IOLs (rigid or foldable) can be used for this method. Ectopia lentis is another indication that poses difficulty in IOL positioning.

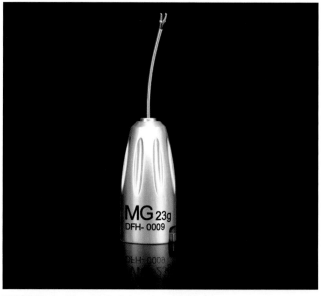

FIGURE 3: The Siebel forceps which has a ruler for rhexis can also be used as a glued IOL forceps (*Courtesy*: Larry Laks, Microsurgical Technology, MST, USA)

Pediatric Eyes

Capsular tension rings[31] (CTR) have been used in cases where zonular weakness is identified. Endocapsular ring-assisted IOL implantation tried in ectopia lentis has induced late postoperative IOL decentration. Secondary lens epithelial proliferation and capsule shrinkage are much more pronounced in young children than in adults and the chance of decentration is observed to increase.[32] Iris-fixated lenses have been tried in deficient capsular support in pediatric eyes.[17] Yen and associates reported dislocation of the iris lenses in pediatric eyes and chances of suture degradation are not eliminated.[17]

Dureau and associates tried suturing the PC IOL to the iris using 10-0 prolene; however, postoperative pupil distortion and endophthalmitis occurred.[18] In congenital aniridia with subluxated cataract where there is zonular dehiscence and deficient iris, AC or iris-fixated IOLs cannot be placed. The glued IOL technique can be easily performed in such conditions. Basti and associates[33] have shown an endothelial loss of 5.28% in pediatric eyes after endocapsular cataract extraction (ECCE) with IOL and 7.5% after primary posterior capsulotomy, anterior vitrectomy with ECCE and IOL implantation. The specular loss (range 1.3-5.94%) in our series does not differ much from the previous reports. Moreover, there was no significant corneal edema seen in the immediate postoperative period. After meticulous treatment for amblyopia, we achieved a visual acuity of 20/20 in 17.1% of the operated eyes. BCVA better than 20/60 was obtained in 46.3% of the operated eyes. Pre-existing posterior segment pathology or corneal scar, as well as amblyopia, are the reasons for decreased postoperative vision in some cases. Eyes with the onset of ocular pathology during the critical period of visual development showed less postoperative visual improvement. None of the patients developed postoperative retinal detachment, spontaneous IOL dislocation, endophthalmitis, or glaucoma. The main objective of our method is to grant good vision so as to impart better "sensual" input to the eye from early childhood. The usual problem in pediatric eyes is with IOL power calculation, as the chance of shift in refraction is known to occur in the growing eye. SRK II formulas have been shown to give predictable refraction and have been used for IOL power calculation.[34] According to Neely and associates,[34] there seems to be no significant difference between SRK II and SRK T formulas in mean prediction error. Another report by Andreo and associates showed that theoretical formulas do not outperform the regression formula.[35] It is known that the greatest rate of refractive growth or change occurs between 1 and 3 years of age. After 3 years, the rate of refractive growth follows a more linear trend.[36]

Conclusion

This method of IOL implantation has shown reasonable results in children.

References

1. Epley KD, Shainberg MJ, Lueder GT, Tychsen L. Pediatric secondary lens implantation in the absence of capsular support. J AAPOS. 2001;5(5):301-6.
2. Hiles DA. Peripheral iris erosions associated with pediatric intraocular lens implants. J Am Intraocul Implant Soc. 1979; 5(3):210-2.
3. Zetterström C, Lundvall A, Weeber H Jr, Jeeves M. Sulcus fixation without capsular support in children. J Cataract Refract Surg. 1999;25(6):776-81.
4. Agarwal A, Kumar DA, Jacob S, Baid C, Agarwal A, Srinivasan S. Fibrin glue-assisted sutureless posterior chamber intraocular lens implantation in eyes with deficient posterior capsules. J Cataract Refract Surg. 2008;34(9):1433-8.
5. Kumar DA, Agarwal A, Prakash G, Jacob S, Saravanan Y, Agarwal A. Glued posterior chamber IOL in eyes with deficient capsular support: a retrospective analysis of 1-year post-operative outcomes. Eye (Lond). 2010;24(7):1143-8.
6. Prakash G, Kumar DA, Jacob S, Kumar KS, Agarwal A, Agarwal A. Anterior segment optical coherence tomography-aided diagnosis and primary posterior chamber intraocular lens implantation with fibrin glue in traumatic phacocele with scleral perforation. J Cataract Refract Surg. 2009;35(4):782-4.
7. Prakash G, Jacob S, Kumar DA, Narsimhan S, Agarwal A, Agarwal A. Femtosecond assisted keratoplasty with fibrin glue-assisted sutureless posterior chamber lens implantation: a new triple procedure. J Cataract Refract Surg. 2009;35(6):973-9.
8. Nair V, Kumar DA, Prakash G, Jacob S, Agarwal A, Agarwal A. Bilateral spontaneous in-the-bag anterior subluxation of PC IOL managed with glued IOL technique: A case report. Eye Contact Lens. 2009;35(4):215-7.
9. Agarwal A, Kumar DA, Jacob S, Prakash G, Agarwal A. Fibrin glue-assisted sutureless posterior chamber intraocular lens implantation in eyes with deficient posterior capsules [Reply to letter]. J Cataract Refract Surg. 2009;35(5):795-6.
10. Kumar DA, Agarwal A, Jacob S, Prakash G, Agarwal A, Sivagnanam S. Repositioning of the dislocated intraocular lens with sutureless 20-gauge vitrectomy. Retina. 2010;30(4):682-7.
11. Kumar DA, Agarwal A, Prakash G, Jacob S. Managing total aniridia with aphakia using a glued iris prosthesis. J Cataract Refract Surg. 2010;36(5):864-5.
12. Wilson ME, Bluestein EC, Wang X-H. Current trends in the use of intraocular lenses in children. J Cataract Refract Surg. 1994;20(6):579-83.
13. Morrison D, Sternberg P, Donahue S. Anterior chamber intraocular lens (ACIOL) placement after pars plana lensectomy in pediatric Marfan syndrome. J AAPOS. 2005;9(3):240-2.
14. Wagoner MD, Cox TA, Ariyasu RG, Jacobs DS, Karp CL; American Academy of Ophthalmology. Intraocular lens implantation in the absence of capsular support: a report by the American Academy of Ophthalmology. Ophthalmology. 2003;110(4):840-59.
15. Buckley EG. Scleral fixated (sutured) posterior chamber intraocular lens implantation in children. J AAPOS. 1999; 3(5): 289-94.
16. Buckley EG. Hanging by a thread: the long-term efficacy and safety of trans-scleral sutured intraocular lenses in children (an American Ophthalmologist Society Thesis). Trans Am Ophthalmol Soc. 2007;105:294-311.

17. Yen KG, Reddy AK, Weikert MP, Song Y, Hamill MB. Iris-fixated posterior chamber intraocular lenses in children. Am J Ophthalmol. 2009;147(1):121-6.

18. Dureau P, de Laage de Meux P, Edelson C, Caputo G. Iris fixation of foldable intraocular lenses for ectopia lentis in children. J Cataract Refract Surg. 2006;32(7):1109-14.

19. Bardorf CM, Epley KD, Lueder GT, Tychsen L. Pediatric transscleral sutured intraocular lenses: efficacy and safety in 43 eyes followed an average of 3 years. J AAPOS. 2004;8(4):318-24.

20. Jongebloed WL, Worst JFG. Degradation of polypropylene in the human eye: a SEM-study. Doc Ophthalmol. 1986;64(1):143-52.

21. Kanigowska K, Gra³ek M, Czarnowska E, Zajaczkowska A. Subluxation of scleral-fixated PC IOL caused by polypropylene suture degradation—case report. Klin Oczna. 2009; 111(4-6):138-41.

22. Price MO, Price FW Jr, Werner L, Berlie C, Mamalis N. Late dislocation of scleral-sutured posterior chamber intraocular lenses. J Cataract Refract Surg. 2005;31(7):1320-6.

23. McAllister AS, Hirst LW. Visual outcomes and complications of scleral-fixated posterior chamber intraocular lenses. J Cataract Refract Surg. 2011;37(7):1263-9.

24. Sewelam A, Ismail AM, El Serogy H. Ultrasound biomicroscopy of haptic position after transscleral fixation of posterior chamber intraocular lenses. J Cataract Refract Surg. 2001; 27(9):1418-22.

25. Sharpe MR, Biglan AW, Gerontis CC. Scleral fixation of posterior chamber intraocular lenses in children. Ophthalmic Surg Lasers. 1996;27(5):337-41.

26. Gabor SG, Pavilidis MM. Sutureless intrascleral posterior chamber intraocular lens fixation. J Cataract Refract Surg. 2007;33(11):1851-4.

27. Scharioth GB, Prasad S, Georgalas I, Tataru C, Pavlidis M. Intermediate results of sutureless intrascleral posterior chamber intraocular lens fixation. J Cataract Refract Surg. 2010;36(2):254-9.

28. Maggi R, Maggi C. Sutureless scleral fixation of intraocular lenses. J Cataract Refract Surg. 1997;23(9):1289-94.

29. Rodríguez-Agirretxe I, Acera-Osa A, Ubeda-Erviti M. Needle-guided intrascleral fixation of posterior chamber intraocular lens for aphakia correction. J Cataract Refract Surg. 2009;35(12):2051-3.

30. Kumar DA, Agarwal A, Gabor SG, et al. Sutureless sclera fixated posterior chamber intraocular lens. Letter to editor. J Cataract Refract Surg. 2011;37(11):2089-90.

31. Konradsen T, Kugelberg M, Zetterström C. Visual outcomes and complications in surgery for ectopia lentis in children. J Cataract Refract Surg. 2007;33(5):819-24.

32. Dietlein TS, Jacobi PC, Konen W, Krieglstein GK. Complications of endocapsular tension ring implantation in a child with Marfan's syndrome. J Cataract Refract Surg. 2000; 26(6):937-40.

33. Basti S, Aasuri MK, Reddy S, Reddy S, Rao GN. Prospective evaluation of corneal endothelial cell loss after pediatric cataract surgery. J Cataract Refract Surg. 1998;24(11):1469-73.

34. Neely DE, Plager DA, Borger SM, Golub RL. Accuracy of intraocular lens calculations in infants and children undergoing cataract surgery. J AAPOS. 2005;9(2):160-5.

35. Andreo LK, Wilson ME, Saunders RA. Predictive value of regression and theoretical IOL formulas in pediatric intraocular lens implantation. J Pediatr Ophthalmol Strabismus 1997;34(4):240-3.

36. Crouch ER, Crouch ER Jr, Pressman SH. Prospective analysis of pediatric pseudophakia: Myopic shift and postoperative outcomes. J AAPOS. 2002;6(5):277-82.

MISCELLANEOUS

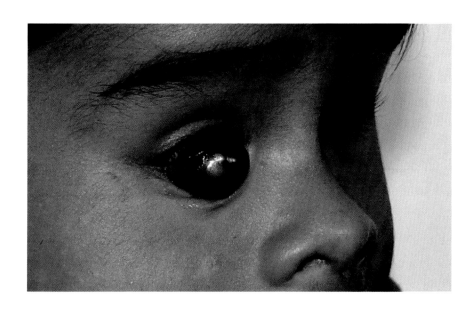

21 Complications of Glued IOL Surgery

Priya Narang

Introduction

Glued IOL is an excellent technique which is aimed at restoring pseudophakia in complicated cases where either the posterior capsule is deficient or is inadequate to support an intraocular lens.[1-4] It can be done both as a primary or as a secondary procedure. Loss of the posterior capsule and its potential support for the IOL is one of the most difficult challenges faced by cataract surgeons. Efficient management of this complication is important for the long-term health of the operative eye. The technique has evolved and extended its application to many different scenarios and as a part of combined surgeries too.[5-8]

Anterior vitrectomy is a crucial tool in the skill set of the anterior segment surgeon. Although a planned anterior vitrectomy may be performed in such settings as traumatic cataract removal, massive subluxated lens or secondary IOL placement, this procedure is most often an unplanned—and unwelcome—addition to a cataract surgery. Even the most experienced surgeon will occasionally be faced with vitreous inadvertently prolapsing into the anterior segment. Thus, a surgeon's comfort with basic anterior vitrectomy principles and techniques can defuse intraoperative stress and improve patient outcomes when complications involving the vitreous occur.

Complications are an inherent part of any surgery and their knowledge is essential; so that they can be avoided and kept at bay. Although this technique is easy; there are norms to be followed and certain nuances of the surgery to be understood. Adhering to the norms makes the surgery very predictable and forgiving. Complications can be broadly divided as:
1. Intraoperative
2. Postoperative.

Intraoperative Complications

Intraoperatively, it is very important to keep a strict vigil on all the proceedings of the surgery. A slight distraction from perfection can prove to be hazardous. Complications do occur; but they can also be anticipated at times depending on the case and can be dealt accordingly.

Scleral Flap Complications

Partial scleral thickness flaps are fashioned approximately 2.5 by 2.5 mm in size and are exactly 180° opposite each other. A scleral marker is stained with a dye and is used to mark the site for the creation of flaps. Variation in the fashioning of the scleral flap can lead to various unfavorable outcomes as stated below:

Eccentric Flaps

When the scleral marking is not appropriate, eccentric flaps do occur **(Figures 1A to D)**. Surgery should not be proceeded with such flaps as sclerotomy is to be done beneath these flaps and a path is created for the externalization of haptics. This eventually leads to decentration of the IOL **(Figures 2A and B)**. A fresh flap should be created diagonally opposite to the previous one and then the surgery should be proceeded to the next level.

Perforation

Perforation at the site of creation of scleral flap can occur when the surgeon fails to create a partial scleral thickness flap and instead goes too deep. In such cases, the scleral flap should be sutured back to its bed; and fresh flaps should be created at a different site after scleral marking.

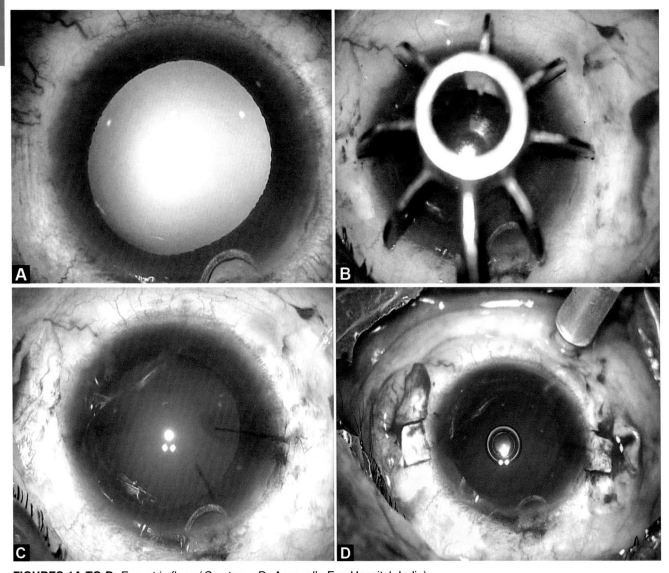

FIGURES 1A TO D: Eccentric flaps (*Courtesy:* Dr Agarwal's Eye Hospital, India)
A. Aphakic eye for glued IOL surgery
B. Scleral flap marker
C. Note the scleral marking (violet mark) is eccentric
D. Scleral flaps created are eccentric. The flaps should be 180 degrees apart. Note the flaps are about 160 degrees apart which will lead to a decentered IOL

Flaps of Irregular Size

The flap size should be nearly 2.5 by 2.5 mm. Too narrow flaps should be avoided as then it may be difficult to create the scleral pocket next to the sclerotomy. Scleral pockets are created at the edge of flap, parallel to the sclerotomy site. Too wide flaps should also be avoided as a greater amount of haptic length is wasted from the sclerotomy site to the entry point of the scleral pocket **(Figure 2C)**. As a result little amount of haptic is available for the tucking. It

is the amount of haptic tucked on either side which is responsible for giving stability to the IOL.

Inadequate Flap Adherence Post-Surgery

This usually occurs if the glue is not properly applied beneath the flap or if the flap is not pressed properly after the application of glue. During the process of application of glue, the scleral bed should be completely dry and the infusion should be either stopped or removed. If the infusion is kept 'ON' then the glue

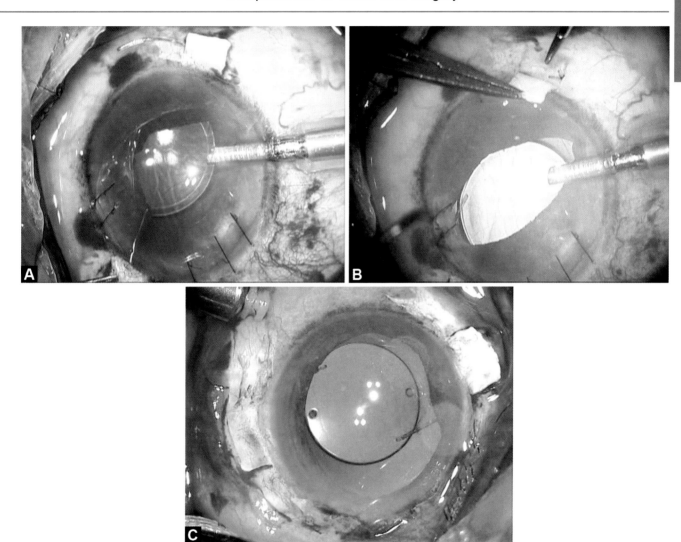

FIGURES 2A TO C: Eccentric flaps solution and too large flaps (*Courtesy:* Dr Agarwal's Eye Hospital, India)
A. Glued IOL decentered. Note the scleral flaps are eccentric and not 180 degrees apart. Note faint violet mark in lower left corner where the flap is but no marker in the upper right corner which led to the eccentric flap
B. Glued IOL centered. A fresh sclerotomy is made in the upper right flap so that the two sclerotomies are 180 degrees apart. The IOL is again passed back into the vitreous cavity and again externalized through the fresh sclerotomy. IOL now centered. If flap was very badly decentered then a fresh flap would have to be made
C. Too large flaps
Too wide flaps should be avoided as a greater amount of haptic length is wasted from the sclerotomy site to the entry point of the scleral pocket. As a result little amount of haptic is available for the tucking

gets washed away by the fluid leaking from the sclerotomy sites. Inadequate flap adherence can lead to; hypotony, exposure of the sclerotomy wound or exposure of the haptic.

Infusion Cannula Hiccups

The success of glued IOL surgery depends a lot on the maintenance of infusion into the eye. The use of anterior chamber (AC) maintainer was first described

by Blumenthal for cataract surgery in 1987.[9] The eye maintains its configuration only with the help of infusion. At no point of time, viscoelastic should be used for inflating the eyeball. The role of viscoelastic should be limited to the loading of the foldable IOL and protection of the endothelium.

Infusion can be maintained in the eye depending on the surgeons choice with the help of an AC maintainer or a trocar cannula.

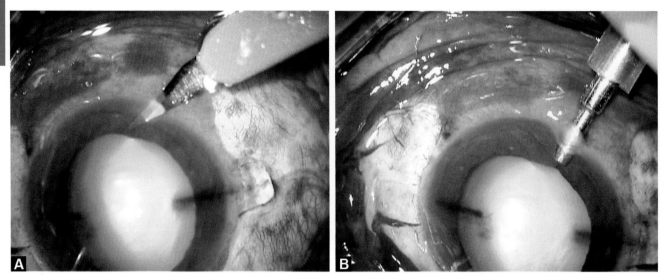

FIGURES 3A AND B: AC maintainer problem (*Courtesy:* Dr Agarwal's Eye Hospital, India)
A. Paracentesis made with a side port knife
B. AC maintainer fixed. Note the iris getting sucked into the AC maintainer. AC maintainer should not be directed vertically down rather should be parallel to the iris plane

AC Maintainer

The advantage with using an AC maintainer is that it is easy to introduce and can be managed easily by an anterior segment surgeon. It should be introduced at a location where it does not interfere with surgery. A stab incision **(Figures 3A and B)** should be created for the introduction of the AC maintainer with an MVR blade or a side port blade. Tight wound helps in preventing leakage and thereby maintaining the anterior chamber properly throughout the surgery. Too lose an AC maintainer can lead to leakage or the AC maintainer coming out. The AC maintainer should be parallel to the iris plane **(Figures 3A and B)**. One problem with the AC maintainer is that it pushes the iris back when the fluid is on which does not happen with a trocar cannula. So if one is using an AC maintainer one can fix the AC maintainer then create the sclerotomy under the scleral flap and then turn on the infusion. Otherwise if the iris is pushed back when one does the sclerotomy the iris can get hit with the 20G needle.

Trocar Cannula

The 23/25 gauge trocar cannula is introduced into the eye at the level of pars plana approximately 3 mm to 3.5 mm from the limbus. It is introduced into the eye by keeping it parallel to the scleral surface and then introducing it vertically into the vitreous cavity. This gives it a good valvular creation and subsequently does not require sutures once removed **(Figures 4A to D)**.

After introduction of the trocar, the entry point into the vitreous cavity should be confirmed before putting 'ON' the infusion. If the tip of the trocar is not seen in the vitreous cavity, the infusion should not be put on and the surgeon should get aware that probably it is in the subchoroidal or subretinal space. Ensure proper placement of trocar cannula to prevent sub-retinal infusion.[10] Putting ON the infusion at this stage can lead to a retinal detachment. Vitreous hemorrhage can also occur at times following the insertion of the trocar cannula.

Sclerotomy Complications

Sclerotomy is done with a 20-gauge needle beneath the scleral flap, approximately 1 to 1.5 mm from the limbus and is obliquely guided into the mid-vitreous cavity. The needle should enter the eye behind the iris and the tip of the needle should be seen in the mid-pupillary area. The needle is then withdrawn out of the eye. Any deviation from this can lead to various complications.

Sclerotomy Plane Anterior to Iris

Sclerotomy is done for creating a passage for the exteriorization of the haptics. When the needle is directed obliquely but anteriorly and when the point of

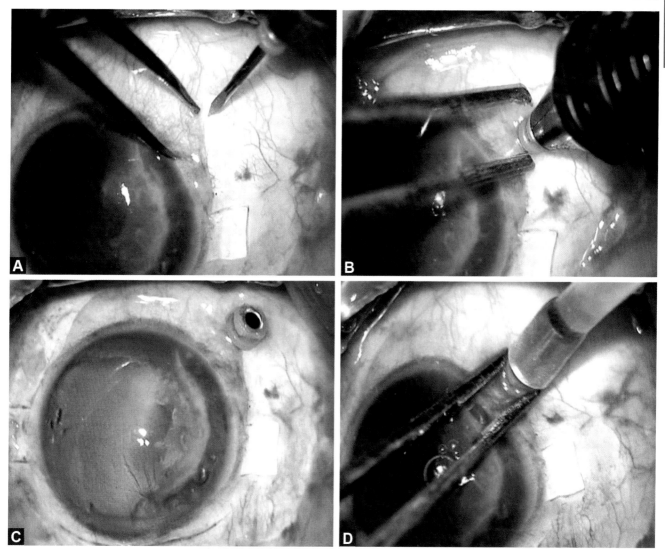

FIGURES 4A TO D: 23G trocar cannula being fixed for a glued IOL surgery (*Courtesy:* Dr Agarwal's Eye Hospital, India)
A. 23G trocar along with scleral guide is placed in the pars plana
B. Trocar is pushed well inside the vitreous cavity with the inserter
C. Scleral guide is seen in place
D. The self-locking infusion cannula is inserted

entry is anterior to 1 mm from the limbus beneath the flap; a plane is created anterior to the iris **(Figure 5)**. The surgeon should redo this step by going slightly posterior to the entry point with the needle directed obliquely into the mid-vitreous cavity; so that a plane is created behind the iris.

Iridodialysis

Any resistance encountered during the procedure of sclerotomy should be taken as a warning sign and the needle should be withdrawn. The probability is that the surgeon has hit the root of the iris. Forceful entry into the eye can lead to detachment of the iris from its root and eventually into a case of full fledged iridodialysis. This complication can be avoided by withdrawing the needle and attempting a fresh entry from a different site.

Hyphema

It usually accompanies iridodialysis or when the anterior ciliary blood vessels are disturbed during the surgical step of sclerotomy. In cases of mild hyphema, the surgery can be continued and the residual blood absorbs within few days. Whereas in cases of moderate

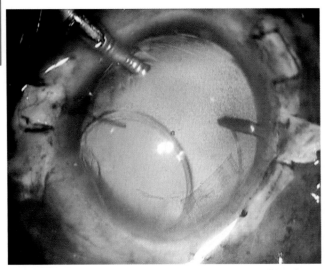

FIGURE 5: Glued IOL forceps is anterior to the iris plane. This is because the sclerotomy has been made anterior to the iris plane (*Courtesy:* Dr Agarwal's Eye Hospital, India)

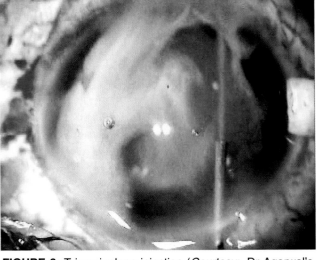

FIGURE 6: Triamcinolone injection (*Courtesy:* Dr Agarwal's Eye Hospital, India)

to severe hyphema, the surgery has to be terminated and should be rescheduled later on. Alternatively a posterior segment surgeon can clear the vitreous hemorrhage on table and proceed with the surgery.

Vitrectomy Complications

Vitrectomy is a very crucial step in this surgery and a lot depends on how well it is done. Perhaps the most challenging aspect of removing vitreous from the anterior chamber is visualizing it. Because of the optical clarity of vitreous and its similarity to cortical fibers, a surgeon often must use indirect clues, such as peaking of the pupil to determine the presence and extent of vitreous prolapse. For this reason, Burke and colleagues have used triamcinolone acetonide to assist in visualization of vitreous in the anterior chamber.[11] Triamcinolone particles "stain" the vitreous gel, making it readily visible for removal **(Figure 6)**.

Triamcinolone can be used to stain the vitreous; this ensures that no vitreous strand is present in the anterior chamber and the pupil is totally free from vitreous. Vitrectomy can be done from the corneal incision (using a 20G cutter) or from the sclerotomy site with a 23G or 25G cutter. The vitreous is removed to a level just posterior to the capsule. When one does vitrectomy through the corneal incision there is a slight dimpling of the cornea as the wound is opened **(Figure 7)**. This does not happen if vitrectomy is done from the sclerotomy site. All phaco-machines have good anterior vitrectomy set ups but they are 20G

probes. So one should use corneal incisions when using them. If one is using a posterior vitrectomy machine which has a 23 or 25G probe then one can use the sclerotomy site.

During vitrectomy iris chewing can occur if the surgeon is too fast or is not cautious enough. Entrapment of the iris can also occur during the withdrawal of the vitrectomy cutter if it is not switched off. This leads to an irregular shape of the pupil postoperatively.

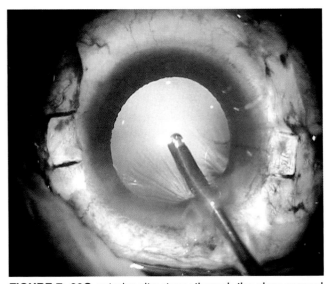

FIGURE 7: 20G anterior vitrectomy through the clear corneal incision. Note the dimpling on the cornea as the main incision is opened. This would not happen if vitrectomy is done from the sclerotomy site (*Courtesy:* Dr Agarwal's Eye Hospital, India)

IOL Complications

IOL Drop

This complication is usually encountered in the early stages of the learning curve of a surgeon. As there is no posterior capsule available for support, any error on the part of the surgeon during the handling of the IOL can lead to an IOL drop. It can be caused by;

Abrupt unfolding of the IOL: The unfolding of the IOL should always be gradual and slow. Abrupt unfolding **(Figure 8)** leads to jerky movement and the surgeon at times misses catching the tip of the leading haptic. Foldable IOL with a 'Pushing' mechanism should be preferred rather than the 'Screwing mechanism'. This gives better control over unfolding **(Figure 9)**.

Slippage of the haptic into the eye: Improper handling of the haptics by a surgeon or an assistant causes the haptic to slip back into the eye and eventually that can lead to an IOL drop.

Faulty glued IOL forceps: The serrations of the forceps are sometimes lost due to continuous reuse and sterilization. This decreases the grip on the haptic which might cause it to slip back into the anterior chamber and if not managed properly can lead to IOL haptic breakage or IOL drop **(Figure 10)**.

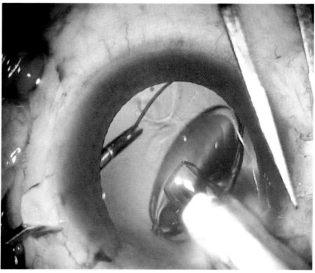

FIGURE 9: Correct implantation of IOL (*Courtesy:* Dr Agarwal's Eye Hospital, India)
One should pass the cartridge into the eye and slowly inject the IOL only after one haptic is caught with the glued IOL forceps

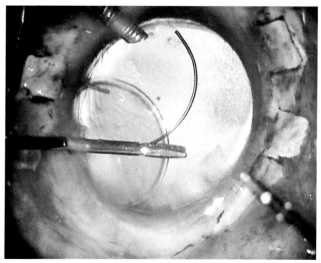

FIGURE 10: Broken IOL haptic (*Courtesy:* Dr Agarwal's Eye Hospital, India)

Haptic Breakage

The haptics of the IOL break when undue pressure is exerted on them or while trying to hold the haptics not from the tip but somewhere midway along the length of the haptic during the process of externalization. This causes kinking of the haptic and when an attempt is made to straighten; it breaks **(Figures 11A and B)**. Apart from kinking, the IOL often breaks from the optic-haptic junction and this happens more frequently with the usage of one-piece IOL, e.g. Aniridia IOL's.

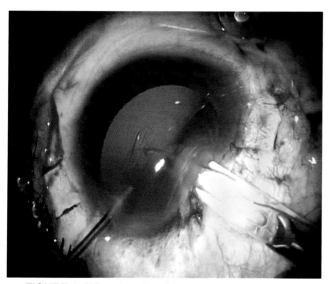

FIGURE 8: Wound assisted implantation in glued IOL surgery (*Courtesy:* Dr Agarwal's Eye Hospital, India)
Note the wound assisted implantation. This should not be done. One can see the dimpling on the cornea hampering visualization. Chances of the IOL falling into the vitreous cavity are high

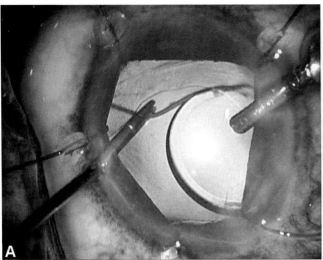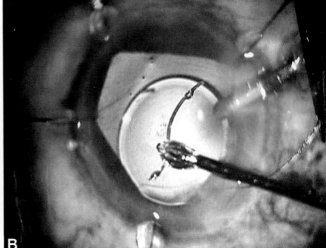

FIGURES 11A AND B: Haptic breakage (*Courtesy:* Dr Agarwal's Eye Hospital, India)
A. IOL haptic deformed with the glued IOL forceps
B. IOL haptic broken

These IOLs are huge one piece IOLs and a certain amount of surgical expertise is needed to tuck them.

Decentration of IOL

This complication can be encountered under certain conditions.

1. **Eccentric scleral flaps:** The partial scleral thickness flaps are to be created exactly 180° opposite one another. Eccentric flaps lead to a decentered IOL as the haptics are externalized beneath the flaps from the sclerotomy site. As the IOL is not positioned along its long axis, continuous stress on the haptics leads to decentration.

   In such cases, fresh flaps should be created exactly opposite each other and the procedure of externalization of haptic should be re-done on one side. This ensures proper centration of the IOL.

2. **Improper tucking of the haptic:** The haptics should be tucked equally on the either side in the scleral pockets. Inadequate or disproportionate tucking of the haptic along its length; leads to decentration. This is especially important where a multifocal IOL is being implanted. Centration of the IOL is the key to success.

IOL Tilt

This can occur once again if the IOL is not centered well.

Postoperative Complications

Vitritis

A slight element of vitritis follows this surgery as these eyes are compromised and they do have vitreous protruding into the anterior chamber. A thorough vitrectomy is advised for all these cases. Undue manipulation of the IOL during the process of externalization of haptic can also lead to significant amount of vitritis in the postoperative period. This usually occurs with beginners as the surgery has its own learning curve. Usage of viscoelastic into the eye gives a significant amount of reaction and can lead to severe vitritis. Apart from loading of the foldable IOL and protection of the endothelium, one should avoid viscoelastic in glued IOL surgery. Oral and topical steroids help to curb vitritis.

Hypotony

A surgeon usually comes across hypotony or choroidal detachment in cases of;
a. Improper closure of the wound
b. Large gauge sclerotomy entry
c. Failure to inject air into the eye after the surgery.

   Hypotony can be prevented by taking all the above measures and using glue to seal all the corneal incisions created during the surgery, e.g. corneal tunnel, side port wound, infusion entry point, etc.

If after air injection the eye is hypotonic, inject some balanced salt solution into the eye through the clear corneal incision. The fluid will go into the vitreous cavity and distend the globe and solve hypotony. After the surgery is done and the speculum removed, one should always check if the eye is hypotonic. If it is then inject the fluid the way just described.

Postoperatively, if eye is still hypotonic, give systemic steroids in a tapering dosage for two weeks. This would prevent any choroidals from forming.

Secondary Glaucoma

Intraocular pressure (IOP) may be elevated postoperatively because of residual viscoelastic or postoperative inflammation. Intraocular pressure needs to be continuously monitored in all the cases that have undergone glued IOL surgery. The eyes which require this surgery are usually compromised.

This complication can manifest in the early postoperative period due to either;
a. Inflammation
b. Vitreous in the anterior chamber following inadequate vitrectomy
c. Steroid responders.

In the published literature, the most common complication of intravitreal triamcinolone acetonide treatment was a transient rise in intraocular pressure, and, very rarely, needed glaucoma surgery.[12-18] In cases of trauma, secondary glaucoma may be pre-existing also due to architectural damage to the trabecular meshwork and the angle structures.

Cystoid Macular Edema (CME)

CME follows when there is lot of disturbance created by mishandling and mismanagement of the vitreous which occurs maximally during the phase of vitrectomy or during the exteriorization of haptics **(Figure 12)**. Pre-existing CME should be ruled out especially in cases where glued IOL is done as a secondary procedure. If cataract extraction is complicated by posterior capsule rupture and vitreous loss, severe iris trauma or vitreous traction at the wound, there is a significantly higher incidence (up to 20%) of clinically apparent CME.[19]Clinically significant CME usually occurs within 3-12 weeks postoperatively, but in some instances its onset may be delayed for months or many years after surgery. Spontaneous resolution of the CME with subsequent visual improvement may occur within 3-12 months in 80% of the patients.[20]

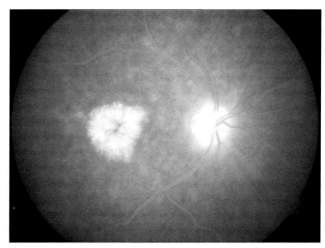

FIGURE 12: Cystoid macular edema (*Courtesy: Dr Agarwal's Eye Hospital, India*) Flower petal appearance on fluorescein angiography

The hypothesis that vitreomacular traction causes CME has been confirmed histopathologically.[21] Other anterior segment changes, such as incarceration of the anterior vitreous to the corneal wound, have been related to CME. This complication is associated not only with increased incidence of CME but also with a worse functional prognosis.[22]

Retinal Detachment

Improper management of the vitreous and traction on the vitreous strands can lead to retinal detachment in the postoperative period. Care should be taken in all cases where this technique is combined with posterior segment surgery requiring pars plana vitrectomy (PPV).

Vitreoretinal traction is responsible for the occurrence of rhegmatogenous RD **(Figure 13)**. In certain eyes, strong vitreoretinal adhesions are present, and the occurrence of PVD can lead to a retinal tear formation. It is this increased incidence of PVD that is a risk factor in the development of retinal breaks and subsequent RD. PPV may also be complicated by iatrogenic retinal breaks, which, if undetected, may lead to RD **(Figures 14 to 16)**. They commonly occur posterior to the sclerotomy site as a result of mechanical traction by the exchange of instruments through the sclerotomy. In patients with retained lens material, higher traction can be induced due to nuclear fragment manipulation. Recommended techniques for these patients include the following: the induction of PVD with maximal vitreous removal before phacofragmentation, lens fragment debulking before fragmentation, use of low energy with

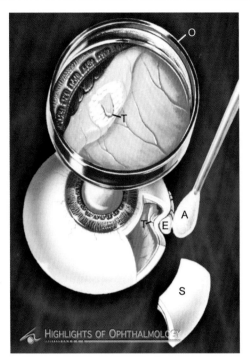

FIGURE 13: Final view of buckle with proper retinal indentation and positioning of the tear

This internal/external conceptual illustration shows a cross-section and the corresponding surgeon's view of the final configuration of a circumferentially placed sponge exoplant (E). The cross-section shows a portion of the globe without sclera (S) to enhance clarity for the reader. The surgeon's view is through the indirect ophthalmoscope (O). Note the indented configuration in both views. The retina is reattached and the tear (T) is flat. Also note that the tear is properly positioned on the anterior slope of the buckle.

(*Courtesy:* Jaypee Highlights of Ophthalmology, "Retinal and Vitreoretinal Surgery—Mastering the Latest Techniques", English Edition, 2002. Editor-in-Chief: Benjamin F Boyd, MD, FACS; Co-Editor: Samuel Boyd, MD)

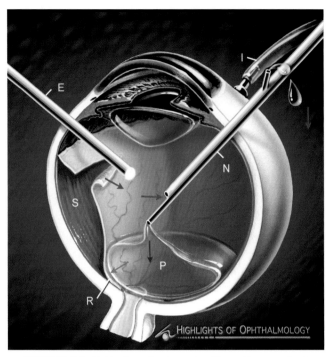

FIGURE 14: Retinal reattachment with perfluorocarbon liquid in case of giant tear

In the case of retinal detachment with giant retinal tear, perfluorocarbon liquid (P) is injected into the vitreous cavity via Chang cannula (N). Because the liquid has a specific gravity greater than water, it gravitates (blue arrow) to the posterior pole. This forces the subretinal fluid (S, red arrows) out through the giant retinal tear and out of the eye via the Chang cannula. The retina (R) is being forced to reattach (green arrow) in this manner. Infusion cannula (I). Endoilluminator (E).

(*Courtesy:* Jaypee Highlights of Ophthalmology, "Retinal and Vitreoretinal Surgery—Mastering the Latest Techniques", English Edition, 2002. Editor-in-Chief: Benjamin F Boyd, MD, FACS; Co-Editor: Samuel Boyd, MD)

high aspiration during the removal of retained lens material, and intraoperative indirect ophthalmoscopic evaluation of the retinal periphery with scleral indentation to diagnose intraoperative retinal breaks. Small-gauge transconjunctival sutureless vitrectomy has also been reported to cause iatrogenic postoperative RD. This is thought to be related to the lack of adequate peripheral vitrectomy with the more flexible instruments and excessive traction at the sclerotomy sites.

Endophthalmitis

This is a complication which is universal and can happen to any intraocular surgery if the sterilization process is not followed stringently. Intraoperative posterior capsule

rupture is associated with an 8- to 11-fold higher risk of acute endophthalmitis, suggesting that these eyes should be closely monitored for signs of infection in the immediate postoperative period.[23] Pseudo-endophthalmitis after an intravitreal injection of triamcinolone acetonide (IVTA) seems to be a distinct clinical entity that may resolve without specific treatment.[24] Acute postoperative endophthalmitis following IVTA occurs rapidly and can result in severe loss of vision.[25]

IOL Subluxation

IOL subluxation could occur. This is basically due to a mistake during surgery. One should tuck the haptics well and glue them in. If the white to white is too

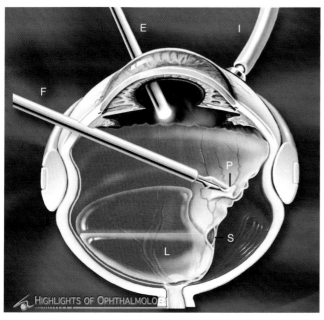

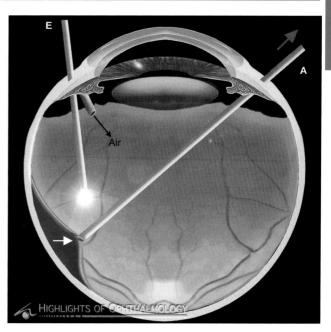

FIGURE 15: Surgical treatment of PVR
Perfluorocarbon liquid (L) is injected. This will reveal any persistent traction from epiretinal membranes (P) which must be removed. A vitreoretinal pic or Grieshaber mini-diamond forceps (F) is used to remove such a membrane (P). Note subretinal membrane (S). Endoilluminator (E) and infusion terminal (I).

(*Courtesy:* Jaypee Highlights of Ophthalmology, "Retinal and Vitreoretinal Surgery—Mastering the Latest Techniques", English Edition, 2002. Editor-in-Chief: Benjamin F Boyd, MD, FACS; Co-Editor: Samuel Boyd, MD)

large, example 12 mm in the horizontal axis then one should do a vertical glued IOL and create the flaps at 12 and 6 o'clock position. This way there will be more haptic externalized to tuck and glue as the vertical cornea is shorter than the horizontal. If the surgery is done well and good amount of haptic is tucked and glued the IOL will not subluxate.

IOL Haptic Extrusion

If the surgeon has not tucked the haptic well into the sclera haptic; extrusion can occur. In such cases, one should take the patient back to the operation theatre and just create a fresh tunnel and retuck and reglue the haptic.

Conclusion

As with any surgery glued IOL surgery also has its own complications and one should be careful in handling them.

FIGURE 16: Air-fluid exchange and internal drainage of sub-retinal fluid (white arrow) with the extrusion needle (A), endoilluminator (E):

(*Courtesy:* Jaypee Highlights of Ophthalmology, "Retinal and Vitreoretinal Surgery—Mastering the Latest Techniques", English Edition, 2002. Editor-in-Chief: Benjamin F Boyd, MD, FACS; Co-Editor: Samuel Boyd, MD)

References

1. Agarwal A, Kumar DA, Jacob S, Baid C, Agarwal A, Srinivasan S. Fibrin glue-assisted sutureless posterior chamber intraocular lens implantation in eyes with deficient posterior capsules. J Cataract Refract Surg. 2008;34(9):1433-8.
2. Kumar DA, Agarwal A, Prakash G, Jacob S, Saravanan Y, Agarwal A. Glued posterior chamber IOL in eyes with deficient capsular support: a retrospective analysis of 1-year postoperative outcomes. Eye (Lond). 2010;24(7):1143-8.
3. Prakash G, Kumar DA, Jacob S, Kumar KS, Agarwal A, Agarwal A. Anterior segment optical coherence tomography-aided diagnosis and primary posterior chamber intraocular lens implantation with fibrin glue in traumatic phacocele with scleral perforation. J Cataract Refract Surg 2009;35(4):782-4.
4. Agarwal A, Kumar DA, Prakash G, et al. Fibrin glue-assisted sutureless posterior chamber intraocular lens implantation in eyes with deficient posterior capsules [Reply to letter]. J Cataract Refract Surg. 2009;35(5):795-6.
5. Prakash G, Jacob S, Kumar DA, Narsimhan S, Agarwal A, Agarwal A. Femtosecond assisted keratoplasty with fibrin glue-assisted sutureless posterior chamber lens implantation: a new triple procedure. J Cataract Refract Surg. 2009;35(6):973-9.
6. Nair V, Kumar DA, Prakash G, Jacob S, Agarwal A, Agarwal A. Bilateral spontaneous in-the-bag anterior subluxation of PC IOL managed with glued IOL technique: A case report. Eye Contact Lens. 2009;35(4):215-7.

7. Kumar DA, Agarwal A, Jacob S, Prakash G, Agarwal A, Sivagnanam S. Repositioning of the dislocated intraocular lens with sutureless 20-gauge vitrectomy. Retina. 2010;30(4):682-7.

8. Kumar DA, Agarwal A, Prakash G, Jacob S. Managing total aniridia with aphakia using a glued iris prosthesis. J Cataract Refract Surg. 2010;36(5):864.

9. Blumenthal M, Moissiev J. Anterior chamber maintainer for extracapsular cataract extraction and intraocular lens implantation. J Cataract Refract Surg. 1987;13:204-6.

10. Kreiger AE. The management of wound-related complications in pars plana vitrectomy. Trans Am Ophthalmol Soc. 1994;92:307-20;discussion 20-4.

11. Burke SE, et al. J Cataract Refract Surg. 2003;29:645-51.

12. Antcliff RJ, Spalton DJ, Stanford MR, et al. Intravitreal triamcinolone for uveitic cystoid macular edema (An optical coherence tomography study). Ophthalmology 2001;108:765-72.

13. Young S, Larkin G, Branley M, Lightman S. Safety and efficacy of intravitreal triamcinolone for cystoid macular oedema in uveitis. Clin Exp Ophthalmol. 2001;29:2-6.

14. Jonas JB, Sofker A. Intraocular injection of crystalline cortisone as adjunctive treatment of diabetic macular edema. Am J Ophthalmol. 2001;132:425-7.

15. Martidis A, Duker JS, Greenberg PB, et al. Intravitreal triamcinolone for refractory diabetic macular edema. Ophthalmology 2002;109:920-7.

16. Danis RP, Ciulla TA, Pratt LM, Anliker W. Intravitreal triamcinolone acetonide in exudative age-related macular degeneration. Retina. 2000;20:244-50.

17. Jonas JB, Hayler JK, Sofker A, Panda-Jonas S. Intravitreal injection of crystalline cortisone as adjunctive treatment of proliferative diabetic retinopathy. Am J Ophthalmol. 2001;131:468-71.

18. Wingate RJ, Beaumont PE. Intravitreal triamcinolone and elevated intraocular pressure. Aust NZJ Ophthalmol. 1999;27:431-2.

19. Bradford JD, Wilkinson CP, Bradford RH Jr. Cystoid macular edema following extracapsular cataract extraction and posterior chamber intraocular lens implantation. Retina. 1988;8(3):161-4.

20. Bonnet S. Repercussions of cataract surgery on the development of cystoid macular edema in the diabetic patient. Bull Soc Belge Ophtalmol. 1995;256:127-9.

21. Wolter JR. Cystoid macular edema in vitreoretinal traction Ophthalmic Surg. 1981;12(12):900-4.

22. Federman JL, Annesley WH Jr, Sarin LK, Remer P. Vitrectomy and cystoid macular edema. Ophthalmology. 1980;87(7):622-8.

23. Tien Yin Wong, Soon-Phaik Chee. The epidemiology of acute endophthalmitis after cataract surgery in an Asian population. Ophthalmology 2004;111(4):699-705.

24. Sutter FKP, Gillies MC. Clinical science. Pseudo-endophthalmitis after intravitreal injection of triamcinolone. Br J Ophthalmol. 2003;87:972-4.

25. Moshfeghi DM, Kaiser PK, Scott IU, Sears JE, Benz M, Sinesterra JP, et al. Acute endophthalmitis following intravitreal triamcinolone acetonide injection. American Journal of Ophthalmology. 2003;136:791-6.

22

IOL Tilt

Dhivya Ashok Kumar, Amar Agarwal

Introduction

The accurate position of an intraocular lens (IOL) in the capsular bag is vital in preventing postoperative tilt and astigmatism. IOL tilt is one of the components of malposition that can lead to astigmatism, change in optical higher-order aberrations, and loss of best-corrected visual acuity.[1-3] Ultrasound biomicroscopy, Scheimpflug images, Purkinje reflections, photographic documentation, anterior segment analysis system are the methods used for evaluation of IOL position.[3-9] Although anterior segment optical coherence tomography (OCT) has been used to image the IOL position, there were no reports of postoperative IOL tilt estimation with OCT in a large population.[10] We used for the first time anterior segment OCT to evaluate the position of IOLs implanted within the capsular bag after uneventful phacoemulsification and correlated the results with visual acuity and refractive outcomes.

IOL Tilt Assessment with the Anterior Segment OCT

OCT is a noninvasive, high-resolution imaging method that provides cross-sectional tomography of the ocular structures *in vivo*. So far, it has many promising clinical applications in cataract and refractive surgery as well as in glaucoma diagnosis and anterior segment tumor imaging.[11-18] Herein we have described the application of anterior segment OCT for IOL tilt examination. The aim was to identify the ability of anterior segment OCT to detect IOL position after IOL implantation. The same has been shown by deriving the position of the IOL with reference to the limbus. We have taken limbus as the anatomic reference point because it can

be delineated easily by any observer. Because structures like the Schlemm canal and the trabecular meshwork have not been visualized readily with the existing time-domain OCT systems, they were not taken as reference.

The examination can be performed in the immediate postoperative period and in eyes with poor corneal clarity resulting from edema. IOL malposition **(Figure 1)** is one of the indications for removal, exchange, or repositioning of a posterior chamber IOL. Although there have been reports on examination of an IOL with OCT, there are no reports on IOL tilt analysis.[10,16,17] We did the first study of IOL tilt using an anterior segment OCT. The idea was conceived by one of us (DAK).

The high-speed OCT with 1310-nm wavelength used in our study has an axial resolution of 18 microns and transverse resolution of 60 microns. It has a scan speed of approximately 8 frames/second. With the anterior segment scan (16 × 6 mm) image, the corneal vertex, limbus, and IOL are visualized. The corneal scan gives a high-resolution, cross-sectional, quantitative image of the IOL position. Ultrasound biomicroscopy has been used to examine the intraocular position of the IOL after phacoemulsification, extracapsular cataract extraction, and transscleral or iris fixation of posterior chamber lenses.[8,10] The main advantage of OCT over ultrasound biomicroscopy is its noninvasive (non-contact) nature, high resolution, and faster execution. There is no need for coupling fluid application. Hence, this can be performed in the early postoperative period and in traumatized corneas. However, it is not possible to visualize the haptic position below the iris, which can be imaged with ultrasound biomicroscopy. Scheimpflug images taken from the Pentacam (Oculus, Inc., Lynnwood, Washington, USA) also have been used for tilt analysis.

Technique of Anterior Segment OCT for IOL Tilt Assessment

The headrest and chin rest of the OCT are adjusted to guarantee a perpendicular position of the patient's head for each examination. Cross-sectional imaging of the IOL is then carried out with the Visante anterior segment OCT (Carl Zeiss Meditec, Dublin, California, USA). The anterior segment single-scan mode is used. Images are obtained in 4 axes, namely 180 to 0 degrees, 225 to 45 degrees, 315 to 135 degrees, and 270 to 90 degrees. The optics of the IOL are imaged with reference to the position of the iris, limbus, and capsule. The images are then analyzed with the caliper tools in the software of the anterior segment OCT for iris vault (distance in millimeters between the iris margin and the anterior surface of the IOL at the papillary plane [D1, D2]; **Figure 1**). Using MatLab software version 7.1 (Mathworks, Natick, Massachusetts, USA), anterior segment single scan images are analyzed. A straight line (L) passing through the limbus on either side of the image is marked as the reference line. A second line (1) passing through the horizontal axis of the IOL **(Figure 2)** is also marked. The horizontal axis of the IOL is determined by the following method. The image from OCT is converted to binary for subsequent extraction of edge coordinates. The selected points on the anterior and posterior arc edges of IOL are obtained. The mathematical representation to fit the anterior and posterior arc of IOL are derived from the equation of the circles passing through the given points

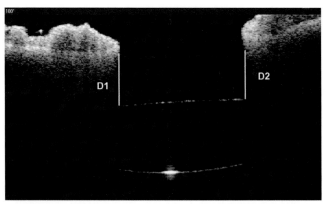

FIGURE 2: Corneal high-resolution optical coherence tomography image showing intraocular lens (IOL) position. D1, D2 = distance in millimeters from iris margin to IOL optic edge at the pupillary plane

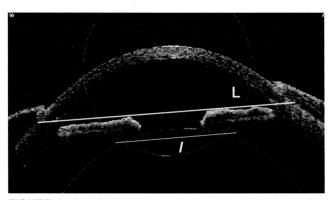

FIGURE 3: Anterior segment optical coherence tomography analysis of intraocular lens (IOL) tilt. L = slope of limbus; l = slope of IOL

(Figure 2). The intersection points of the 2 circles are joined to form the horizontal axis of the IOL. This is executed in all the 4 quadrants (180 to 0 degrees, 225 to 45 degrees, 315 to 135 degrees, and 270 to 90 degrees). The slopes are calculated for both the straight lines (L,1). When the reference line along the limbus and the IOL optic are parallel, the optic is not considered to be tilted. The angle (thetha) in degrees between the 2 lines (L and 1) is determined. The slope ratio is calculated by dividing the slope of the IOL by the slope of the limbus **(Figure 3)**.

IOL Tilt Assessment with UBM

Decentered IOLs **(Figures 4A and B)** can be assessed with the UBM. Ultrasound biomicroscopy (UBM) can also be used to note the position or tilt of an IOL **(Figure 5)**. Ectopia lentis **(Figures 6A and B)** or subluxated cataract is often associated with zonular

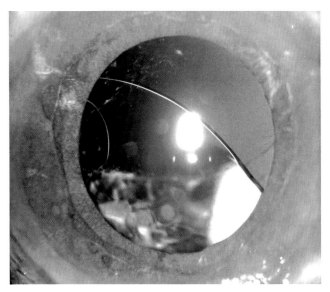

FIGURE 1: Malpositioned IOL

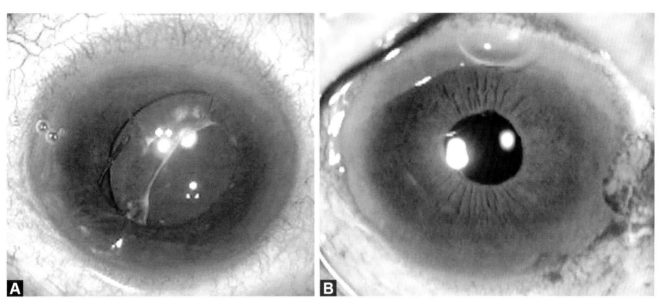

FIGURES 4A and B: Preoperative picture of decentered IOL (A) and postoperative picture (B) showing glued IOL centeration without explantation. This was a case of an Iraqi ophthalmologist who had in his eye a decentered IOL

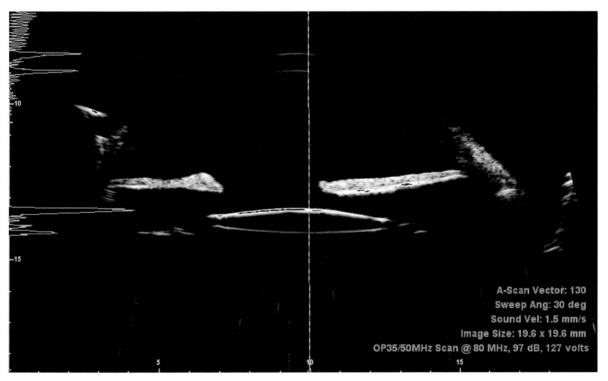

A-Scan Vector: 130
Sweep Ang: 30 deg
Sound Vel: 1.5 mm/s
Image Size: 19.6 x 19.6 mm
OP35/50MHz Scan @ 80 MHz, 97 dB, 127 volts

FIGURE 5: Ultrasound biomicroscopy (UBM) image of glued IOL

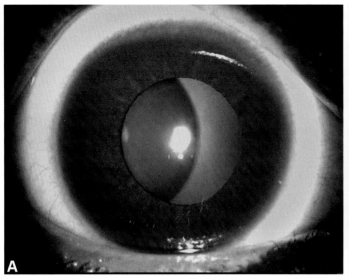 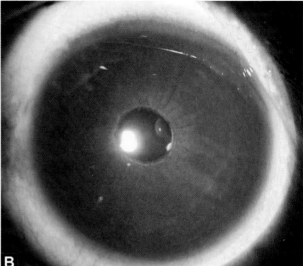

FIGURES 6A AND B: Ectopia lentis
A. Ectopia lentis in a pediatric eye
B. One year postoperative picture with a glued IOL

weakness, which makes surgery with lens extraction and implantation of an intraocular lens (IOL) challenging. Moreover, posterior capsule rupture can prevent normal IOL implantation in the capsular bag.

Discussion

The change in the properties of the biomaterial when the IOL is placed in a stretched position is a major concern. There are 2 factors that contribute to the ability of IOL loops to maintain their original symmetrical configuration. One is the loop rigidity (the resistance of the haptic to external forces that bend the loops centrally) and the other is the loop memory (the ability of the loops to reexpand laterally to their original size and configuration). These 2 factors can be demonstrated by compressing or stretching the haptics *in vivo*. *In vivo*, the centrifugal force vector due to resistance to compression by the capsular bag keeps the IOL stable. Similarly, with glued IOL, the stretch creates a centripetal resistance force. Along with the intralamellar scleral tuck, this stabilizes the IOL. Spontaneous IOL dislocation is one of the main problems associated with trans-scleral fixation of suture-fixated IOLs. However, this is known to occur due to suture degradation or disintegration.

In the glued IOL since the haptics are snugly tucked into the scleral tunnel the chance is reduced. When the eye moves, it acquires kinetic energy from its muscles and attachments and the energy is dissipated to the internal fluids as it stops. Thus pseudophacodonesis is the result of oscillations of the fluids in the anterior and posterior segment of the eye. These oscillations, initiated by movement of the eye, result in shearing forces on the corneal endothelium as well as vitreous motion leading to permanent damage. Although complete scleral wound healing with collagen fibrils may take up to 3 months, since the haptic is snugly placed inside a scleral pocket, the IOL remains stable. There are no clinical pseudophacodonesis observed in glued IOLs due to good stability of the IOL.

Pseudophakic posterior iris chaffing syndrome which results from the haptics of the sulcus-fixated IOL in direct contact with the posterior surface of the overlying iris causes focal iris atrophy and pigment dispersion. Microhyphemas, intermittent spikes in intra-ocular pressure or pigment dispersion on a long-term leads to Uveitis-Glaucoma-Hyphema (UGH) syndrome. Recurrent redness and pain is the common presentation in these eyes with UGH syndrome. IOL rotation and recurrent irritation of iris are known to cause late UGH syndrome. Moreover, rubbing between the IOL optic and iris seems to contribute to the high flare counts in eyes with a sulcus-to-sulcus IOL fixation. In our series, consistent vault was maintained as seen in UBM **(Figures 7A to D)** between the iris and the IOL which is one factor for less postoperative uveitis and pigment dispersion. We need to assess the IOL tilt to rule out any UGH syndrome.

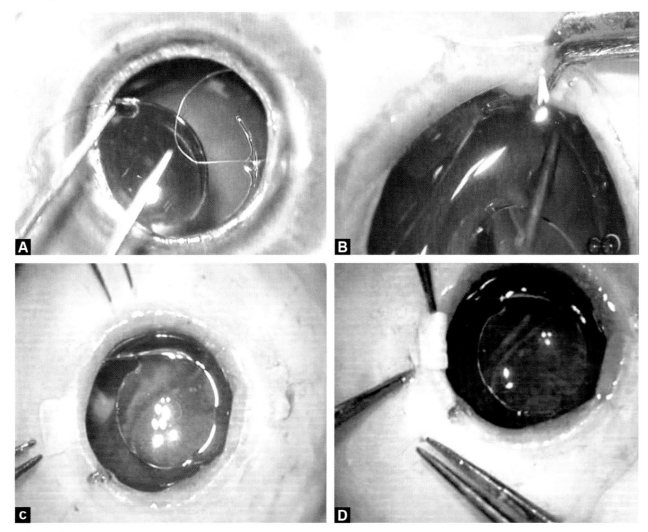

FIGURES 7A TO D: Cadaver eye studies
A. Sutured scleral fixated (SF) IOL
B. SF IOL showing iris shaffing
C. Glued IOL in cadaver eye
D. Haptic is externalized and tucked with less chance of uveal irritation

Conclusion

High speed anterior segment OCT or UBM can be used in analysis of tilt and position in eyes with sulcus fixated, glued IOLs and sutured scleral fixated IOLs as well.

References

1. Takei K, Hommura S, Okajima H. Optimum form of posterior chamber intraocular lenses to minimize aberrational astigmatism. Jpn J Ophthalmol. 1995;39(4):390-401.
2. Taketani F, Matuura T, Yukawa E, Hara Y. Influence of intraocular lens tilt and decentration on wavefront aberrations. J Cataract Refract Surg. 2004;30(10):2158-62.
3. Oshika T, Sugita G, Miyata K, et al. Influence of tilt and decentration of scleral-sutured intraocular lens on ocular higher-order wavefront aberration. Br J Ophthalmol. 2007;91(2):185-8.
4. Mester U, Sauer T, Kaymak H. Decentration and tilt of a single-piece aspheric intraocular lens compared with the lens position in young phakic eyes. J Cataract Refract Surg. 2009;35(3):485-90.
5. Schaeffel F. Binocular lens tilt and decentration measurements in healthy subjects with phakic eyes. Invest Ophthalmol Vis Sci. 2008;49(5):2216-22.
6. Sasaki K, Sakamoto Y, Shibata T, Emori Y. The multipurpose camera: a new anterior eye segment analysis system. Ophthalmic Res. 1990;22(Suppl 1):3-8.
7. Akkin C, Ozler SA, Mentes J. Tilt and decentration of bag-fixated intraocular lenses: a comparative study between capsulorrhexis and envelope techniques. Doc Ophthalmol. 1994;87(3):199-209.

8. Loya N, Lichter H, Barash D, Goldenberg-Cohen N, Strassmann E, Weinberger D. Posterior chamber intraocular lens implantation after capsular tear: ultrasound biomicroscopy evaluation. J Cataract Refract Surg. 2001;27(9):1423-7.

9. Hayashi K, Hayashi H. Comparison of the stability of 1-piece and 3-piece acrylic intraocular lenses in the lens capsule. J Cataract Refract Surg. 2005;31(2):337-42.

10. Detry-Morel ML, Van Acker E, Pourjavan S, Levi N, De Potter P. Anterior segment imaging using optical coherence tomography and ultrasound biomicroscopy in secondary pigmentary glaucoma associated with in-the-bag intraocular lens. J Cataract Refract Surg. 2006;32(11):1866-9.

11. Alpins NA, Goggin M. Practical astigmatism analysis for refractive outcomes in cataract and refractive surgery. Surv Ophthalmol. 2004;49(1):109-22.

12. Li Y, Shekhar R, Huang D. Corneal pachymetry mapping with high-speed optical coherence tomography. Ophthalmology. 2006;113(5):792-9.

13. Tang M, Li Y, Avila M, Huang D. Measuring total corneal power before and after laser *in situ* keratomileusis with high-speed optical coherence tomography. J Cataract Refract Surg. 2006; 32(11):1843-50.

14. Memarzadeh F, Li Y, Chopra V, Verma R, Francis BA, Huang D. Anterior segment optical coherence tomography for imaging the anterior chamber after laser peripheral iridotomy. Am J Ophthalmol. 2007;143(5):877-9.

15. Bakri SJ, Singh AD, Lowder CY, et al. Imaging of iris lesions with high-speed optical coherence tomography. Ophthalmic Surg Lasers Imaging. 2007;38(1):27-34.

16. Wolffsohn JS, Davies LN. Advances in anterior segment imaging. Curr Opin Ophthalmol. 2007;18(1):32-8.

17. Garcia JP Jr, Rosen RB. Anterior segment imaging: optical coherence tomography versus ultrasound biomicroscopy. Ophthalmic Surg Lasers Imaging. 2008;39(6):476-84.

18. Mutlu FM, Bilge AH, Altinsoy HI, Yumusak E. The role of capsulotomy and intraocular lens type on tilt and decentration of polymethylmethacrylate and foldable acrylic lenses. Ophthalmologica. 1998;212(6):359-63.

23

Results of Glued IOL

Dhivya Ashok Kumar, A Sathiya Packialakshmi, Amar Agarwal

Introduction

Intraocular lens implantation (IOL) in eyes that lack posterior capsular support is a problem for cataract surgeons for a long time. It is not only due to the visual outcome but also to the related complications they face in the postoperative period. We have performed glued IOL since 2007 with **(Figure 1)** good results.[1-10]

IOL Stability in Glued IOL Surgery

IOL dislocation is one of the main problems associated with transscleral fixation of suture-fixated IOLs.[11] However, in our technique, the IOL haptic is secured inside scleral pockets **(Figure 1)** at the site where the tip is externalized. We routinely tuck the haptic tip inside a scleral tunnel made with a 26-gauge needle. Another concern is the change in the properties of the biomaterial when the IOL is placed in a stretched position. According to Izak et al,[12] the 2 factors that contribute

to the ability of IOL loops to maintain their original symmetrical configuration are loop rigidity (the resistance of the haptic to external forces that bend the loops centrally) and loop memory (the ability of the loops to reexpand laterally to their original size and configuration). These 2 factors can be demonstrated by compressing or stretching the haptics *in vivo* **(Figures 2A and B)**. *In vivo*, the centrifugal force vector due to resistance to compression by the capsular bag keeps the IOL stable **(Figure 3A)**. Similarly, stretch creates a centripetal resistance force. Along with the intralamellar scleral tuck, this stabilizes the IOL **(Figure 3B)**.

Although complete scleral wound healing[13] with collagen fibrils may take up to 3 months, since the haptic is snugly placed inside a scleral pocket, the IOL remains stable. Intraocular lens centration/tilt was followed both clinically and with anterior segment optical coherence tomography. The difference between the topographic (Orbscan) and manifest refraction was constant in all eyes during the entire postoperative period, which suggests minimal new IOL-induced

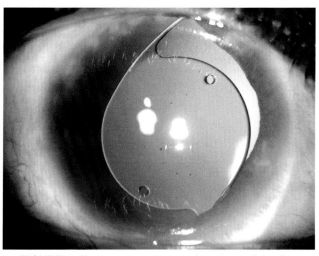

FIGURE 1: Four years postoperative photo of the first pediatric glued IOL case. The child had a cracker injury

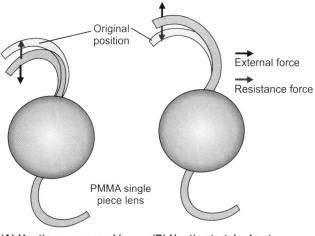

(A) Haptic compressed in **(B) Haptic stretched out**

FIGURES 2A AND B: The *ex vivo* vector diagram shows the effect of compression and stretching on the IOL haptic

172

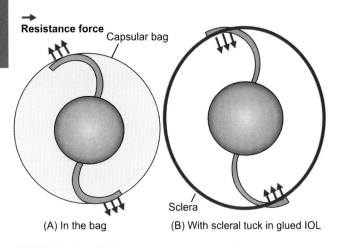

FIGURES 3A AND B: *In vivo* force vector diagram
A. Centrifugal force vector due to resistance to the compression by the capsular bag keeps the IOL stable
B. In the glued IOL, the stretch creates a centripetal resistance force; along with the intralamellar scleral tuck, this stabilizes the IOL

astigmatism. Moreover, the stability of the IOL is well maintained by the tucking procedure.

Results

Total 210 eyes of glued IOL were retrospectively analyzed from December 2007 to August 2010. Out of this 152 eyes had single piece rigid glued IOL, 21 eyes had monofocal three piece foldable IOL and 5 eyes had multifocal foldable IOL. There were 12 eyes with pediatric glued IOL, 5 eyes with 20G sutureless vitrectomy, 2 eyes with glued iris prosthesis and 3 eyes with transposition

of posterior chamber IOL into anterior chamber. In the combined surgeries, 5 eyes had optical penetrating keratoplasty, 2 eyes had Descemet's stripping and endothelial keratoplasty and 3 eyes had iridoplasty. The mean follow-up of 152 eyes with PMMA glued IOL was 9.7± 3.2 months. Fifty-nine (38.8%) out of 152 eyes completed ≥12 months follow-up. Hundred and sixteen (76.3%) and 36 (23.68%) eyes out of 152 eyes underwent the surgery as primary and secondary procedure, respectively. The most common indication was posterior capsular rupture with no sulcus support (56%) followed by subluxated cataract (21%). Eight out of 152 eyes underwent IOL exchange, out of which 6 eyes had AC IOL and 2 eyes had sutured scleral fixated IOL.

The most common indication for IOL exchange was uveitis and significant improvement noted in the postoperative period with a subjective questionnaire **(Table 1)**. Single piece PMMA IOL with optic size 6.5 mm and overall diameter of 13 mm was implanted in all the eyes. The mean preoperative UCVA in decimal equivalents was 0.024 ± 0.02 and the mean postoperative UCVA at the last follow-up was 0.53 ± 0.26. There was significant improvement in UCVA (Paired t-test p = 1.00×10^{-51}). Mean BCVA preoperatively was 0.71 ± 0.26 and is 0.80 ± 0.21 postoperatively (p = 1.35×10^{-5}). Seventy-nine out of 152 eyes (52%) gained 20/20 visual acuity at one month postoperatively. Multi-piece foldable IOL were implanted in 58 eyes, however, results were analyzed only in 21 eyes that finished minimum 6 months follow-up. The mean postoperative UCVA was 0.26 ±

TABLE 1: SYMPTOMATIC IMPROVEMENT IN EYES WITH IOL EXCHANGE OVER A PERIOD FOLLOW-UP (9.7 ± 2.7 MONTHS)

Category score	Symptom scale	Patient history	Preoperative n=6	Postoperative n=6
0	Asymptomatic	No symptoms	0	5
1	Mild	Occasional uveitis responding to medications	2	0
2	Moderate	Recurrent uveitis (repeated episode of uveitis separated by periods of inactivity without treatment, in which these periods of inactivity without treatment are at least 3 months in duration)	2	0
3	Severe	Persistent uveitis characterized by prompt relapse (in less than 3 months) after discontinuation of therapy	2	0

0.15 and BCVA was 0.51 ± 0.25. There was significant change in both postoperative BCVA and UCVA (Friedman test, p = 0.000). The mean preoperative and one year postoperative endothelial densities were 2872.7 ± 216.3 cells/mm^2 and 2750.2 ± 194.3 cells/mm^2, respectively. Five eyes of 5 patients underwent sutureless 20G vitrectomy with fibrin glue assisted PC IOL implantation without explantation. The mean preoperative UCVA was 0.08 ± 0.07 and postoperative mean UCVA was 0.53 ± 0.13. There was significant difference in the UCVA (p = 0.043). The mean postoperative best corrected visual acuity (BCVA) was 0.76 ± 0.22. The mean postoperative central foveal thickness measured in spectral domain optical coherence tomography (OCT) (Cirrus OCT, Carl Zeiss Meditec, Dublin, California, USA) was 281 microns at one year follow-up. Ultrasound biomicroscopy with 50 MHz frequency and 50 micron resolution showed no vitreous traction or uveal incarceration in pars plana ports in the postoperative period. The serial images taken at the pars plicata region showed good wound closure. Five eyes of 5 patients underwent multifocal (three refractive and two diffractive) glued IOL procedure. The indication was aphakia in all the 5 eyes. The mean preoperative spectacle BCVA was 0.60 ± 0.25 and the mean postoperative BCVA was 0.77 ± 0.34. There was no significant difference in BCVA (p = 1.000). The postoperative mean additional add for best near corrected vision was 0.5 ± 1.1 D. There was significant decrease in the near addition (p = 0.000). The mean postoperative intraocular pressure (IOP) as noted with non contact tonometry was 12 ± 1.7 mm Hg. There was no significant change in IOP (p = 0.083). The mean postoperative specular count was 2355 ± 277 cells/mm^2. Good patient satisfaction was seen as the subjective dysphotopic phenomenon like glare or ghost images are observed to be less.

Complications

Table 2 gives the complication profile in PMMA IOL's at one year follow-up. In foldable glued IOL, subconjunctival haptic was seen in 4 eyes. Decentration was seen in one eye and repositioning was done for the same. Resolving vitreous hemorrhage was seen in 3 eyes. No endophthalmitis was seen in any of the eyes. Recurrent uveitis was noted in 4 out of 58 eyes with foldable IOL. Optic capture was observed in 4 PMMA IOL and 3 foldable glued IOL. Chronic macular edema

TABLE 2: INTRA- AND POSTOPERATIVE COMPLICATIONS ANALYSIS

	Number of eyes (%) (out of 152) Mean follow-up = 9.7±2.7 months
Intraoperative	
Hyphema	n = 2 (1.31%)
Postoperative	
Early (< 1 month)	
Grade 2 anterior uveitis	n = 0 (0%)
Decentration	n = 3 (1.97%)
Macular edema	n = 3 (1.97%)
Late (> 1 month)	
Optic capture	n = 4 (2.63%)
Pigment dispersion	n = 3 (1.97%)
Endophthalmitis	n = 0 (0%)
Chronic macular edema	n = 3 (1.97%)

was seen in 3 eyes with PMMA IOL. There was no postoperative secondary glaucoma in any of the eyes.

Conclusion

The glued IOL procedure can be done as a primary procedure or secondary IOL implantation in eyes with deficient capsular support. Monofocal (single piece/multipiece), multifocal or aniridia IOLs can be implanted. The suture related and corneal endothelial complications are prevented via this procedure. Recently introduced modifications in the glued IOL (Handshake technique, use of 23G infusion, foldable glued IOL) help in easy learning and wider use of the technique for various indications.

References

1. Gabor SG, Pavilidis MM. Sutureless intrascleral posterior chamber intraocular lens fixation. J Cataract Refract Surg. 2007;33(11):1851-4.
2. Agarwal A, Kumar DA, Jacob S, Baid C, Agarwal A, Srinivasan S. Fibrin glue-assisted sutureless posterior chamber intraocular lens implantation in eyes with deficient posterior capsules. J Cataract Refract Surg. 2008;34(9):1433-8.
3. Kumar DA, Agarwal A, Prakash G, Jacob S, Saravanan Y, Agarwal A. Glued posterior chamber IOL in eyes with deficient capsular support: a retrospective analysis of 1-year postoperative outcomes. Eye (Lond). 2010;24(7):1143-8.
4. Prakash G, Kumar DA, Jacob S, Kumar KS, Agarwal A, Agarwal A. Anterior segment optical coherence tomography-aided diagnosis and primary posterior chamber intraocular lens implantation with fibrin glue in traumatic phacocele with scleral perforation. J Cataract Refract Surg. 2009;35(4):782-4.
5. Prakash G, Jacob S, Kumar DA, Narsimhan S, Agarwal A, Agarwal A. Femtosecond assisted keratoplasty with fibrin glue-assisted sutureless posterior chamber lens implantation: a new triple procedure. J Cataract Refract Surg. 2009;35(6):973-9.

173

6. Nair V, Kumar DA, Prakash G, Jacob S, Agarwal A, Agarwal A. Bilateral spontaneous in-the-bag anterior subluxation of PC IOL managed with glued IOL technique: A case report. Eye Contact Lens. 2009;35(4):215-7.

7. Agarwal A, Kumar DA, Prakash G, et al. Fibrin glue-assisted sutureless posterior chamber intraocular lens implantation in eyes with deficient posterior capsules [Reply to letter]. J Cataract Refract Surg. 2009;35(5):795-6.

8. Kumar DA, Agarwal A, Jacob S, Prakash G, Agarwal A, Sivagnanam S. Repositioning of the dislocated intraocular lens with sutureless 20-gauge vitrectomy Retina. 2010;30(4):682-7.

9. Kumar DA, Agarwal A, Prakash G, Jacob S. Managing total aniridia with aphakia using a glued iris prosthesis. J Cataract Refract Surg. 2010;36(5):864-5.

10. Kumar DA, Agarwal A, Gabor SG, et al. Sutureless sclera fixated posterior chamber intraocular lens. Letter to editor. J Cataract Refract Surg. 2011;37(11):2089-90.

11. Price MO, Price FW Jr, Werner L, Berlie C, Mamalis N. Late dislocation of scleral-sutured posterior chamber intraocular lenses. J Cataract Refract Surg. 2005;31:1320-6.

12. Izak AM, Werner L, Apple DJ, Macky TA, Trivedi RH, Pandey SK. Loop memory of haptic materials in posterior chamber IOL implantation. J Cataract Refract Surg. 2002;28: 1229-35.

13. Lee KH, Kim MS, Hahn TW, Kim JH. Comparison of histologic findings in wound healing of rabbit scleral homografts with fibrin glue (Tisseel_) and suture material. J Refract Surg. 1995;11:397-401.

24 High-Speed Imaging of the Glued IOL

Samaresh Srivastava, Vaishali A Vasavada,
Viraj A Vasavada

Introduction

Pseudophacodonesis is a relatively less understood phenomenon. It is not uncommon to see fine IOL movements with movements of the eye even following uneventful in-the-bag IOL implantation. Oscillations induced by saccadic eye movements cause turbulences in the aqueous humor and the vitreous cavity. Under normal conditions the crystalline lens-capsular bag-zonular complex has a stabilizing barrier effect against these micromovements in the eye. However, when this natural barrier is lost, endophthalmodonesis is a continuing trauma to the eye.

Mechanism of Pseudophacodonesis

Studies of high-speed motion pictures of the eyes of patients after extracapsular and intracapsular cataract extraction show that pseudophacodonesis and iridodonesis are the result of oscillations of the fluids in the anterior segment of the eye. These oscillations, initiated by movement of the eye, result in shearing forces on the corneal endothelium which may result in damage. Similar motion of the vitreous causes shearing forces which may damage the retina.[1]

Thus, a potential concern with IOL fixation in the absence of capsular bag support could be IOL tilt, decentration and pseudophacodonesis that could lead to constant motion in the vitreous and ultimately to retinal damage. Intraocular lens (IOL) implantation in eyes that lack posterior capsule support has been accomplished with an iris-fixated IOL,[2] an anterior chamber IOL, transscleral IOL fixation through the ciliary sulcus or pars plana intrascleral fixation and glued IOL fixation.[3]

Glued IOL technique has the advantage that there is externalization of the greater part of the haptics along their curvature, which stabilizes the axial positioning of

the IOL, thereby preventing IOL tilt.[4] Moreover, placing the IOL haptic beneath the flap prevents further movement of the haptic, reducing the pseudophacodonesis[1] that leads to constant motion in the vitreous.

Studying Pseudophacodonesis

Previously, Jagger and Jacobi[1] described an indirect method of analyzing pseudophacodonesis by filming the movement of light reflex from the front of the lens implant. Clinically, the best indication of pseudophakodonesis is "shimmering" from mobile Purkinje-Sanson images III and IV from the anterior and posterior IOL surfaces, which can be observed during examination of subtle eye movements at the slit lamp (Holladay J: personal communication, 1996). Miller and Doane and Jacobs et al used high-speed cinematography to demonstrate pseudophakodonesis with corneal touch associated with iris supported IOLs.[5]

We employed high-speed photography to study pseudophacodonesis following glued IOL implantation. Imaging with a high-speed camera has been utilized for slow motion analysis in various fields, including automotive vehicle safety testing, military test ranges, fluid dynamics and solid mechanics. It allows us to visualize dynamics of fast moving objects which are beyond the limits of normal human perception without blur. In the field of ophthalmology, several authors[6-11] have utilized high speed cameras to evaluate and understand different processes including role of cavitation and jack hammer effect in phacoemulsification, fluid movement and phacotip movements during phacoemulsification and dynamics in the choriocapillaris.

We evaluated patients with glue fixation of IOLs in the absence of capsular support for IOL donesis and compared them with patients with adequate capsular support who had undergone in-the-bag IOL implantation (both single piece and three piece IOL).

High-speed Imaging—Technique

A high-speed camera mounted on the slit lamp was used to study the IOL position and stability.

A Pike F-032B VGA (video graphics array) camera (Allied Vision Technology, Germany) was used for the current study **(Figure 1)**. At full resolution, it runs 208 frames per second (fps). The camera was mounted on an adapter to a beam splitter on the slit lamp (SL130, Zeiss, Germany). The camera was then connected to a laptop. The Raw 8 mode was used to capture images.

The software used for image capture was the AVT (Allied Vision Technology) universal package. The trigger for image capture was controlled on the laptop using this software. The camera's 200 fps speed and good image quality allowed us to analyze all clinical events with complete exactitude.

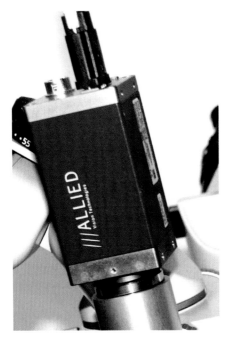

FIGURE 1: A high-speed imaging camera mounted on a slit lamp using a C mount on a 50-50 beam splitter

Eliciting Pseudophacodonesis

The patient was positioned on the slit lamp and asked to fixate straight ahead. The third and fourth Purkinje images (from the anterior and posterior IOL surfaces) were identified. The patient was then asked to perform voluntary horizontal eye movements as rapidly as

he/she could. During this several sequences of movement were filmed for the patient, focusing on the third Purkinje image formed at the anterior surface of the IOL. The fine oscillations of the third and fourth Purkinje images and their separation from each other were observed.

Image Analysis

Images were captured at 200 frames/second (fps). For purpose of viewing and analysis, they were converted into a video at 30 fps (PAL format). These images were replayed as a super slow motion movie **(Figure 2)**. Pinnacle 14 software was used for this purpose. Analysis was performed for several sequences in 10 patients with glue fixated IOL and 10 patients with in the bag implantation. With the patient's eye steady, the positions of the third and fourth Purkinje images were noted. Fine oscillations along with displacement of the third and fourth Purkinje image in relation to each other was suggestive of IOL donesis when the patient made eye movements.

Observations

In patients with glue fixated IOLs, on viewing the third and fourth Purkinje images, we found that there was no flutter in the images on induction of saccades. The images were steady and moved as the eyes moved without any oscillations whatsoever, indicating a non-donetic IOL. These observations were not noticeable on viewing the normal speed video, but were high-lighted with high speed imaging. On analyzing the patients with in-the-bag IOL implant, we found that as the eyes moved, there were fine low frequency oscillations seen on the third and fourth Purkinje images on the IOL. There was also a persistence of these oscillations after the eye came to a halt, suggesting pseudophacodonesis.

Discussion

When a human eye moves it acquires kinetic energy from its muscles, and when it stops it must somehow give up its energy. Since the eye is not completely rigid, one expects fluid friction to dissipate part of its kinetic energy.[1] Moreover, in real-life conditions much more vigorous movements may occur, like shaking the head, participating in active sports or driving a motor vehicle.

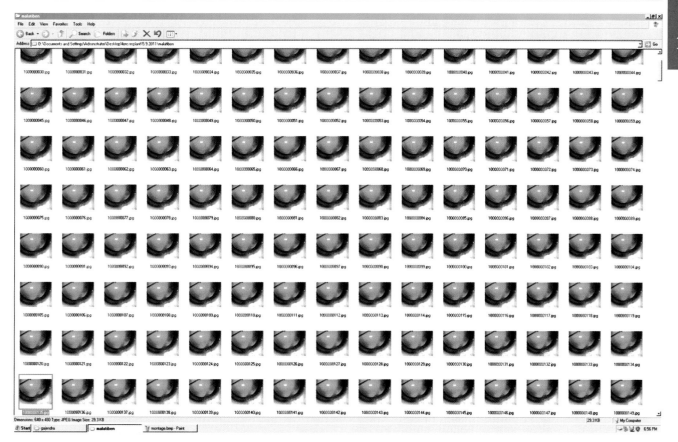

FIGURE 2: Images captured at 200 frames per second stored in a laptop to be converted into super slow motion video. On inducing saccadic movements of the eye, there is no visible donesis or flutter of the third and fourth Purkinje mages in a glued IOL, suggesting a stable IOL without donesis. In an eye with an intact capsular bag and in the bag foldable IOL a visible donesis is seen as persistent flutter of the third and fourth Purkinje images after the saccades have come to a halt, suggestive of pseudophacodonesis

Removal of the crystalline lens deprives the eye of the stabilizing effect of the lens-zonule barrier and makes the eye susceptible to damage by continuous endophthalmodonesis.[12] The incidence of pseudophakic retinal detachment following current surgical techniques of cataract extraction is lower than that found after intracapsular cataract extraction[13] because PC IOL reduces the frequency of retinal detachment by stabilization of the eye and limiting the ophthalmodonesis.

Glued IOL fixation is an extremely useful technique in myriad clinical situations in which capsular support is not available, such as a subluxated IOL, a dislocated IOL, zonulopathy, or secondary IOL implantation. However, these are situations where the natural compartmentalization is lost, and therefore IOL donesis over a long-term could have potentially serious effects on the posterior segment. As opposed to conventional techniques of scleral fixation of IOL, glued IOL involves placing the haptic beneath the flap. The

intrascleral fibrosis that eventually occurs would prevent further movement of the haptic, reducing pseudophacodonesis that leads to constant motion in the vitreous and, ultimately, to retinal damage.[14]

Recently, we described the realtime, intraoperative use of high-speed imaging to study minute details during phacoemulsification (Srivastava S, Vasavada AR, Realtime, Intraoperative High-Speed Imaging during Phacoemulsification, JCRS). Extending its application, we found that mounting this camera on a slit lamp allowed us to make detailed observations of very rapid movements of the IOL, which are difficult to perceive on normal videography. Thus, it provides an objective and user-friendly method to document IOL stability in a clinical setting. This technology can be used to study surgical techniques and technologies, to understand split second phenomena occurring during surgical procedures and for training purposes. Additionally, high-speed imaging can also provide valuable insights into several clinical phenomena like subtle IOL donesis, which are otherwise difficult to detect on routine examination or videography techniques.

Conclusion

To conclude, using high-speed photography we could confirm our clinical impression that glued IOLs are extremely stable not only as regards to tilt or decentration but it also prevents micromovements of the IOL.

References

1. Jacobi KW, Jagger WS. Physical forces involved in pseudophacodonesis andiridodonesis. Albrecht Von Graefes Arch Klin Exp Ophthalmol. 1981;216(1):49-53. PubMed PMID: 6909024.
2. Zeh WG, Price FW Jr. Iris fixation of posterior chamber intraocular lenses. J Cataract Refract Surg. 2000;26:1028-34.
3. Agarwal A, Kumar DA, Jacob S, Baid C, Agarwal A, Srinivasan S. Fibringlue-assisted sutureless posterior chamber intraocular lens implantation in eyes with deficient posterior capsules. J Cataract Refract Surg. 2008;34(9):1433-8. PubMed PMID: 18721701.
4. Teichmann KD, Teichmann IAM. The torque and tilt gamble. J Cataract Refract Surg. 1997;23:413-8.
5. Jacobs PM, Cheng H, Price NC. Pseudophakodonesis and corneal endothelialcontact: direct observations by high-speed cinematography. Br J Ophthalmol. 1983;67(10):650-4. PubMed PMID: 6615750; PubMed Central PMCID: PMC1040157.
6. Miyoshi T, Yoshida H. Ultra-high-speed digital video images of vibrations of an ultrasonic tip and phacoemulsification. J Cataract Refract Surg. 2008;34:1024-8.
7. Fernandez de Castro L, Dimalanta R, Solomon K. Bead-flow pattern: Quantitation of fluid movement during torsional and longitudinal phacoemulsification. J Cataract Refract Surg. 2010;36:1018-23.
8. Miyoshi T, Yoshida H. Emulsification action of longitudinal and torsional ultrasound tips and the effect on treatment of the nucleus during phacoemulsification. J Cataract Refract Surg. 2010;36:1201-6.
9. Zacharias J. Role of cavitation in the phacomeulsification process. J Cataract Refract Surg. 2008;34:846-52.
10. Bond LJ, Cimino WW. Physics of ultrasonic surgery using tissue fragmentation: part II. Ultrasound Med Biol. 1996;22:101-7.
11. Koyama T. Experimental studies of the choroidalmicrocirculation. III. High speed cinematographic analysis of choriocapillary blood flow. Nippon Ganka Gakkai Zasshi. 1981;85:1420-5.
12. Binkhorst CD. Corneal and retinal complications after cataract extraction. The mechanical aspect of endophthalmodonesis. Ophthalmology. 1980;87(7):609-17. PubMed PMID: 7402593.
13. Lois N, Wong D. Pseudophakic retinal detachment. Surv Ophthalmol. 2003;48(5):467-87. Review. PubMed PMID: 14499816.
14. Nicula C, Nicula D. Etiopathogenic consideration in the development ofretinal detachment in aphakic and pseudoaphakic eye. Oftalmologia. 2000;50(4):28-31. Romanian. PubMed PMID: 11392824.

Bryce Radmall, Zack Oakey,
Brian Stagg, Balamurali Ambati

Introduction

Alternative IOL fixation in the absence of capsular support can be accomplished through one of the two following generalized approaches: utilization of support from the anterior chamber angle with an AC IOL or a posterior chamber approach. In addition to glued, intrascleral haptic fixation **(Figure 1)**, PC IOLs may be secured by suturing the IOL to either the iris or the sclera. Although a review from the American Academy of Ophthalmology has proven each method of IOL fixation to be safe and effective,[1] each situation dictates which method is best, as each differs in technical demand, intraoperative time, structural prerequisite, and associated surgical complications. A detailed review of each surgical technique is beyond the scope of this chapter; however, technical reviews of the major extracapsular approaches have been described by Por and Lavin.[2]

Sutured IOLs

Introduction

The glued IOL technique is most similar to the sutured scleral technique. Utilizing sutures, rather than fibrin glue, to anchor an IOL to the sclera has traditionally been a common method to stabilize an IOL in the setting of poor capsular support. Malbran et al first described suture-fixated IOL placement in 1986, and since that time several modifications have been made to the originally described method.[3] Today a sclera-sutured IOL **(Figure 2)** is placed using one of two general methods: *ab extreno* method where the suture is passed from the exterior to interior of the eye or *ab interno* method performed by passing the suture from inside to out. Scleral grooves,[4,5] tunnels,[6,7] or flaps[8-10] are created to gain access to the ciliary sulcus and the PC IOL may be secured using one-point,[11] two-point,[12] three-point,[13]

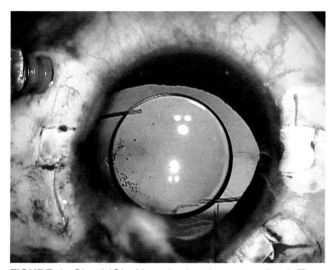

FIGURE 1: Glued IOL. Note the haptics externalized. They will be tucked and glued to the sclera (*Courtesy:* Dr Agarwal's Eye Hospital, India)

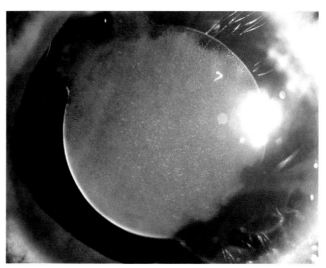

FIGURE 2: Sutured opacified PC IOL (*Courtesy:* Dr Agarwal's Eye Hospital, India). Note the PC IOL is opacified

or four-point,[4] scleral-sutured fixation. In contrast, sutureless or glued sclera-fixated IOLs involve externalization of IOL haptics for fixation within the sclera.

Alternatively, a PC IOL may be placed by suturing it to the iris. Iris suturing is less technically demanding than scleral suturing while still offering the benefits of posterior chamber positioning. The IOL may be positioned by tethering the haptics[14] or by suturing the optic itself to the iris.[15]

Indication

The basic indication for a sutured PC IOL is similar to that of any other form of IOL fixation—namely, lack of capsular support. This may be a result of damage due to blunt trauma or cataract surgery complications. Inherent weakness of capsular fibers may be caused by conditions such as Marfan's syndrome or homocystinuria. Infections such as endophthalmitis or uveitis may also compromise capsular integrity.

As there exists multiple viable options for IOL fixation, the anterior segment surgeon must be aware of certain situations when particular extracapsular approaches are relatively contraindicated. Iris-sutured PC IOLs would be a poor choice in the setting of marked iris tissue loss, atrophy, or instability.[16] Recent studies have reported the use of fibrin-glue-assisted techniques as a means for fixation of IOL-iris prosthesis in aniridia.[17] A PC IOL, located farther away from the angle structures of the eye and closer to the native position of the natural lens, theoretically causes less irritation to the cornea, iris, and angle structures. This decreases the risk of corneal decompensation or glaucoma when compared to an AC IOL.[18,19] A scleral-sutured IOL approach may be a prudent choice when performing extracapsular IOL fixation in a patient who has shallow anterior chamber depth or pre-existing damage to the corneal endothelium. Secondary to the anatomy of their anterior chamber, it has been suggested that scleral fixation of the IOL is preferred in patients suffering from Marfan's syndrome.[20] Scleral-sutured IOLs typically require longer intraoperative time and are thought to be technically the most demanding.

Prognosis/Outcomes

Iris-sutured PC IOLs and scleral-sutured PC IOLs have been shown to be safe and effective options for IOL fixation in a setting that lacks capsular support.[1] However, it is difficult to compare outcomes among the sutured PC IOL, glued IOL, and AC IOL approaches as there have been few studies that directly compare the different fixation techniques. Furthermore, most comparative studies that have been conducted are retrospective in nature and lack comparisons that include the glued IOL technique, given that it was pioneered in 2007.[21] The only prospective randomized study comparing AC IOLs, scleral-attached PC IOL, and iris-attached PC IOL occurred in the setting of penetrating keratoplasty. It showed that iris-fixated IOLs demonstrated a statistically significant decrease in risk of complications (cystic macular edema), though no difference in visual acuity across the groups was detected.[22] PC IOLs are thought to possess a theoretic advantage when compared to AC IOLs because they are located near the nodal point of the eye and in the eye's rotational axis.[2] However, a prospective study of patients with Marfan's associated lens subluxation demonstrates no difference in visual outcomes at 1 year when comparing iris-sutured PC IOLs to iris-claw AC IOLs.[23]

A review of recent case series suggests that in general, patients undergoing IOL fixation in the absence of capsular support experience improved visual acuity independent of the technique employed. Poorer visual outcomes are often related to ocular comorbidities associated with the underlying pathology necessitating extracapsular fixation. In a study specifically investigating outcomes of scleral-fixated vs iris-fixated IOLs, statistically similar results were attained, and both methods were considered successful.[20]

An important distinction between the sclera-sutured and glued IOL approaches is that the glued IOL technique is devoid of suture related complications.[24] Suture associated inflammation, loose suture, or a broken suture may lead to malpositioning of the IOL and subsequently poorer visual outcomes. It is essential to remember that regardless of IOL fixation approach, important indicators for prognosis are as follows: minimization of IOL tilt, centration of the IOL, correct location of the IOL haptics, and proper concealment of any utilized suture knot to avoid erosion.[5-7]

AC IOLs

Introduction

The modern AC IOL, first conceived in the 1950s, is an alternative in cases where capsular support is inadequate. In order for an AC IOL **(Figure 3)** to be a viable alternative, it must be vaulted sufficiently to

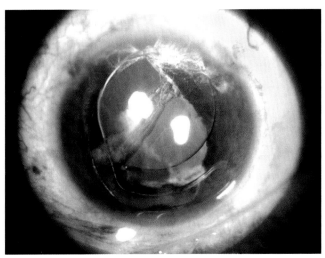

FIGURE 3: AC IOL (*Courtesy:* Dr Agarwal's Eye Hospital, India)

minimize IOL-iris contact, possess flexible open-looped haptics that resist increased vaulting under compression, and establish multi-point fixation.[2]

Prerequisites for implantation include the presence of an anatomically normal anterior chamber and accurate sizing of its horizontal with optical coherence tomography.[25] This is a critical step in placement and classically a serious disadvantage as inaccurate measurement will lead either to excessive movement if size is overestimated or anterior vaulting if size is underestimated. Once adequate measurement is achieved, the goal is to place the AC IOL in the anterior chamber with the footplates resting against the scleral spur, without capturing any iris tissue or interfering with any existing iridectomies.

Indication

To date there is insufficient evidence to support superiority of one lens system or fixation site.[1] Several researchers have contributed case studies and series pointing to particular advantages and disadvantages of the AC IOL and patterns have begun to emerge. Prominent considerations that argue for or against AC IOLs are dependent on patient condition. In particular the status of anterior curvilinear capsulorhexis (CCC) is important. In those cases where the CCC is intact and a previously implanted C-loop IOL is compromised, reverse optic capture is the preferred method. However, if a previous C-loop IOL is dislocated and the CCC is not intact, IOL exchange is considered and an AC IOL becomes the alternative of choice.[1]

Despite AC IOLs having the clear advantage over any PC IOL in ease of insertion, PC IOLs are still preferred in most circumstances. This is because of PC IOL nodal position, giving optimal optic benefits as well as its theoretical safety advantages with a safe distance away from the trabecular meshwork and corneal endothelium. These advantages possibly reduce risk of glaucoma, uveitis, and corneal decompensation.[1]

Prognosis/Outcomes

Since its development, the AC IOL has been controversial for its side effect profile with some noting dramatic adverse outcomes; yet others suggest that AC IOLs could replace competing techniques.[26] Despite technical improvements, considerations should still be made concerning the long-term effects of placing a lens in the anterior chamber given its unique anatomical relationship to surrounding structures.

Recognition of the possibility of adverse corneal effects has been with AC IOL literature since its inception, most prominent among these is pseudophakic bullous keratopathy. Indeed, several groups have reported their efforts for correcting this specific side effect.[27,28] However, if keratoplasty procedure frequency is used as a quality meter, it appears that PC IOLs are more often associated with need for penetrating keratoplasty than use of AC IOLs; despite intuitive assumptions and other objective evidence, one might expect the opposite to be true.[29,30] Because PC IOL placement is more often the procedure selected, some have suggested that disproportionate representation in correction keratoplasty may be due to use phenomenon rather than anything specific to IOL mechanics.[29] Supporting evidence is found in other studies "linking corneal edema to AC IOL use".[31]

Uveitis-glaucoma-hyphema syndrome, uveitis alone, and cystoid macular edema have been identified as prominent noncorneal adverse outcomes associated with use of an AC IOL.[31] However, these complications are similar to those found with PC IOL use; and therefore, prognosis is considered equivalent until future large-scale studies are conducted.

Conclusion

There exist many viable surgical solutions for IOL replacement in the setting of inadequate capsular support. Fortunately, the vast majority of patients

182

experience improved visual outcomes following extracapsular fixation. In the absence of complicating factors and comorbidities, several different surgical approaches may be equally likely to result in an excellent visual outcome. Varying individual circumstance and situation may dictate which approach would most likely yield the best possible outcome for the patient. Anterior chamber, iris-fixated, scleral-sutured, and glued IOL techniques are all practical surgical solutions when used appropriately in the setting of compromised capsular support. Most reports in the literature describe a series of patients who have undergone one specific fixation technique making it difficult to compare outcomes among the many different techniques. Additional research and prospective studies are needed to determine if, over the long-term, all options are equally tolerated and effective.

References

1. Wagoner MD, Cox TA, Ariyasu RG, Jacobs DS, Karp CL. Intraocular lens implantation in the absence of capsular support: a report by the American Academy of Ophthalmology. Ophthalmology. 2003;110:840-59.

2. Por YM, Lavin MJ. Techniques of intraocular lens suspension in the absence of capsular/zonular support. Surv Ophthalmology. 2005;50:429-62.

3. Malbran ES, Malbran E Jr, Negri I. Lens guide suture for transport and fixation in secondary IOL implantation after intracapsular extraction. Int Ophthalmol. 1986;9:151-60.

4. Almashad GY, Abdelrahman AM, Khattab HA, Samir A. Four-point scleral fixation of posterior chamber intraocular lenses without scleral flaps. Br J Ophthalmol. 2010;94:693-95. DOI 10.1136/bjo.2009.161349.

5. Lin CP, Tseng HY. Suture fixation technique for posterior chamber intraocular lenses. J Cataract Refract Surg. 2004;30:1401-4. DOI 10.1016/j.jcrs.2003.11.044.

6. Hoffman RS, Fine IH, Packer M. Scleral fixation without conjunctival dissection. J Cataract Refract Surg. 2006;32:1907-12. DOI 10.1016/j.jcrs.2006.05.029.

7. Hoffman RS, Fine IH, Packer M, Rozenberg I. Scleral fixation using suture retrieval through a scleral tunnel. J Cataract Refract Surg. 2006;32:1259-63. DOI 10.1016/j.jcrs.2006.02.065.

8. Caca I, Sahin A, Ari S, Alakus F. Posterior chamber lens implantation with scleral fixation in children with traumatic cataract. J Pediatr Ophthalmol Strabismus. 2011;48:226-31. DOI 10.3928/01913913-20100719-01.

9. Ma KT, Kang SY, Shin JY, Kim NR, Seong GJ, Kim CY. Modified Siepser sliding knot technique for scleral fixation of subluxated posterior chamber intraocular lens. J Cataract Refract Surg. 2010;36:6-8. DOI 10.1016/j.jcrs.2009.07.048.

10. Zhang ZD, Shen LJ, Liu XQ, Chen YQ, Qu J. Injection and suturing technique for scleral fixation foldable lens in the vitrectomized eye. Retina. 2010;30:353-6 DOI. 10.1097/IAE.0b013e3181c7021d.

11. Bas AM, Bulacio JL, Carrizo R. Monoscleral fixation for posterior chamber intraocular lenses in cases of posterior capsule rupture. Ann Ophthalmol. 1990;22:341-5.

12. Malbran ES, Malbran E Jr., Negri I. Lens guide suture for transport and fixation in secondary IOL implantation after intracapsular extraction. Int Ophthalmol. 1986;9:151-60.

13. Berger RR, Kenyers AM, Van Coller B, Pretorius CF. Vertical tripod fixation (VTF) simplifies transscleral approaches. Ophthalmic Surg. 1995;26:367-71.

14. McCannel MA. A retrievable suture idea for anterior uveal problems. Ophthalmic Surg. 1976;7:98-103.

15. Navia-Aray EA. Suturing a posterior chamber intraocular lens to the iris through limbal incisions: results in 30 eyes. J Refract Corneal Surg. 1994;10:565-70.

16. Boerman H, Chu Y. IOL Implantation without capsular supportCataract and Refractive Surgery Today. 2006;23-6.

17. Kumar DA, Agarwal A, Prakash G, Jacob S. Managing total aniridia with aphakia using a glued iris prosthesis. J Cataract Refract Surg. 2010;36:864-5.

18. Solomon K, Gussler JR, Gussler C, Van Meter WS. Incidence and management of complications of transsclerally sutured posterior chamber lenses. J Cataract Refract Surg. 1993;19:488-93.

19. Apple DJ, Price FW, Gwin T, Imkamp E, Daun M, Casanova R, Hansen S, Carlson AN. Sutured retropupillary posterior chamber intraocular lenses for exchange or secondary implantation. The 12th annual Binkhorst lecture, 1988. Ophthalmology. 1989;96:1241-7.

20. Zheng D, Wan P, Liang J, Song T, Liu Y. Comparison of clinical outcomes between iris fixated anterior chamber intraocular lenses and scleral fixated posterior chamber intraocular lenses in Marfan's syndrome with lens subluxation. Clin Experiment Ophthalmol. 2011. DOI 10.1111/j.1442-9071.2011.02612.x.

21. Agarwal A, Kumar DA, Jacob S, Baid C, Agarwal A, Srinivasan S. Fibrin glue-assisted sutureless posterior chamber intraocular lens implantation in eyes with deficient posterior capsules. J Cataract Refract Surg. 2008;34(9):1433-8.

22. Schein OD, Kenyon KR, Steinert RF, Verdier DD, Waring GO, 3rd, Stamler JF, Seabrook S, Vitale S. A randomized trial of intraocular lens fixation techniques with penetrating keratoplasty. Ophthalmology. 1993;100:1437-43.

23. Hirashima DE, Soriano ES, Meirelles RL, Alberti GN, Nose W. Outcomes of iris-claw anterior chamber versus iris-fixated foldable intraocular lens in subluxated lens secondary to Marfan syndrome. Ophthalmology. 2010;117:1479-85 DOI 10.1016/j.ophtha.2009.12.043.

24. Kumar DA, Agarwal A, Gabor SG, et al. Sutureless scleral fixated posterior chamber intraocular lens. Letter to editor. J Cataract Refract Surg. 2011;37(11):2089-90.

25. Goldsmith JA, Li Y, Chalita MR, et al. Anterior chamber width measurement by high-speed optical coherence tomography. Ophthalmology. 2005;112:238-44.

26. Aydin E, Bayramlar H, Totan Y, Daglioglu MC, Borazan M. Dislocation of a scleral-fixated posterior chamber intraocular lens into the anterior chamber associated with pseudophakic bullous keratopathy. Ophthalmic Surg Lasers Imaging 2004; 35(1):67-9.

27. Gupta PK, Bordelon A, Vroman DT, AFshari NA, Kim T. Early outcomes of descemet stripping automated endothelial keratoplasty in pseudophakic eyes with anterior chamber intraocular lenses. Am J Ophthalmol. 2011;151(1):24-28.e1. Epub 2010 Oct 20.

28. Wylegala E, Tarnawka D. Management of pseudophakic bullous keratopathy by combined descemet-stripping endothelial keratoplasty and intraocular lens exchange. J Cataract Refract Surg 2008;34(10):1708-14.

29. Cosar CB, Sridhar MS, Cohen EJ, Held EL, Alvim Pde T, Rapuano CJ, Raber IM, Laibson PR. Indications for penetrating keratoplasty and associated procedures, 1996-2000. Cornea. 2002;21(2):148-51.

30. Numa A, Nakamura J, Takashima M, Kani K. Long-term corneal endothelial changes after intraocular lens implantation. Anterior vs posterior chamber lenses. J Ophthalmol. 1993;37(1):78-87.

31. Sawada T, Kimura W, Kimura T, Suga H, Ohte A, Yamanishi S, Ohara T. Long-term follow-up of primary anterior chamber intraocular lens implantation. J Cataract Refract Surg. 1998;24:1515-20.

26 | Complications of Transscleral Sutured Posterior Chamber Intraocular Lenses

Andrew S McAllister, Peter Beckingsale

Introduction

The implantation of an intraocular lens into the intact capsular bag after removal of the crystalline lens provides stable fixation at a position closest to the nodal point of the eye. When the posterior capsule ruptures **(Figure 1)** or there is a lack of zonular support **(Figures 2 and 3)**, an intraocular lens (IOL) can be placed into the anterior chamber (AC) or posterior chamber (PC) rather than leave the patient aphakic. Fixation options in the AC include an iris fixated lens, the previously used closed loop AC IOLs or the modern style of open loop AC IOLs. In the PC an IOL can be fixated into the posterior chamber (PC) by transscleral suturing or intrascleral gluing within the ciliary sulcus or fixated to the posterior surface of the iris by the haptics, the optic or by clips.[1-3]

Because of their anatomic location, PC IOLs have a theoretical advantage over AC IOLs. They provide better visual acuity, binocularity and a lower incidence

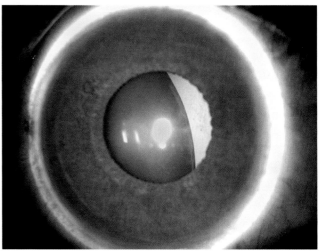

FIGURE 2: Subluxated crystalline lens (*Courtesy:* Dr Agarwal's Eye Hospital, India)

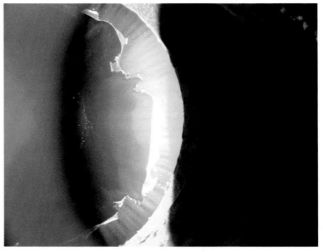

FIGURE 3: Pseudoexfoliation (*Courtesy:* Dr Agarwal's Eye Hospital, India)

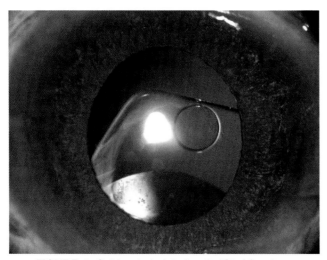

FIGURE 1: Subluxated plate haptic IOL (*Courtesy:* Dr Agarwal's Eye Hospital, India)

of strabismus than contact lenses and they avoid the complications of AC IOLs **(Table 1)**, seen more in the rigid closed loop lenses than the open loop and iris

TABLE 1: INDICATIONS, ADVANTAGES AND DISADVANTAGES OF AC IOLS COMPARED TO TSS PC IOLS[1,2]

IOL type	Indications	Advantages	Disadvantages
AC IOL	• Bleeding disorders • Extensive scleroconjunctival scarring (e.g. after trauma) • Intact anterior vitreous face	• Technically less demanding • Shorter operating time • Easier to remove, manipulate or replace • No suture associated problems • Placement far away from ciliary body (reduced risk of hemorrhage)	• Need for iridectomy/iridotomy • Requires mostly intact iris diaphragm • Concerns regarding long-term effects on corneal endothelium and blood aqueous barrier
TSS PC IOL	• Corneal endothelial protection; endothelial disorders (cornea guttata), PBK after AC-IOL implantation; in conjunction with PK or DSEK • Anterior chamber: Peripheral synechiae, shallow (<3.0 mm); abnormal angle • Defects of the iris; aniridia • Glaucoma; surgery in combination with glaucoma filtering operation	• Physiological position near the nodal point of the eye • IOL placement separated from the corneal endothelium • Preserves the eye's anatomy (minimises aniseikonia) • Independent of presence of iris tissue	• Technically more complex • Longer operating time • Extensive vitrectomy often required • Long-term dependence on fixation of IOL by sutures • Ciliary body erosion from haptics • Risk of hemorrhage and retinal detachment • Late suture erosion and exposure • Risk of suture endophthalmitis

AC IOL—anterior chamber intraocular lens; DSEK—Descemet stripping endothelial keratoplasty; IOL—intraocular lens; PK—penetrating keratoplasty; PBK—pseudophakic bullous keratopathy; TSS PC IOL—transscleral sutured posterior chamber intraocular lens

fixated lenses.[4-8] Complications of the AC IOLs include irreversible corneal endothelial cell loss, pseudophakic bullous keratopathy, peripheral anterior synechia and glaucoma caused by long-term anterior chamber irritation.[8-11] PC IOLs are indicated where these conditions are preexisting and in situations where an AC IOL may be at higher risk of complications such as diabetic patients, corneal guttata, shallow anterior chambers (<3.0 mm), anterior segment disruption, aniridia, and IOL implantation with penetrating keratoplasty and endothelial keratoplasty.[1,8,11,12]

The issues that surround the use of transscleral sutured (TSS) PC IOLs include a more demanding technique of introduction and fixation of the IOL, longer duration of surgery than other IOL implantations, sutures tracking into the eye and surgical manipulation in the region of the ciliary body which can cause hemorrhage and retinal detachment.[11-13] Serious postoperative complications of TSS PC IOLs are also relatively common, such as knot and suture erosion,[14-16] lens tilt,[15] suture breakage,[17,18] endophthalmitis,[18] retinal detachment,[17,18] choroidal hemorrhage,[15,17] elevated intraocular pressure (IOP)[9,13,17,19-22] and open angle glaucoma.[6,15,23]

Surgical Technique

Implant Design

Recommendations for TSS PC IOL implants are: the lens should be well polished and have a smooth edge to minimize chafing of the epithelium of the posterior iris and ciliary body; the ciliary ring has a mean diameter of 11.15 ± 0.5 mm so the total haptic diameter is to be 12.5 mm to 13.0 mm;[24,25] the optic diameter should be 6 mm or more to compensate for lens tilt or decentration which occurs in 5 to 10% of patients; the haptics should have 10° angulation and eyelets to prevent slippage of sutures; in children the pupil may have a diameter of 7.0 mm or more in darkness, therefore, a IOL with a large optical diameter is needed.[1] The Alcon (Alcon, Fort Worth, Texas, USA) CZ 70 BD polymethyl methacrylate (PMMA) IOL with a 7 mm optic diameter is a commonly used TSS PC IOL, with one eyelet on each haptic to allow easy and secure suture fixation to the sclera. Other lenses available include the Bausch and Lomb 6190B (Bausch and Lomb, San Dimas, California) and Pharmacia U152S (AMO, Santa Ana, California) which have one eyelet, and the Opsia (Chauvin Opsia, Labege Cedex, France) Grenat IOL which has two eyelets per haptic.

Rigid versus Foldable Implants

Using a foldable IOL is preferred as it requires a smaller incision but none are available with eyelets; foldable optics have an insertion diameter of 3.5 mm compared to rigid polymethyl methacrylate (PMMA) optics which have a diameter of more than 6 mm.[26] The smaller incision for foldable IOLs is usually self-sealing, and with the use of viscoelastics, allows better maintenance of the anterior chamber during IOL insertion and suturing.[27] This achieves greater intra-operative control, allows for a shorter operative time, minimizes surgically induced astigmatism, and visual rehabilitation may occur sooner.[26]

The larger incision for the PMMA optics often results in egress of intraocular fluids causing intra-operative hypotony; increasing the risk of choroidal hemorrhage, making the procedure more difficult and time consuming due to the frequent need to pressurise the globe, working with a soft eye, and necessity of ensuring a watertight wound closure with sutures.[1,12] Three percent of patients may develop postoperative hypotony with PMMA lenses, which can be corrected early on by resuturing the leaking corneal incision.[17] For chronic leaks around scleral sutures, an injection of autologous blood and placement of a bandage contact lens at the site may be sufficient.[17]

Methods of Lens Implantation

TSS PC IOLs are typically fixed into the ciliary sulcus with a 10/0 polypropylene suture through scleral and conjunctival incisions. Different techniques have been described, and the optimal lens placement method remains controversial.[2,8,28,29] Technique variations include the method of introducing the suture needle (ab externo (outside-in) or ab interno (inside-out)), of securing the haptic to the fixating suture, the number of points of fixation and the methods used to avoid suture and/or knot erosion.[2,28,29] Needles recommended include the ¼ circle tapercut double armed Ethicon CIF-4 (preferred for the ab interno method), and straight transchamber SABRELOC spatula double armed Ethicon STC-6 (Ethicon, Somerville, New Jersey).[2,28]

Prior to the introduction of the implant, a thorough anterior or pars plana vitrectomy around the surgical and suture insertion site, and removal of at least the anterior third of the vitreous is recommended.[12] This is to prevent vitreous-implant contact and subsequent tractional retinal detachment or cystoid macular edema.[12] Additional vitreoretinal surgery is also necessary in cases such as subluxated lenses or subluxated IOLs.[19]

The risk of intraoperative and postoperative complications increases if needle and/or haptic placement is too anterior (at the iris base) or too posterior (beyond the pars plicata) from the ciliary sulcus.[30] It is estimated that the ciliary sulcus is 0.8 to 0.9 mm posterior to the limbus in the vertical meridian, and 0.4 to 0.5 mm posterior to the limbus in the horizontal meridian.[25,31,32]

Because needle placement is obscured by the iris, suture fixation of the IOL is a blind procedure and the final position of the lens is not entirely predictable.[2] This was demonstrated in a study assessing TSS PC IOL position with ultrasound biomicroscopy.[33] Using intraoperative endoscopic sulcus verification localizes more precisely the ciliary sulcus for haptic and suture placement but this is not routinely used.[30,34] In patients with postoperative visual or other symptoms suggesting TSS PC IOL dislocation, ultrasound biomicroscopy can be used as a diagnostic test.[12]

Ab externo needle introduction provides more precise positioning and is most likely to achieve sulcus fixation.[30,35] This method of suture introduction also produces better visual acuity and reduced rates of astigmatism, cystoid macular edema, pupil distortion, suture exposure, IOL decentration and hemophthalmos when compared with results from the *ab interno* approach.[32] Inserting the needle *ab externo* obliquely, midway between perpendicular to the eye wall and parallel to the iris, has a wide safety zone and is the most reproducible compared to other needle insertion approaches.[36] To reduce the amount of tissue penetrated and the risk of bleeding, a perpendicular needle insertion away from the ciliary vessels located in the horizontal meridian, such as 2 and 8 or 4 and 10 o'clock, is best.[12]

For hypotonic eyes and open sky implantation of the IOL during penetrating keratoplasty, *ab interno* suture introduction is recommended to avoid pars plicata fixation, as prolapse of the ciliary processes may occur in front of the needle tip when attempting the *ab externo* approach.[30]

Once the IOL haptic is positioned into the ciliary sulcus, the sutures are transfixed through scleral linear incisions, tied and either left long or cut short. The conjunctival incisions are then closed with absorbable sutures. Traditional methods to avoid suture exposure and risk of endophthalmitis are to place suture knots covered by Tenon's and conjunctiva or under a partial thickness scleral flap.[12] Long-term erosion of knots for the subconjunctival method is 5 to 50%,[7,14,15,20,37,38] and 14.7 to 73% for scleral flaps.[14-16] To reduce knot erosion, two point scleral fixation using a continuous-loop suture with knot rotation can be used; this has exposure rates of 6.7% after twenty-four months of patient follow-up.[39] Suture fixation through a corneoscleral pocket with a double-pass 4-point fixation avoids conjunctival dissection, the need for knot rotation and reduces the risk of knot exposure.[28]

Visual Outcomes

Using TSS PC IOLs with an anterior vitrectomy can result in either the same or improved visual outcomes in 71.9% of eyes, with a mean improvement of 2 Snellen chart lines of vision.[40] Other studies have similar results and showed poorer visual outcomes for eyes with preoperative pathology, previous complicated surgery and those requiring removal of an AC IOL.[17-19]

For primary insertion of implants, open loop AC IOLs are reported to have better visual outcomes than TSS PC IOLs, with postoperative Snellen BCVA of 6/12 or better in 71.1% compared to 47.1% respectively, which may be due to longer operating time for TSS PC IOL insertion (89.5 ± 27.6 minutes compared to 62.9 ± 15.1 minutes) resulting in more light-induced cystoid macular edema (CMO).[13,41] A complete anterior vitrectomy and postoperative topical nonsteroidal anti-inflammatory can help prevent the occurrence of CMO, which commonly occurs 1-3 months after surgery in 5.5%[5] of secondary TSS PC IOLs.[2] Nd:YAG laser vitreolysis or repeat vitrectomy may be necessary if there is postoperative vitreous incarceration. The sutures passing through the ciliary body and uveal contact by the IOL may also cause chronic low-grade inflammation responsible for late onset CMO.[1]

Lens tilt greater than 5 degrees will also result in refractive error and poorer visual outcomes,[42] with IOL tilt or decentration occurring in 5 to 10% of patients.[1]

Decline in postoperative corneal endothelial cell counts and visual acuity is comparable in TSS PC IOL and open loop AC IOL insertions for up to three months postoperatively.[19] It is suggested that postoperative endothelial cell loss may be due to surgical trauma rather than the presence of an IOL.[13]

Complications

Generally there are few intraoperative complications during placement of a TSS PC IOL.[40] In the post-operative period complications are relatively common, with 53.7% (95% CI: 42.3 to 64.7%) of cases having at least one postoperative complication and 15.8% requiring at least one postoperative surgical procedure.[40]

Ocular hypertension is the most encountered complication, affecting 30.5% of eyes at a mean of 106 days postoperatively; 48% of within 1 week following IOL insertion, and 44% having a past history of glaucoma (Relative risk = 2.3, 95% confidence interval: 1.2 to 3.9, Fishers exact p = 0.026).[40] The effect can be transient (28%), ongoing and treated with medication (60%), or not controlled (12%). These results were slightly less than one large study evaluating post-operative IOP and glaucoma with TSS PC IOL insertion;[19] and the incidence of glaucoma between open loop AC IOLs and TSS PC IOLs is said to be similar.[8] Risk factors for postoperative ocular hypertension include a past history of glaucoma, ocular trauma, treatment of RD with silicone oil, use of intraoperative viscoelastic substances, hyphema and corticosteroid use.[17]

Ocular hypotension can occur (6.1%), and leakage from the surgical wound is important to identify and correct.[40] Postoperative corneal edema may also occur (6.1%) as well as hyphema (9.8%) which mostly resolves without treatment.[40]

Choroidal hemorrhage has been reported to occur in up to 3.2%.[15,17] Risk factors for hemorrhage are prolonged procedure duration, sutures placed at 3 and 9 o'clock and/or 2 mm posterior to the limbus, double suture passes, hypotony, removal of residual lens material, extensive vitrectomy, repair of large iris defects, or iridoplasty.[2,12] Patient factors that contribute include older age, bleeding disorders or anticoagulation, hypertension, peripheral vascular disease, glaucoma, aortic stenosis, emphysema, and prior eye surgery.[12]

Retinal detachment (RD) following TSS PC IOLs is said to be higher in young patients due to attached posterior hyaloids and ocular pathology; the risk of RD from ectopia lentis and axial myopia ranges from 9% to 19%.[17,43] RD after TSS PC IOL insertion without vitrectomy occurs in 1.1-6.0% of patients;[8] with a pars plana vitrectomy 8.2% may experience a RD;[17] and with an anterior vitrectomy the rate is 4%[18] to 4.9% at an average of 53 weeks.[40] Retinal tears commonly occur near the axis of fixation sutures, and risk factors include previous trauma, myopia greater than −1D, vitreous hemorrhage, and traction to the vitreous base which is reduced by intraoperative vitrectomy.[2]

Studies with long follow-up have shown that there are high rates of postoperative suture related complications.[8,17,18,40] Exposure of the sutures are common (11% at an average of 81.6 weeks); and rupture of the 10/0 polypropylene suture is a significant long-term problem, though the incidence reported varies. For instance, 27.9% of eyes may have suture rupture on average four years after surgery; 49% of young patients may require further surgery, 57% for suture breakage.[17] Another study where 40.2% of eyes had more than four years of follow-up showed rupture of the polypropylene sutures occurred in 6% of eyes at a mean of 4.9 years; four were of patients under 40 years, or 30.7% of the eyes in this age group with a relative risk of 21.2 compared to older patients.[40] In other studies suture breakage occurred in 24% of patients after seven to ten years of follow-up,[18] compared to no suture ruptures after more than 12 years follow-up.[44] It has been postulated that patients with primary familial bilateral ectopia lentis may carry an enzyme which degrades polypropylene or have some other effect on polypropylene sutures.[3] However, higher breakage rates in younger patients is more likely due to active lifestyle associated with continuous microtrauma, combined with biodegradation of the polypropylene and gravitational forces.[17] From a histological study, implant stability was due to intact scleral sutures and not to fibrous encapsulation or correct placement of the haptic in the ciliary sulcus.[37] As a result, IOL dislocation is likely to occur if sutures are inadvertently removed or if suture fatigue occurs.[17,45] In eyes where dislocation of the TSS PC IOL has occurred, insertion of an AC IOL may provide better long-term visual outcomes.[46] To increase the durability of implants, 9-0 polypropylene weighed against the possible increased risk of endophthalmitis associated with a larger knot, and other suture materials such as Gore-Tex can be used.[2,47] Late endophthalmitis at an incidence of 4%[18] from exposed sutures can be reduced by covering the sutures with scleral flaps, leaving suture ends long, rotating knots into the sclera, tying the knot in the depths of a partial thickness scleral incision or creating a corneoscleral pocket.[2,28]

Conclusion

Despite the relatively common rates of complications associated with TSS PC IOLs, patients with aphakia report that surgery improves their quality of life; therefore, they are prepared to accept the risks of surgery rather than use contact lens or spectacle correction.[17]

Implant location is a major advantage of TSS PC IOLs and can provide favorable visual outcomes, with loss of vision due to serious, severe and progressive conditions. However, the difficulty of insertion, duration of surgery, complication rates and evidence that modern open loop and iris claw AC IOLs, iris fixated[8] and scleral glued IOLs have similar outcomes have resulted in much debate over which is the safest and most efficacious implant for patients without posterior capsular support. Long-term follow-up is required of patients following insertion of a TSS PC IOL. Suture erosion and rupture, particularly in young patients, can occur years after implantation, and patients need to be counselled of potential complications during the consent process.

References

1. Dick HB, Augustin AJ. Lens implant selection with absence of capsular support. Curr Opin Ophthalmol. 2001;12(1):47-57.
2. Por YM, Lavin MJ. Techniques of intraocular lens suspension in the absence of capsular/zonular support. Surv Ophthalmol. 2005;50(5):429-62.
3. Michaeli A, Assia EI. Scleral and iris fixation of posterior chamber lenses in the absence of capsular support. Curr Opin Ophthalmol. 2005;16(1):57-60.
4. Smith P, Wong S, Stark W. Complications of semiflexible, closed loop anterior chamber intraocular lenses. Arch Ophthalmol. 1987;105:52-7.
5. Stark W, Gottsch J, Goodman D, Goodman G, Pratzer K. Posterior chamber intraocular lens implantation in the absence of capsular support. Arch Ophthalmol. 1989;107:1078-83.
6. Smiddy W, Sawusch M, O'Brian T, Scott D, Huang S. Implantation of scleral-fixated posterior chamber intraocular lenses. J Cataract Refract Surg. 1990;16(6):691-6.
7. Price Jr FW, Wellemeyer M. Transscleral fixation of posterior chamber intraocular lenses. J Cataract Refract Surg. 1995;21(5):567-73.
8. Wagoner MD, Cox TA, Ariyasu RG, Jacobs DS, Karp CL. Intraocular lens implantation in the absence of capsular support: A report by the American Academy of Ophthalmology. Ophthalmol. 2003;110(4):840-59.
9. Buckley EG. Scleral fixated (sutured) posterior chamber intraocular lens implantation in children. J AAPOS 1999;3(5):289-94.

10. Furuta M, Tsukahara S, Tsuchiya T. Pupillary elongation after anterior chamber lens implantation after cataract surgery in children. J Cataract Refract Surg. 1986;12:273-5.

11. Epley K, Shainberg M, Lueder G, Tychsen L. Pediatric secondary lens implantation in the absence of capsular support. J AAPOS 2001;5:301-6.

12. Hannush SB. Sutured posterior chamber intraocular lenses: Indications and procedure. Curr Opin Ophthalmol. 2000;11(4): 233-40.

13. Kwong YY, Yuen HK, Lam RF, Lee VY, Rao SK, Lam DS. Comparison of outcomes of primary scleral-fixated versus primary anterior chamber intraocular lens implantation in complicated cataract surgeries. Ophthalmol. 2007;114(1):80-5.

14. Holland EJ, Daya SM, Evangelista A, Ketcham JM, Lubniewski AJ, Doughman DJ, et al. Penetrating keratoplasty and transscleral fixation of posterior chamber lens. Am J Ophthalmol. 1992;114(2):182-7.

15. Solomon K, Gussler JR, Gussler C, Van Meter WS. Incidence and management of complications of transsclerally sutured posterior chamber lenses. J Cataract Refract Surg 1993;19(4):488-93.

16. Uthoff D, Teichmann KD. Secondary implantation of scleral-fixated intraocular lenses. J Cataract Refract Surg. 1998;24(7): 945-50.

17. Vote BJ, Tranos P, Bunce C, Charteris DG, Da Cruz L. Long-term outcome of combined pars plana vitrectomy and scleral fixated sutured posterior chamber intraocular lens implantation. Am J Ophthalmol 2006;141(2):308-12.e1.

18. Asadi R, Kheirkhah A. Long-term Results of Scleral Fixation of Posterior Chamber Intraocular Lenses in Children. Ophthalmol. 2008;115(1):67-72.e1.

19. Krause L, Bechrakis NE, Heimann H, Salditt S, Foerster MH. Implantation of scleral fixated sutured posterior chamber lenses: a retrospective analysis of 119 cases. Int Ophthalmol. 2009;29(4): 207-12.

20. Heidemann DG, Dunn SP. Transsclerally sutured intraocular lenses in penetrating keratoplasty. Am J Ophthalmol. 1992; 113(6):619-25.

21. Johnston RL, Charteris DG, Horgan SE, Cooling RJ. Combined pars plana vitrectomy and sutured posterior chamber implant. Arch Ophthalmol. 2000;118(7):905-10.

22. Heidemann DG, Dunn SP. Visual results and complications of transsclerally sutured intraocular lenses in penetrating keratoplasty. Ophthalmic Surg. 1990;21(9):609-14.

23. Robin J, Gindi J, Kohl K. An update of the indications for penetrating keratoplasty. Arch Ophthalmol. 1986;104:87-9.

24. Apple DJ, Price FW, Gwin T, Imkamp E, Daun M, Casanova R, et al. Sutured retropupillary posterior chamber intraocular lenses for exchange or secondary implantation: The 12th Annual Binkhorst Lecture, 1988. Ophthalmol. 1989;96(8):1241-7.

25. Davis RM, Campbell DM, Jacoby BG. Ciliary sulcus anatomical dimensions. Cornea. 1991;10(3):244-8.

26. Oshima Y, Oida H, Emi K. Transscleral fixation of acrylic intraocular lenses in the absence of capsular support through 3.5 mm self-sealing incisions. J Cataract Refract Surg. 1998;24: 1223-9.

27. Dick HB, Schwenn O. Viscoelastics in Ophthalmic Surgery. New York: Springer; 2000.

28. Hoffman RS, Fine IH, Packer M. Scleral fixation without conjunctival dissection. J Cataract Refract Surg 2006;32:1907-12.

29. Chen SX, Lee LR, Sii F, Rowley A. Modified cow-hitch suture fixation of transscleral sutured posterior chamber intraocular lenses: long-term safety and efficacy. J Cataract Refract Surg. 2008;34(3):452-8.

30. Althaus C, Sundmacher R. Intraoperative intraocular endoscopy in transscleral suture fixation of posterior chamber lenses: Consequences for suture technique, implantation procedure, and choice of PCL design. Refract Corneal Surg. 1993;9(5):333-9.

31. Duffey RJ, Holland EJ, Agapitos PJ, Lindstrom RL. Anatomic study of transsclerally sutured intraocular lens implantation. Am J Ophthalmol. 1989;108(3):300-9.

32. Gabric N, Henc-Petrinovic L, Dekaris I. Complications following two methods of posterior chamber intraocular lens suturing. Documenta Ophthalmologica. 1996;92(2):107-16.

33. Pavlin CJ, Rootman D, Arshinoff S, Harasiewicz K, Foster FS. Determination of haptic position of transsclerally fixated posterior chamber intraocular lenses by ultrasound biomicroscopy. J Cataract Refract Surg. 1993;19(5):573-7.

34. Jurgens I, Lillo J, Buil JA, Castilla M. Endoscope-assisted transscleral suture fixation of intraocular lenses. J Cataract Refract Surg. 1996;22(7):879-81.

35. Althaus C, Sundmacher R. Transscleral suture fixation of posterior chamber intraocular lenses through the ciliary sulcus: endoscopic comparison of different suture techniques. Ger J Ophthalmol. 1992;1(2):117-21.

36. Yasukawa T, Suga K, Akita J, Okamoto N. Comparison of ciliary sulcus fixation techniques for posterior chamber intraocular lenses. J Cataract Refract Surg. 1998;24(6):840-5.

37. Lubniewski AJ, Holland EJ, Van Meter WS, Gussler D, Parelman J, Smith ME. Histologic study of eyes with transsclerally sutured posterior chamber intraocular lenses. Am J Ophthalmol. 1990; 110(3):237-43.

38. Epstein E. Suture problems. J Cataract Refract Surgl 1989;16:116.

39. Walter KA, Wood TD, Ford JG, Winnicki J, Tyler ME, Reed JW. Retrospective analysis of a novel method of transscleral suture fixation for posterior-chamber intraocular lens implantation in the absence of capsular support. Cornea. 1998; 17(3):262-6.

40. McAllister A, Hirst L. Visual outcomes and complications of scleral-fixated intraocular lenses. J Cataract Refract Surg. 2011; 37(7):1263-9.

41. Bergman M, Laatikainen L. Long-term evaluation of primary anterior chamber intraocular lens implantation in complicated cataract surgery. Int Ophthalmol. 1996-97;20:295-9.

42. Tsai YY, Tseng SH. Transscleral fixation of foldable intraocular lens after pars plana lensectomy in eyes with a subluxed lens. J Cataract Refract Surg. 1999;25(5):722-4.

43. Johnston RL, Charteris DG. Pars plana vitrectomy and sutured posterior chamber lens implantation. Curr Opin Ophthalmol. 2001;12:216-21.

44. Mimura T, Amano S, Sugiura T, Funatsu H, Yamagami S, Araie M, et al. Refractive change after transscleral fixation of posterior chamber intraocular lenses in the absence of capsular support. Acta Ophthalmol Scand. 2004;82(5):544-6.

45. McCluskey P, Harrisberg B. Long-term results using scleral-fixated posterior chamber intraocular lenses. J Cataract Refract Surg. 1994;20(1):34-9.

46. Sarrafizadeh R, Ruby AJ, Hassan TS, et al. A comparison of visual results and complications in eyes with posterior chamber intraocular lens dislocation treated with pars plana vitrectomy and lens repositioning or lens exchange. Ophthalmol. 2001; 108:82-9.

47. Price FW Jr, Wellemeyer M. Transscleral fixation of posterior chamber intraocular lenses. J Cataract Refract Surg. 1995;21(5): 567-73.

27 Glued Endocapsular Hemi-Ring Segment for Sutureless Transscleral Fixation of the Capsular Bag

Soosan Jacob, Amar Agarwal

Introduction

Subluxated cataracts and IOLs are generally dealt with depending on the degree of subluxation. For subluxations of upto 3-4 clock hours, a capsular tension ring is often sufficient but for subluxations of a larger extent, stabilization of the capsular bag by reattaching it to the scleral wall becomes essential in order to avoid continued decentration and subluxation. This aim has been traditionally achieved by the use of sutures to fixate the bag to the sclera. Sutural fixation has the disadvantages of requiring a greater degree of surgical skill and expertise and a longer surgical time. It involves the need to pass long, thin and difficult to maneuver needles through the eye, thus making the procedure challenging to perform. The role of sutures in long term stability has also been questioned with issues secondary to suture degradation, suture erosion, exposure, knot unraveling and late IOL subluxation/ dislocation known to occur with 10-0 prolene. Though this has been attempted to be resolved by using 9-0 prolene or even 8-0 Goretex sutures, the need still remains to determine an alternate mode of capsular bag fixation to the scleral wall.

Glued Endocapsular Hemi-Ring Segment

The Glued Endocapsular Hemi-Ring Segment (Glued ECHR)[1-5] or the Glued Endocapsular Ring (ECR), designed by one of us (SJ) and manufactured by Mateen Amin (Epsilon Eye Instruments), aims at fulfilling this need for sutureless transscleral fixation of the capsular bag and its contents. It is manufactured using PVDF (polyvinylidene fluoride), the material used for manufacturing IOL haptics. This material is known to be biocompatible and inert within the eye, is flexible,

has better memory and shape recovering capability than other IOL haptic materials, especially prolene and is, therefore, an ideal material for the intended use. It has also been found to be inert and stable within the scleral wall as a similar tuck has been used for the glued IOL technique and the Scharioth technique for transscleral secondary fixation of IOL in the absence of a capsular bag.

The glued ECHR is manufactured in the same gauge as the haptics of IOLs. It has an open segment design **(Figure 1A)**. The two arms of the device lie within the capsular fornix, the double scroll Malyugin type locking mechanism **(Figure 1B)** engages the rhexis rim atraumatically and the haptic of the device anchors the entire capsular bag transsclerally **(Figures 2A to I)**. The device can be inserted either by introducing the haptic first and then fish-tailing the rest into the eye or by inserting the arms first under the rhexis followed by the haptic. It is manufactured in different sizes and can, therefore, extend 180 degrees around the capsular bag or can be smaller in size depending on surgeon preference. The double scrolls and the haptic provide vertical and horizontal support to the bag during and after surgery whereas the arms provide equatorial fornix expansion.

Surgical Technique

The surgeon constructs a lamellar scleral flap in the area of dialysis **(Figures 3 and 4)**. The rhexis is then constructed followed by a gentle hydrodissection. A sclerotomy is created under the scleral flap just as in glued IOL and a Scharioth intrascleral tunnel is created at the edge of the scleral flap using a 26 gauge needle. The tunnel is created from the outer corner of the scleral bed and pointing towards the limbus so as to be able to anchor the device intrasclerally in a coat-

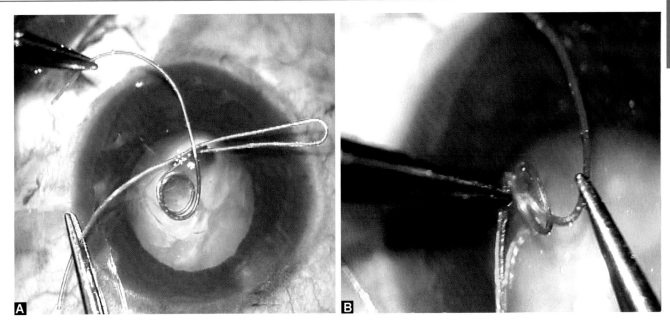

FIGURES 1A AND B

A. Open segment design of the glued endocapsular hemi-ring segment makes it suitable for smaller as well as bigger capsular bags though caution would be recommended in very small eyes such as microspherophakia till further studies are carried out. The glued endocapsular ring (ECR) is manufactured in different sizes

B. The Malyugin type double scrolls engage the rhexis rim in an atraumatic manner

hanger like manner. The device is then inserted into the anterior chamber as described earlier. Care should be taken to verify that it is inserted the right side up. The haptic of the device is externalized through the sclerotomy using intraocular end-gripping microforceps via the handshake technique. The haptic is then cut to the desired length and after making sure that the double scrolls are engaging the rhexis, the haptic is tucked into the intrascleral tunnel. This centers and stabilizes the bag transsclerally and avoids the need for any other stabilization techniques both intra- and postoperatively. The haptic being an extension of the intraocular device and being of a broader gauge (130 microns—the same gauge as IOL haptic) offers more robust and stable long-term fixation, more rotational stability and less pseudophacodonesis than transscleral suturing of the capsular bag as in sutured segments and rings. Phacoemulsification, cortex aspiration and in the bag IOL implantation are carried out as usual. At the end of surgery, centration is again checked for and adjusted real time by adjusting the degree of tuck of the haptic within the scleral tunnel. This is in contrast to sutured capsular bag fixation where once the suture is tied down to the scleral wall, it is difficult to adjust the degree of centration. Once centered, fibrin glue is used

to hermetically seal the flap as well as to close the conjunctiva just as in the glued IOL procedure. Glue may also be used to seal clear corneal incisions.

The device was also found to provide sufficient capsular support in anterior capsular tear occurring after insertion and it was possible to continue with careful phacoemulsification, cortex aspiration and IOL implantation. We would, however, not recommend implanting the device in a pre-existing anterior capsular tear for fear of extension of the capsular tear during the insertion maneuvers. This device can also be used in subluxated IOLs where the capsular bag is intact. Surgery is done in following the same principles. The lamellar scleral flap is made centered on the area of dialysis. The capsular bag is expanded using viscoelastic. A 20 G sclerotomy is made under the scleral flap. The device is introduced into the anterior chamber so that the arms lie within the expanded capsular fornix and the double scroll mechanism engages the rhexis rim. Pulling the exteriorized haptic centers the bag **(Figure 5)**.

Just as in scleral fixation via sutures, with this device too, accurate placement of the flap so as to lie centered on the zone of dialysis is important to avoid decentration of the bag-IOL complex. A flap that is decentered on the area of dialysis can lead to a

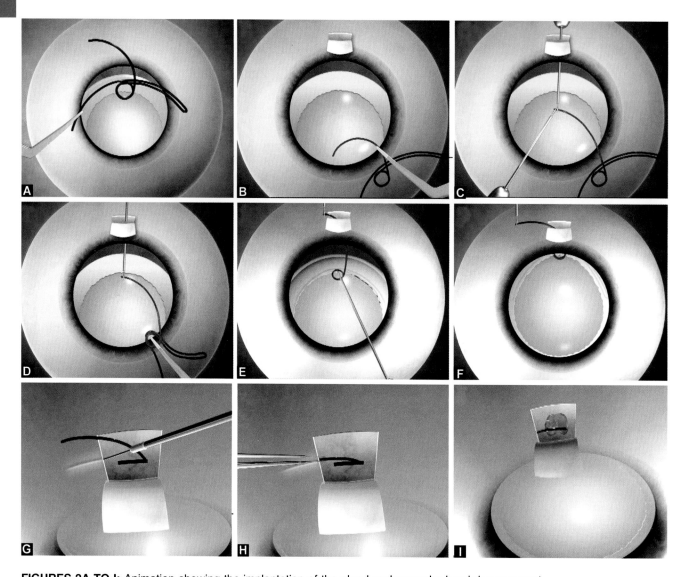

FIGURES 2A TO I: Animation showing the implantation of the glued endocapsular hemi-ring segment
A. The design of the glued ECHR is seen as well as its positioning in the direction of dialysis
B. Lamellar scleral flap and sclerotomy are created in the area of dialysis. The haptic of the device is introduced into the anterior chamber
C. It is caught by an end gripping microforceps introduced through the sclerotomy
D. The rest of the glued ECHR is flexed in using a single handed fish-tailing technique
E. The circular scrolls engage the rhexis rim
F. The capsular bag is centered
G. A scleral tunnel is created at the edge of the scleral flap with a 26 G needle
H. The haptic is tucked into the tunnel
I. Fibrin glue is applied and the flap is sealed down over the haptic

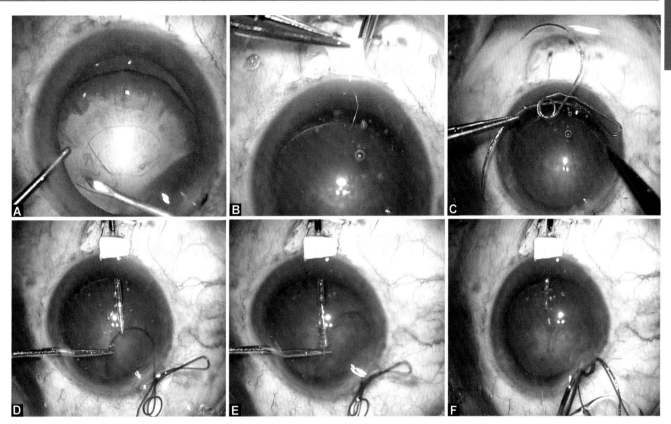

FIGURES 3A TO F: Surgical technique for implanting the glued endocapsular hemi-ring segment
A. 180 degrees subluxation is seen. A scleral flap has been created inferiorly and a rhexis is being created
B. A sclerotomy is made under the scleral flap with a 20 gauge needle taking care that the needle emerges in the space between the iris and the anterior lens capsule
C. A glued ECHR segment is planned to be inserted in the orientation shown
D. The haptic of the glued ECHR segment is caught by an MST forceps introduced from the side port and transferred into the jaws of a waiting end gripping microforceps introduced through the sclerotomy
E. Using the handshake technique, the haptic is transferred between the two hands until the surgeon is holding the haptic at its extreme tip with the forceps passed under the scleral flap
F. The haptic is then exteriorized while at the same time fishtailing/flexing the rest of the ring segment into the anterior chamber using the other hand

decentered IOL. In this case, the glued ECHR offers the advantage of ease of adjustment as compared to sutured segments. A new lamellar scleral flap is constructed in the desired area and a 20 G sclerotomy is made under the flap. The haptic is interiorized into the AC by simply pulling it back in using the end-gripping microforceps. It is then again re-exteriorized via the newly constructed sclerotomy and is then tucked into the intrascleral tunnel. Both flaps are then glued down using fibrin glue as also the conjunctiva. The Glued ECHR thus not only offers good long-term stability and ease of surgery but also the ability to easily adjust centration. Explantation of the glued ECHR segment for any reason during surgery is also relatively simple and being flexible, it only needs to be pulled

out under cover of a viscoelastic after interiorizing the haptic.

Conclusion

To conclude, subluxated cataracts have been a surgical challenge and surgeons around the world have paved the path towards overcoming hurdles associated with surgery and successful implantation of IOL. We now describe this new glued endocapsular hemi-ring segment for sutureless fibrin glue assisted transscleral fixation of the capsular bag and hope to be part of this continuing effort to overcome subluxation and to obtain better and better results for these cases. The glued ECHR provides good and robust fixation of the capsular bag

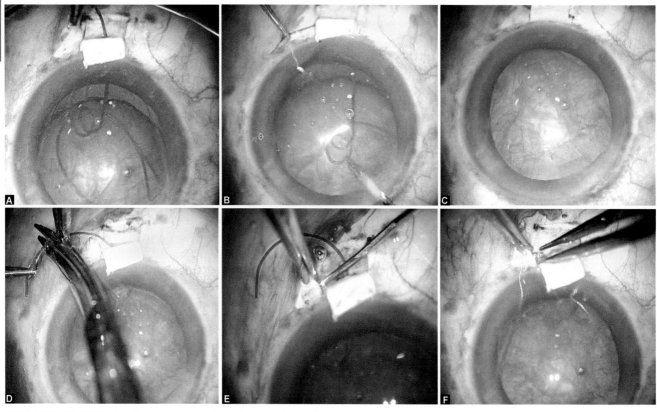

FIGURES 4A TO F: Implanting the glued endocapsular hemi-ring segment

A. The two arms of the ring segment are then inserted under the rhexis using an MST forceps

B. The circular scrolls are then caught by the microforceps and maneuvered so as to engage the rhexis margin in the plane between two circular loops of the scrolls

C. Once the rhexis rim is engaged by the scrolls, pulling on the exteriorized haptic pulls the entire capsular bag complex and centers it

D. The haptic is then cut taking care that a sufficient length is retained

E. A 26 gauge needle is used to create a sclera tunnel at the edge of the sclera flap

F. The tangentially oriented haptic is then tucked into the scleral tunnel parallel to the limbus

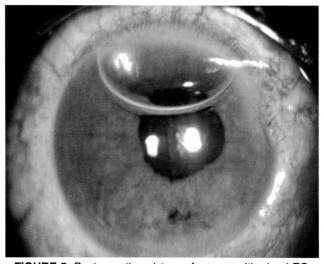

FIGURE 5: Postoperative picture of a case with glued EC hemi-ring segment

complex to the sclera wall while also providing horizontal and vertical support and centrifugal expansion of the capsular bag. It offers ease and rapidity of surgery as well as ease of adjustability while doing away with suture related complications. Even in case of malpositioned flap, it is easy to create a new flap, interiorize and then re-exteriorize the haptic of the device through the new, correctly positioned sclerotomy.

References

1. Jacob S, Agarwal A, Agarwal A, Sathish K, et al. Glued endocapsular hemi-ring segment for fibrin glue-assisted sutureless transscleral fixation of the capsular bag in subluxated cataracts and intraocular lenses. JCRS. 2012;2(38):193-201.
2. Jacob S. Glued Endocapsular Hemi-Ring Segment for Fibrin Glue-Assisted Sutureless Transscleral Fixation of Capsular Bag in Subluxation (Presented as Free paper in ASCRS 2012).
3. Jacob S. Glued Endocapsular Hemi-Ring Segment for Fibrin Glue-Assisted Transscleral Fixation of the Capsular Bag (Awarded Runner up in category of Instruments and Devices at the ASCRS Film Festival).
4. Glued Endocapsular Hemi-Ring: EuroTimes Jan 31 2012 (http://m.eurotimes.org/870/general-news/glued-endocapsular-hemi-ring/).
5. Jacob S, Agarwal A. Glued endocapsular hemi-ring segment makes surgery easier, faster. (Ocular Surgery News U.S. Edition, January 10, 2012).

Index

Page numbers followed by *f* refer to figure